HEALING, PERFORMANCE AND CEREMONY IN THE WRITINGS OF THREE EARLY MODERN PHYSICIANS: HIPPOLYTUS GUARINONIUS AND THE BROTHERS FELIX AND THOMAS PLATTER

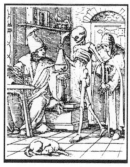

The History of Medicine in Context

Series Editors: Andrew Cunningham and Ole Peter Grell

Department of History and Philosophy of Science
University of Cambridge

Department of History
Open University

Titles in this series include

The Body Divided
Human Beings and Human 'Material' in Modern Medical History
Edited by Sarah Ferber and Sally Wilde

Medicine, Government and Public Health in Philip II's Spain
Shared Interests, Competing Authorities
Michele L. Clouse

Nursing before Nightingale, 1815–1899
Carol Helmstadter and Judith Godden

Secrets and Knowledge in Medicine and Science, 1500–1800
Edited by Elaine Leong and Alisha Rankin

Henri de Rothschild, 1872–1947
Medicine and Theater
Harry W. Paul

The Anatomist Anatomis'd
An Experimental Discipline in Enlightenment Europe
Andrew Cunningham

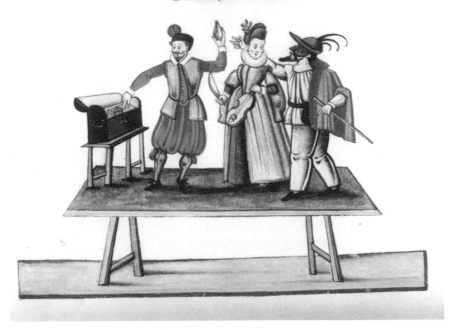

Charlatano, c.1620, 13x19cm, coloured drawing from a friendship album
(*album amicorum*). New York art market, 1968.

Healing, Performance and Ceremony in the Writings of Three Early Modern Physicians: Hippolytus Guarinonius and the Brothers Felix and Thomas Platter

M.A. KATRITZKY
The Open University, UK

Translations by M.A. Katritzky and Verena Theile

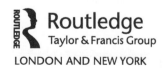

Routledge
Taylor & Francis Group

LONDON AND NEW YORK

First published 2012 by Ashgate Publishing

2 Park Square, Milton Park, Abingdon, Oxon OX14 4RN
711 Third Avenue, New York, NY 10017, USA

Routledge is an imprint of the Taylor & Francis Group, an informa business

First issued in paperback 2016

British Library Cataloguing in Publication Data
Katritzky, M.A.
  Healing, performance and ceremony in the writings of three
  early modern physicians : Hippolytus Guarinonius and the
  brothers Felix and Thomas Platter. -- (The history of
  medicine in context)
  1. Guarinoni, Hippolyt, 1571-1654. 2. Platter, Felix,
  1536-1614. 3. Platter, Thomas, 1574-1628. 4. Physicians as
  authors--Europe--History. 5. Literature and medicine--
  Europe--History. 6. Medicine in literature. 7. Traveling
  theater--Europe--History. 8. Quacks and quackery--
  Europe--History. 9. European drama--History and
  criticism.
  I. Title II. Series
  792'.08861-dc22

Library of Congress Cataloging-in-Publication Data
Katritzky, M.A.
  Healing, performance, and ceremony in the writings of three early modern
  physicians : Hippolytus Guarinonius and the brothers Felix and Thomas
  Platter / M.A. Katritzky.
      p. cm. -- (The history of medicine in context)
  Includes bibliographical references and index.
  ISBN 978-0-7546-6707-0 (hardcover) 1. Guarinoni, Hippolyt,
  1571-1654. 2. Platter, Thomas, 1574-1628. 3. Platter, Felix, 1536-1614. 4.
  Physicians--Austria. 5. Physicians--Switzerland I. Title.
  R128.6.K28 2011
  610.92'2--dc23

                                                                      2011033886

ISBN 978-0-7546-6707-0 (hbk)
ISBN 978-1-138-25411-4 (pbk)

Contents

List of Diagrams and Plates

Diagrams

Plates

For

Erika and †Brian Jackson
Rupert and Katharina Katritzky
Freda and Xavier Gonot Schoupinsky

Acknowledgements

I am deeply grateful to the Trustees of the Barbara Wilkes and Elizabeth Howe Foundations for endowing and contributing to The Barbara Wilkes Research Fellowship in Theatre Studies, to The Open University for confirming the Fellowship's permanence and supporting it, and wish to thank all my colleagues in the OU English Department and Arts Faculty. My special thanks to Richard Danson Brown, Hannah Lavery and the OU Early Modern Literature Research Group, and to Shaf Towheed and the OU Book History and Bibliography Group, Nicky Watson and The Arts and their Audiences, Anne Laurence, Gill Perry and GiTH (OU Gender in the Humanities Group), Paul Lawrence and the Arts Faculty Research Committee, Caitlin Adams, Anne Ford and the REST team, and Andrew Tinson and Arts Faculty IT support. For external funding, I thank the Directors, Trustees and staff of the Herzog August Library, Arts and Humanities Research Council and British Academy.

My research depends on the documentary and human resources of libraries, archives, museums, salerooms and collections. I thank all the past and present librarians, curators, archivists and private collectors who have supported this study. Particular thanks to those in Avignon (Musée Calvet), Basle (University Library), Berlin (Staatliche Museen Preussischer Kulturbesitz), Dijon (Archives Municipales), Frankfurt (Stadtarchiv), Innsbruck (Tiroler Landesmuseum Ferdinandeum, University Library), Langres (Musée), London (British Library, Christies, Courtauld Institute, Sotheby's, Warburg Institute), Milan (Biblioteca Teatrale, Teatro alla Scala), Milton Keynes (The Open University Library), Montpellier (Archives Municipales), Munich (Bayerisches Hauptstaatsarchiv & Geheimes Haus Archiv, Bayerisches Nationalmuseum, Bayerische Staatsbibliothek, Bayerische Staatsgemäldesammlungen), Nürnberg (Germanisches Nationalmuseum, Stadtarchiv), Oxford (Ashmolean Museum; Bodleian, Sackler and Taylorian Libraries; Corpus Christi, New, St Catherine's and St John's College Libraries), Paris (Bibliothèque Nationale), Sigmaringen (Stadt Archiv), Stuttgart (Württembergisches Landesbibliothek), Weimar (Stiftung Weimarer Klassik), Wien (Österreichische Nationalbibliothek) and Wolfenbüttel (Herzog August Bibliothek).

My thanks and appreciation go to Jasper Becker, Asaph Ben-Tov, Jim Davis, Verena Theile, Helen Watanabe-O'Kelly and Nicky Watson for their invaluable comments on draft chapters, and to the organizers and members of the research groups and conferences within whose auspices aspects of this research have been presented, discussed and published, and especially Andy Spong and Andrew Stott (University of Hertfordshire, 1997); Claude Schumacher (*Theatre Research*

International, 1998 and 2000); Piermario Vescovo (*Quaderni veneti*, 1999); Christopher Cairns (*The Renaissance Theatre*, 1999); Roger Mettam, Philip Broadhead and Robert Frost (London University, Institute of Historical Research, 1999); Helen Watanabe-O'Kelly, Ronnie Mulryne and the European Science Foundation (Castelvecchio Pascoli, 2003); Klaus Amann and Max Siller (*Akten des 5. Symposium der Sterzinger Osterspiele*, 2008); Natalia Filatkina, Ane Klein, Birgit Münch and Martin Przybilski (University of Trier, 2008); Margaret Healy (University of Sussex, 2009); Pavel Drábek (Masaryk University Brno, 2009, 2011); Pam Brown, Rob Henke, Susanne Wofford and my friends and colleagues in Theater Without Borders (NYU in Florence 2009, Venice RSA 2010, NYU in Madrid 2011); Alberto Martino and Fausto de Michele (*La ricezione della commedia dell'arte*, 2010); Honza Petružela and David Drozd (*Divadelní Revue*, 2010); Hiram Kümper and Vladimir M. Simić (*Practicing New Editions*, 2011); Laurie Maguire and Peter Friend (University of Oxford, Green-Templeton College, January 2012). I wish to record my deep gratitude to Dr Werner Wilhelm Schnabel for drawing my attention to Jacob Praun's friendship album and providing me with images. As always, my very special thanks go to the staff and Fellows of the Herzog August Library; most especially Ulrike Gleixner, Jill Bepler and Volker Bauer, and all those Fellows with whom I have been privileged to discuss aspects of this work (HAB Visiting Fellows' Colloquium 2011).

Otherwise unattributed translations are mine, as are all errors. Of which there would be very many more, were it not for the remarkable and very greatly appreciated patience, dedication and professionalism of my co-translator Verena Theile (North Dakota), my illustrator Martin Michette (Berlin) and my Ashgate editors, Erika Gaffney, Emily Yates, Aimée Feenan and Gail Welsh, and series editors Ole Grell (OU) and Andrew Cunningham (Cambridge).

Images are courtesy of: Archives de Montpellier (2); Art market and private collectors (20, 39); Bayerisches Nationalmuseum (9, 15); Bayerische Staatsbibliothek (8, 11, 23); Bibliothèque Nationale (3); Bodleian Library and Ashmolean Museum (University of Oxford) (30, 33, 40); British Library (21, 36); David Allen (frontispiece); Gemäldegalerie Kassel (37); Germanisches Nationalmuseum (12, 13, 17, 27–8); Herzog August Bibliothek (4, 5, 26, 29, 31); Musée Calvet (32); Museum of Fine Arts, Budapest (37); Österreichische Nationalbibliothek (14, 18, 35); Stiftung Preussischer Kulturbesitz (1, 38); Stadtarchiv Nürnberg (16, 19, 34); Stiftung Weimarer Klassik (7, 10) and Württembergisches Landesbibliothek (22, 24, 25).

PART I
Introduction

Chapter 1

Healing, Performance and Ceremony in the Writings of Three Physicians

This book examines aspects of performance culture, and of the practice of healthcare and medicine, and some of the complex interconnections between these two fundamental areas of human endeavour. The published and unpublished early modern documents it draws on include substantial and rarely cited German-language writings by three physicians. One has achieved worldwide recognition as a physician, one is better known as a traveller, and the third is little known even within the German-speaking regions. This book focuses on how they engaged with and recorded the theatrical and festival culture of their time, and what their writings communicate about it in general, and also about healing performers, the performance of healing, and influences between healthcare and the stage, in its widest sense.

The three physicians, whose writings have not previously been studied together, are Hippolytus Guarinonius[1] and the half-brothers Felix and Thomas[2] Platter. The Platter brothers were Lutherans who practiced medicine in their home city of Basle. Guarinonius was a devout Catholic born in Trent, who grew up in Prague and Vienna. He chose to practice in Hall, then already in gentle decline from its medieval status as a major salt-mining centre and the largest and most prosperous city on the Tirol's North-South trade route, to a modest provincial town in the shadow of nearby imperial Innsbruck.[3] The medical schools at which they qualified, those of the universities of Montpellier and Padua, were then

---

[1]   The first volume of the longest vernacular medical treatise by Guarinonius (1571–1654) was published in 1610 as *Die Grewel der Verwüstung Menschlichen Geschlechts* (here cited throughout as Guarinonius, *Grewel*). The second volume survives only as an unfinished, unpublished manuscript (Innsbruck UL, Cod.110).

[2]   This son of Thomas Platter the Elder (1499–1582), generally referred to as Thomas Platter the Younger (1574–1628), and here referred to throughout simply as Thomas Platter, is the half-brother of Felix Platter (1536–1614). The journal of Platter the Elder is here cited from Otto Fischer's 1911 edition (Platter the Elder, 'Thomas Platters Lebensbeschreibung'). The journals of his sons Felix (Basle UL, Codex A λ III.3) and Thomas Platter (Basle UL, Ms.A λ V.7–8) are here quoted in translation from the original German language manuscripts. For ease of reference, most footnote references are to the comprehensive, scholarly editions of Valentin Lötscher (here cited as *Felix Platter Tagebuch*) and Rut Keiser (here cited as *Thomas Platter d.J*), rather than to the manuscripts themselves. Non-German synonyms placed in brackets in Thomas Platter's manuscript are here left untranslated.

[3]   Brandstätter, 'Hall', 33.

Europe's most renowned, respectively attracting large communities of Protestant and Catholic German-speaking students, enjoying special privileges (Plates 2, 4–5).[4] Felix Platter left Basle for Montpellier in 1552, returning in 1557. His much younger half-brother Thomas Platter, brought up by Felix after the death of their father Thomas Platter the Elder, left the University of Basle in 1595 to continue his medical studies in Montpellier, returning to Basle in 1600. Hippolytus Guarinonius, born three years before Thomas Platter and outliving him by a quarter of a century, boarded at Prague's Jesuit College for 11 years before completing his medical studies in Padua between 1594 and 1597.

Felix Platter was an ambitious, highly successful physician who published numerous medical treatises. His unfinished manuscript life writings, compiled in his seventies and never intended for publication, mainly cover the period from his earliest childhood to the mid-1560s. The only published works of the much shorter-lived Thomas Platter are posthumous editions of some of Felix's writings. The fair copy of his manuscript travel journal, covering the period 1595–1600, was completed by 1605. By no means all of Hippolytus Guarinonius's numerous Latin and vernacular German medical and theological treatises, tracts and translations have been published even since his lifetime, and the considerable scholarship on him is largely in German. Felix and Thomas Platter attract an international scholarship excellently served by the magisterial editions of their life writings respectively edited by Valentin Lötscher in 1976 and Rut Keiser in 1968, and less so by partial and sometimes unreliable seventeenth-century and modern translations into English of several medical publications, and selected sections of their life writings.[5] Several passages of theatrical interest in the three physicians' writings are well known, notably a brief reference by Hippolytus Guarinonius to English actors, and Thomas Platter's impressions of an itinerant performing and healing

---

   [4]   Such as 'the German Freedom': the right to carry weapons within the city (on which see *Felix Platter Tagebuch*, 203: 26 August 1554, Montpellier).

   [5]   *Felix Platter Tagebuch* (ed. Lötscher); *Thomas Platter d.J* (ed. Keiser). Partial edited transcriptions and translations of Thomas Platter's account of his 1599 visit to England include those of Binz ('Londoner Theater'), Hecht (Platter the Younger, *Englandfahrt*) and Williams (*Thomas Platter's travels in England*). Jennett (*Beloved son Felix* and *Journal of a younger brother*) engagingly compress the accounts of Felix Platter's five years in Montpellier and Thomas Platter's studies and travels in France and Spain, into two slim, readable volumes with minimal scholarly apparatus). An anonymous French translation publishes selected sections of both brothers' Montpellier accounts (Platter, *Félix et Thomas Platter*). The first volume of Le Roy Ladurie's three-volume engagement with the Platter journals (Platter, *Le siècle des Platter*) paraphrases extensive extracts from Platter the Elder and Felix Platter's journals (English translation: Le Roy Ladurie, *The beggar and the professor*); the remaining two introduce and provide French translations of Rut Keiser's edition of Thomas Platter's journal in its entirety, complete with Keiser's scholarly apparatus and footnotes. For seventeenth-century English translations of Felix Platter's medical treatises, see: Plat[t]er, Cole and Culpeper, *A golden practice* (=*Praxis medica*); Plat[t]er, Culpeper and Cole, *Platerus histories* (=*Observations*).

troupe in Avignon in 1598, and of his visit to a performance of *Julius Caesar* on London's South Bank a year later. Most are unavailable in English translation. My title reflects a new perspective on a new selection of primary documents. As such, it prompts immediate questions. Why healing, performance and ceremony? Why physicians? Why these three?

Why Healing, Performance and Ceremony?

Traces of ancient shamanic and other links between healing, performance and ceremony persisted into the early modern period – and beyond – at many levels. Most obviously, they informed the activities of religious faith healers and the class of itinerant traders known as quacks, mountebanks or charlatans. They contributed to the renaissance revival of classical health therapies for melancholy based on music, laughter and comedy, and are a factor in the early modern period's heightened medical, theatrical and popular interest in supernatural phenomena and wondrous humans: magic and monsters.[6] These links also profoundly shaped the interlocking hierarchical power networks underpinning Europe's social and political frameworks, in which spectacle is widely utilized to promote and enhance legally-binding as well as symbolic performed rituals or ceremonies (as compellingly demonstrated by the Europe-wide tradition of the Royal Touch). Recognizing the power of performance and healing to attract the respect, money and compliance of individuals, build and bind communities, and forge perceptions of physical and mental norms, early modern Church, court and city all competed for their control. Their confrontations highlight the interdependence of the practice of medicine and theatre, at a time when the boundaries between them were still porous and flexible.

Early modern healthcare and performance encroached on and enriched each other in many ways. Physicians performed public dissections to spectators in anatomy theatres; monstrous humans were eagerly examined by physicians as well as being collected by aristocrats and viewed by fairground visitors; religious centres and leaders drew crowds by staging exorcisms or other spectacular procedures associated with healing powers. Itinerant quacks pioneered many theatrical trends. Strongly incentivized to attract clients and promote their medical products and services, their stage routines often involved magic and medicine. From the beginnings of Western drama, popular theatrical trends crossed fluidly between quack and non-quack stages, in a lively culture of Europe-wide interchange. During the medieval period, the medical activities of actual quack troupes were promoted by professional performers, and medicine-peddling quacks became the earliest secular characters in the religious plays then at the heart of the Christian festive year. Their 'merchant scene', as it became known, dominated the central

---

[6]   This term is here used in its early modern sense of congenitally, physically abnormal human (or animal).

third of certain late medieval Easter mystery plays. It provided a public forum for ridiculing and debating popular medical practices, and initiated the surprisingly high medical content of the performing arts (which continues to flourish unabated in the age of television).

Researches into the interdependencies between early modern healing and performing do not reflect a unified field of enquiry. Generally, they follow discipline-led concerns and approaches of one or another academic field. Unremarkably, theatre historians traditionally foreground spectacle; medical historians concentrate on healthcare activities. One fruitful approach treats literary play texts as a primary documentary source for enquiries into early modern medical practice.[7] Some are general, others focus on specific questions.[8] Despite the heavy pressures of disciplinary agendas, increasingly holistic approaches are being pioneered by scholars publishing in several languages on another developing area: performing quacks.[9] Groundbreaking collaborative ventures are contributing towards the goal of achieving fruitful new approaches and findings in this field.[10] This book builds on these findings. In order to contextualize key texts and their English translations within the overview of early modern theatrical culture offered by the chosen three physicians, it interrogates their descriptions of spectacle and ceremony, performers, and performance strategies for insights into theatrical and medical practice, and their interfaces, and for evidence concerning specific healers and performers.

Why Physicians?

In order to maintain their position at the top of the early modern healthcare provision pyramid, qualified physicians were required to safeguard their economic interests in a precarious balancing act that postmodern medical history is only now beginning to fully explore. As well as apothecaries, surgeons and barber-

---

[7]   The pioneer in this field is Silvette (*The doctor on the stage*). See also: Moss and Peterson, *Disease, diagnosis, and cure*; Kerwin, *Beyond the body*; Pettigrew, *Shakespeare and the practice of physic*.

[8]   Such as the need 'to address one of the thorniest problems facing the history of Spanish medicine: bridging the gap between the elite world of academic medicine and its popular reception' (Slater and Terrada, 'Scenes of mediation', 227).

[9]   Kröll, 'Spectacles de foire' and 'Kurier die Leut auf meine Art'; Hattori, *Performing cures*; King, *The making of the dentiste*; Feinberg, 'Quacks and mountebanks'; Jones, 'Pulling teeth'; Porter, *Quacks, fakers & charlatans*; Park, 'Country medicine'; Hädge, 'Meß-Ärtzte'; Henke, 'The Italian mountebank'; Gentilcore, *Medical charlatanism*; Katritzky, *Women, medicine and theatre*.

[10]   See, for example, collaborative publications edited by Katritzky ('The commedia dell'arte'), Jütte ('The doctor on the stage'), Nutton ('Medicine in the renaissance city'), or Hädge and Baumbach (*Theaterkunst & Heilkunst*).

surgeons, midwives, hangmen and other professional colleagues with officially recognized healthcare expertise, they competed with various less clear-cut categories of unlicensed religious, supernatural and itinerant rivals. In the medical arena, practitioners of faith healing, magic and quackery integrated performance into their commercial and medical practice, in multifarious ways that qualified healthcare professionals increasingly ridiculed and undermined. Fortune-tellers, potion sellers, snake charmers, wise women and astrologers drew extensively on spectacle and ceremony in the service of health enhancement and promotion. A close relationship between healthcare provision and performance was central to early modern itinerant medical practice, and contributed materially to the effectiveness of its cures. Many quacks were actual performers themselves, using theatricality, in its widest possible sense, to attract customers and to promote and advertise their pharmaceuticals and healthcare services.

Qualified physicians were unusually informed and articulate observers of such activities. The privileged multiple viewpoints available to those who contributed to religious or secular performances staged within their own communities, or whose medical responsibilities took them to courts or foreign regions where they could experience performances and ceremonies inaccessible to most commoners or non-locals, greatly enriched their theatrical perceptions. As well as aiding assessment of genuine and false symptoms, diagnosis and cure, their professional training and medical experience supported accurate interpretation and communication of on and offstage healthcare practices, magic, and acrobatic routines. Keenly aware of the competitive threat of unlicensed healthcare practitioners, early modern physicians have left some of the most insightful observations on overlaps between medical and theatrical culture. No historical record is uncoloured by personal bias. The passages examined here are taken from the writings of three individuals whose social, religious and geographical backgrounds, and medical training and practice, offer contrasts as well as parallels.

Why these Three Physicians?

The decision to focus this book on passages of theatrical interest in the writings of Felix Platter, his younger half-brother Thomas Platter, and Hippolytus Guarinonius arises out of my long-term researches into German sources for the commedia dell'arte. Felix Platter has left a festival account featuring prominent and early use of commedia dell'arte costumes at a German court tournament. Thomas Platter and Hippolytus Guarinonius, familiar to theatre historians since the nineteenth century through much debated brief allusions to English actors, are the authors of several accounts of Italian commedia dell'arte quack troupes, of which the most informative are an extended passage in the manuscript travel journal of Thomas Platter and some three dozen theatrical descriptions in Guarinonius's published medical treatise of 1610. As well as representing substantial sources for stage practice, both clarify links between quack practice and the commedia dell'arte. Unlike most other early modern texts and images documenting quacks, they not only confirm interactions between itinerant healing and performance, but illuminate the details of how they functioned.

Having previously examined each of these three accounts individually, my aim here is to study them together, contextualized within the three physicians' rich range of theatrically relevant writings. In this book, considerations of the Christian festive year, Jewish culture, English actors, quacks, magic and monsters, use this approach to address general questions regarding these physicians' records of theatre and ceremony. An examination of Jacobean drama with reference to Thomas Platter's description of the ceremony of magical impotence provides a case study for exploring previously unnoted theatre-historical connections of one particular account. This approach also contributes new findings specifically relating to the three commedia dell'arte passages, as when the stage roles noted by Felix Platter and the quack troupe described by Thomas Platter are identified, or the literary strategies that impelled the deeply devout Guarinonius to pepper his serious medical treatise with detailed descriptions of scatological itinerant stage routines are clarified.[11]

Researches into German sources for the commedia dell'arte received a tremendous boost in the 1980s, when Jean-Marie Valentin initiated in depth investigations into the lengthy vernacular medical treatise containing Guarinonius's fleeting comment on the English actors, as an exceptional source of descriptions of commedia dell'arte lazzi, or pre-rehearsed units of transferable, expandable, stage business.[12] The characteristic stock roles, improvisational methods and lazzi of the commedia dell'arte were developed in sixteenth-century Italy, by itinerant troupes. They pioneered mixed-gender acting as a viable profession, and from around 1570, their commercial success enabled them to export it across the Alps to Spain, France, German-speaking Europe, and even London. A few of the most renowned early modern commedia dell'arte troupes were regularly financed by court invitations. Most relied on door takings from indoor, public performances in enclosed hired venues, often heavily supplemented by marketplace trading. Weather permitting, this usually involved free outdoor performances on trestle stages, in combination with the sale of medical goods or services. The commedia dell'arte was the earliest form of fully professional theatre, and the first to publicly flaunt the break from all-male drama, and from harsh restrictions imposed on year-round performing by the Christian festive year. Close attention to links between quackery and the commedia dell'arte illuminates the fundamental contribution made by this alliance to the development of year-round professional mixed-gender theatre in early modern Europe. Alberto Martino's comprehensive overview of the commedia dell'arte's early German sources considers Guarinonius's lazzi descriptions in detail, adding a further lazzo to those identified by Valentin and by

---

[11]   See this volume: Felix Platter (Chapters 7 and 16); Thomas Platter (Chapters 12 and 17); Hippolytus Guarinonius (Chapters 13–15 and 18).

[12]   Valentin, 'Herr Pantalon', 'Bouffons ou religieux?' and *Theatrum Catholicum*.

the present author.[13] In an updated version of his article, again concentrating on theatre-historical and literary issues, Martino confirms the writings of Guarinonius and Thomas Platter as among the most valuable of all German sources for the early commedia dell'arte.[14]

As well as representing informative early modern German-language records relating to the Italian professional actors, the commedia dell'arte descriptions of these three physicians are of wider documentary significance. They are of interest as contrasting and complementary theatre-historical records, and Thomas Platter and Hippolytus Guarinonius's descriptions of professional performances in the context of medical activities, concerning itinerants who earned their living by combining performance and healing, are of considerable medical-historical relevance. Thomas Platter here provides the most detailed early modern account of the commercial strategies of commedia dell'arte quack troupes. Taken as a group, they offer rich insights into both the medical and the theatrical practice of early modern quacks. Their documentary value is enhanced by contextualization within longer texts, and within each physician's writings as a whole, which afford a cumulative overview of festival and performance culture, and yield numerous further passages relevant to interdependencies between early modern performing and healing.

The writings of Guarinonius and the Platter brothers reveal a shared interest in performance and theatre coloured by their own individual experiences of performing, religious beliefs, and medical expertise. Felix Platter's instrumental and dancing talents, and Hippolytus Guarinonius's contributions to local religious drama and music, reflect contrasting strategies for utilizing theatrical skills to enhance medical careers and advance social standing, even while, in the case of Guarinonius, censuring professional performers in deeply negative terms. Thomas Platter's most revealing theatrical descriptions draw on the latest ethnographical advances in the science of apodemics, involving searching personal interviews with the performers themselves, often carried out over several visits. This book approaches these three male Christian physicians' writings with reference to their personal, professional and socio-religious contexts. It is concerned to acknowledge special insights brought by early modern medical professionals to an understanding of theatrical culture per se, and with respect to synergies between medicine and performance. Part I introduces the physicians. Part II focuses on festival culture.

---

[13]   Katritzky, 'Hippolytus Guarinonius' descriptions', 'Comic stage routines' and 'Guarinonius' lazzi'; Martino, 'Fonti tedesche degli anni 1585–1615', 684.

[14]   Martino acknowledges the present author's researches into Guarinonius's and Thomas Platter's theatrical descriptions, but neither the medical-historical importance of their descriptions, nor Felix Platter's account of commedia dell'arte costumes in a court festival masquerade ('Fonti tedesche degli anni 1565–1615', 21, 32, 43: Katritzky, 'Was commedia dell'arte performed by mountebanks?', 'Mountebanks, mummers and masqueraders', 'Marketing medicine', 'Hippolytus Guarinonius' descriptions', 'Comic stage routines', The art of commedia).

Part III examines the three physicians' accounts of English actors, marketplace performing and healing, magic and monsters. The subject of Part IV is itinerant performing quacks. Part V provides English translations of selected source texts.

Part II focuses on the three physicians' writings on religious, civic and court festivals, performances often combining spectacle with ceremony. Taken as a whole, major passages, but also countless brief comments, demonstrate how fundamentally these depended on the annual cycle of local, regional and Europe-wide holy-day feasts and fasts. While this is by no means a new insight, these particular records build up a vivid impression of the crucial role represented by this venerable tradition, not just at communal level, but in the everyday personal and professional lives of three specific individuals. The theatrical culmination of this dominant – Christian – early modern festive year was carnival. The Platter brothers' accounts of this, based on extensive participation in France and Spain as well as in their native Basle, represent some of the most informative descriptions of their time, illuminating medical as well as theatrical aspects of carnival tradition (Chapter 4). In multi-cultural early modern Europe, not everyone participated in the Christian festive year. Chapter 5 surveys the physicians' descriptions of some festivals, ceremonies and customs of the greatest minority religious group, the Jews, with a particular focus on Thomas Platter's uniquely detailed record of Jewish life in Avignon in the 1590s.

Chapter 6 considers the physicians' references to court festivals. Largely confined to their unpublished life writings and mostly dating to the 1590s, those of the Platter brothers, despite attracting little scholarly attention, are highly informative, ranging from brief allusions at second hand, to illustrated eyewitness accounts rivalling official printed descriptions in length and detail. Several record festivals unknown from other sources. Relevant to the present enquiry are the special perspectives offered by the Platter brothers' status as trained medical practitioners, and their freedom to illuminate aspects habitually ignored, glossed over, even deliberately misrepresented in the official accounts published in conjunction with the grander court festivals. These include the major and minor injuries and accidents routinely resulting from tournaments and other performances involving martial arts or hunting, journeys to and from festivals, and the impact of adverse weather conditions. Guarinonius's references to festivals are not factual descriptions. They support specific arguments in his medical writings. One of the longest purports to record his dialogue with a merchant who has recently attended a tournament in Stuttgart. The subject of this previously unrecognized account is here identified as a tournament parade at a founding court festival of the Protestant Union, staged only days before this dialogue was written. It provides fresh and detailed insights into the Catholic reception of this groundbreaking festival, well known from the official Protestant records, and raises questions concerning modern theatre-iconographical methodologies. The subject of Chapter 7 is Felix Platter's account of theatrical costumes at a German court wedding of 1598. Unlike the festival's official chronicler, Jakob Frischlin, Platter here correctly identifies 10 tournament masquerade characters significant for the early diffusion of the commedia dell'arte. This passage is here examined as a valuable, under-recognized record of the commedia dell'arte's considerable impact on sixteenth-century German festival culture.

Parts III and IV consider performers and healers, and their use of medicine and theatre. They examine the role of healing, and medical marketing, in the commercial strategies of performing troupes, and the particular insights physicians bring as spectators and critics of itinerant theatre. The subject of Part III is Thomas Platter's well known account of English actors and London's theatres and other tourist attractions, here set in the context of his visit to England, and of his account of Spanish theatre. It also considers Guarinonius's most discussed theatrical comments, on itinerant English players who, in contrast to Italian commedia dell'arte troupes, typically performed and toured independently of medical activities (Chapter 8). The physicians' writings are interrogated to provide an overview of the roles of healthcare and performing in the economic strategies of itinerant quacks, and how and where they traded (Chapter 9). Their references to two supernatural categories, magic and monsters, are considered. Magicians, necromancers and witches, but also some faith healers and quacks, professed, or were accused of, supernatural healing and other powers. They variously drew on magic, superstition, medicine and theatre in support of a wide range of occult practices, from card tricks to the ritual of magical impotence, this latter here considered with reference to a description of the practice by Thomas Platter, and its relevance to English drama (Chapter 10). During the early modern period, monsters, widely regarded as supernatural omens, were increasingly studied as indicative medical phenomena. The three physicians' writings advance our understanding of the diverging theatricalization and medicalization of human monstrosity. The case of Pedro Gonzales and his family is revisited in the light of newly identified archival evidence. This supports previously contested details of Felix Platter's account of his personal medical examination of two Gonzales children who inherited their father's hairy face and body, and brings into sharp focus the exceptional value of humans with rare, congenital, physical abnormalities as spectacular 'tokens' in the aristocratic gifts-for-patronage exchange economy (Chapter 11).

Part IV investigates quacks' medical and theatrical strategies, through close examination of Thomas Platter's account of a quack troupe in 1598 (Chapter 12), and Guarinonius's descriptions of professional comic stage routines (Chapters 13–15). The integration of medical practice and performance typically offered by Italian commedia dell'arte quack troupes, is an obvious manifestation of the intertwinement of early modern theatrical and medical culture. The quack-related descriptions of Guarinonius and Thomas Platter contribute to a growing body of documentary evidence suggesting that quacks did not always simply passively borrow from mainstream theatrical practice. Successful quacks adapted spectacular routines to suit their own economic and medical agendas, and their modifications in turn influenced developments in dramatic literature and stage practice. The complex, symbiotic relationship between certain professional healers and performers is a major factor in, and informs the specifics of, the high medical content of early modern drama. Reassessment of an account by Thomas Platter, describing the combination of medicine and performance offered by one specific Italian quack troupe he observed in Avignon in 1598, offers unprecedented insights into this relationship, and facilitates detailed consideration of an individual performer and his longterm career. Newly-discovered archival documents allow me to identify the actor whose stage name Platter gives as Zan Bragetta. He is Giovanni Paulo Alfieri, an Italian troupe leader never previously connected to medical or healthcare activities, and until now known only for having acted in Paris with the renowned French performer Valleran-le-Conte, on the stage of the Hôtel de Bourgogne in 1612. This new identification advances our understanding of the fluid overlaps between theatre and medicine on early modern European itinerant stages.

An examination of the commedia dell'arte descriptions of Hippolytus Guarinonius further illuminates questions regarding these interfaces. Almost wholly uncited by specialists outside the German-speaking regions, they are unusually informative regarding lazzi, the comic set-piece routines of the commedia dell'arte, and Guarinonius's treatise confirms that they were acted by professional quacks dependent on the sale of healthcare products and services (Chapter 13). His descriptions of some three dozen lazzi, ranging from fleeting allusions to lengthy detailed accounts, are examined in the context of other known records of lazzi, textual and visual, and with respect to what they can tell us about quack performances (Chapter 14). Didactic, literary, therapeutic and promotional explanations for Guarinonius's extensive use of lazzi descriptions in his medical treatise are explored. Their inclusion was intended as a medical marketing strategy offering a textual therapy for melancholy. As a vehicle for contrasting the unhealthy folly of sinful Italian stage fools with the healthy lifestyle of devout southern German Catholics, they also exemplify specific 'deadly' sins viewed by Guarinonius as being life-threatening in the medical as well as theological sense. Literary responses to these lazzi (not least Guarinonius's own), are considered in Chapter 15. Here, they are identified as a major element in a serious medical treatise's impact as a counter-Reformational contribution to the tradition of 'folly literature'; not random, medically inappropriate add-ons, but integral components of Guarinonius's holistic literary attempt to cure the bodies, minds and souls of his readers.[15]

Part V presents English translations of some source texts, including Felix Platter's account of a court festival of 1598, and Thomas Platter and Hippolytus Guarinonius's most substantial records of quack activities.[16] Before moving on to a detailed consideration of their theatrical writings, it is time to take a closer

---

[15]   Initiated in 1494 by the publication of the original German-language edition of Sebastian Brant's *Ship of fools*.

[16]   Discussed below, in Chapter 7 (Chapter 16), Chapters 5 and 12 (Chapter 17) and Chapters 13–15 (Chapter 18).

look at the three physicians themselves. They are the subject of the remaining two chapters of this introductory section, overviewing the travels, and medical and performing interests, practice and skills informing their writings.

Chapter 2

The Brothers Felix Platter (1536–1614) and Thomas Platter (1574–1628)

Felix and Thomas Platter are known to early modern historians far beyond the German-speaking regions. Felix, whose three older sisters[1] died in Basle plague epidemics, was the much-loved only surviving child of Thomas Platter the Elder's marriage to Anna Dietschi, the housemaid of his mentor, the Zurich humanist Oswald Myconius.[2] Thomas was one of six children from the second marriage Platter the Elder entered into when it seemed clear that Felix would remain childless.[3] Raised in great poverty in the rural Alpine Valais and effectively educated only in his twenties by Myconius and other mentors, Platter the Elder converted to Lutheranism and established himself as a Humanist in Basle. Here he ran a printing press and, with Anna Dietschi, a boarding house for local scholars and students. From the 1530s to 1578 he was also a teacher of ancient languages, then head teacher at the Münsterplatz grammar school. Felix Platter was born in Basle, studied medicine at the universities of Basle and Montpellier, and toured Europe before returning home to marry, set up his own practice and take the posts of Basle's public health officer, professor of medicine, dean of the medical school and vice-chancellor of Basle University. All these stages were mirrored some four decades later by his half-brother Thomas.[4]

Felix's high professional ambitions had early roots. Only poverty prevented his father from formal medical study. A central chapter in the memoirs of Platter the

---

[1]   Margaretlein 1 (1530–1), Margaretlein 2 (1533–6) and Ursel (1534–51).

[2]   Platter the Elder, 'Thomas Platters Lebensbeschreibung', 90–1, 106–7, 133–4, 141, 154, 161.

[3]   On 24 April 1572, two months after the death of Anna (1495 to 20 February 1572), Platter the Elder married Esther Gross (c.1555–1612, see Platter the Elder, 'Thomas Platters Lebensbeschreibung', 164–5). Felix Platter's medical writings supplement autobiographical information in his journals, e.g. regarding his father's second family (Platter, *Obseruationum*, 256). The most authoritative secondary sources of information on the Platter family and their immediate circle, not always further acknowledged in the present footnotes, are Valentin Lötscher and Rut Keiser's notes to their monumental editions of the journals (*Felix Platter Tagebuch* and *Thomas Platter d.J*) and Lötscher's biographical monograph (*Felix Platter und seine Familie*). Hippolytus Guarinonius considers noteworthy that Christoph Faber's 20-year fourth and final marriage, entered into at the age of 60, produced eight children (*Grewel*, 49).

[4]   Platter, *Englandfahrt*, XVIII–XXI.

Elder relates his entry into the service of a medical mentor, Giovanni Epiphanius.[5] This Venetian alcoholic, banished from the Bavarian court for contravening fasting regulations, took Platter with him from Zurich to Pruntrut, when he became personal physician to Jakob Philipp von Gundelsheim, Bishop of Basle. He promised to support Platter's 'special interest in practicing medicine', but died only a few months later, in the plague epidemic of 1531 that claimed Platter the Elder's oldest child. As a publisher and teacher, Platter the Elder became a great collector of medical publications, and regularly took the young schoolboy Felix to witness public executions and dissections of human corpses.[6] Despite struggling with several phobias, not least a nauseous reaction to all rings and ring-shaped objects and human physical nonconformity, however minor, Felix was then already studying herbals, collecting and dissecting plants and insects, keenly observing the butchering of farm animals, and expressing a strong desire to fulfil his father's frequently articulated wish for him to study medicine.[7]

On 29 September 1551, shortly before his fifteenth birthday, Felix Platter successfully underwent the University of Basle's traditional pre-matriculation ceremony and commenced his medical studies there.[8] On 10 October 1552, Felix Platter left plague-ridden Basle for Montpellier, where he continued his medical studies on arrival three weeks later, even before immatriculating on 4 November (Plate 2). At the start of his fourth year of medical study in Montpellier, Felix Platter received a letter from Basle from his childhood friend Balthasar Hummel, who had studied and lodged with him in Montpellier in 1554.[9] Having returned to Basle to practice as an apothecary, Hummel sent Felix a damning report of medical practice in their home city, that was in stark contrast to parental warnings concerning the powerful professional competition facing him on his return.[10] Felix paraphrased Hummel's letter in his journal, noting his friend's concerns that Basle's physicians were being poached by courts, spa resorts and schools, and that the incompetence and ignorance of those that remained were seriously devaluing the healing – and earning – power of his own profession of pharmacist:

---

[5]   Platter, *Obseruationum*, 95; Platter the Elder, 'Thomas Platters Lebensbeschreibung', 104–14.

[6]   *Felix Platter Tagebuch*, 96–8, 103–5 (1546, Basle).

[7]   *Felix Platter Tagebuch*, 101, 111, 127 (1548–52, Basle); Hochlenert, 'Das "Tagebuch" des Felix Platter', 120–1, 154. On his 'ring phobia', see Frenken, *Kindheit und Autobiographie*, 488–9, 499–504, 536; Bumiller, 'Selbstsanalyse', 308–10.

[8]   On the ceremony of 'Deponieren', a ritual cleansing of the would-be student typically involving shaving the head, filing the nails and pulling a tooth, see Lötscher (in *Felix Platter Tagebuch*, 119n556).

[9]   Hummel's daughter Margaretha was one of five children to whom the newly-qualified physician Felix became godfather in 1557. *Felix Platter Tagebuch*, 206, 252, 311 (11 November 1554 and August 1556, Montpellier; November 1557, Basle).

[10]   See, for example, *Felix Platter Tagebuch*, 186, 193 (September 1553 and 26 February 1554, Montpellier).

Dr Zonion has no patients, Dr Pantaleon is in Plombières-les-Bains, Dr Huggelin is with the margrave, Dr Huber is a schoolmaster. He [Hummel] complained bitterly how difficult it was for him to stay solvent, he had no business at his apothecary, and there were few orders. Prescriptions were not highly regarded in Basle, and more often written in German than Latin. The physicians mostly prescribe purgatives based on cassia, liquorice root, or other foolish stuff. Dr Isaac [Keller] makes up his own cheap rubbish for his patients. He [Hummel] would rather be a beggar than a pharmacist in Basle. These physicians know nothing apart from purging, and unlike those of Montpellier, don't use any properly prepared medicines. He consoled himself by thinking of me, and how I would turn things around.[11]

Felix Platter's journal entry continues by recalling his emotions on reading Hummel's words: 'This letter inspired me to think that I possessed better knowledge than some others, and could introduce many practices then unknown there, such as enemas and other *topica*, all sorts of useful remedies. And with the help of God, this is what happened'.[12] In January 1557, while preparing for the tour of France that brought him home to Basle, he sent the last of many letters to his father from Montpellier. His journal's paraphrase of this filial letter reiterates his ambition even more forcefully: 'I was well aware how difficult it would be for me to establish a practice, how much effort and work it involved. But I hoped that by God's grace it would go well for me, because I have already practiced a lot, and I intend to establish my reputation by making use of much more effective methods for healing than are customary with us [in Basle]'.[13]

Felix Platter returned to Basle in May 1557 preoccupied with two goals: becoming a fully qualified physician, and marrying Madlen Jeckelmann.[14] The marriage negotiations had begun only after Madlen Erbßlin, a distant relative by marriage to whom he had been betrothed as a 10-year-old, succumbed to the plague. Acting on rumours spread by friends who discovered the teenage Felix's secret love poems to Madlen Jeckelmann, and desperate for a daughter-in-law to replace Ursel, the daughter he had just lost to the plague, Platter's father approached the widowed Franz Jeckelmann, whose reluctance to part with the daughter who ran his household was not lost on Felix.[15] Twenty-year-old Felix was concerned to publicly celebrate his achievement of his twin goals in his home city, in a manner appropriate to his professional ambitions. Although University of Basle regulations then required candidates for the medical doctorate to have

---

[11]   *Felix Platter Tagebuch*, 223–4 (11 September 1555, Montpellier). The original letter of 18 August 1555 is one of many to Felix in Basle (BUL Frey-Grynaeum I, 8, p.150).

[12]   *Felix Platter Tagebuch*, 224.

[13]   *Felix Platter Tagebuch*, 262 (12–14 January 1557, Montpellier).

[14]   1534–1613.

[15]   Platter the Elder, 'Thomas Platters Lebensbeschreibung', 156–7; *Felix Platter Tagebuch*, 78, 112–14, 120–1, 215, 314 (1545–57, Basle and Montpellier).

reached the age of 24, exceptionally, he was permitted to qualify shortly before his 21st birthday. His journal describes his ostentatious and costly doctoral ceremony, and his more modest wedding a few weeks later, in November 1557. The couple then moved in with his parents for three years, while he struggled to become economically independent by establishing a viable medical practice.

Felix Platter's journal adds 17 further sedentary rivals, male and female, to the five local medical practitioners named in Hummel's letter of August 1555:

> When I came to Basle, there were many doctors there who had adopted medicine as their profession and practiced. Those who had qualified were:
>
> 1. Dr Oswald Bacr, public health officer
> 2. Dr Johannes Huber
> 3. Dr Isaac Keller
> 4. Dr Adam Bodenstein, known as Carlistat
> 5. Dr Heinrich Pantaleon
> 6. Dr Caspar Petri, known as Mellinger
> 7. Dr Guilelmus Gratarolus [of Bergamo], known as Pergomast
> 8. Dr [Johann] Jacob Huggelin
> 9. Dr Jakob Wecker
> 10. the licentiate Philippus Bechius
> 11. *dominus* Johannes Bauhin
>
> Additionally, there were Dr Jacob Myconius[16] and Dr [Johann] Jacob Zonion, both of whom however soon moved away. Then there were the empirics, Ziliochs of St Alban, who was consulted as if he were a doctor, and the widow of Otto Brunfels,[17] who was also much in demand. Then there was me, Dr Felix Platter, and a year later Dr Theodor Zwinger. So around the years 1557 to 1558 there were seventeen doctors in Basle. I had to apply considerable skills if I wanted to earn my living by my practice, and was supported in this by God's rich blessings. Also very famous at this time was Amman, the so-called peasant of Utzendorf, to whom considerable numbers of people went. He could read fortunes by divining water and practiced strange arts for many years, through which he had acquired a considerable estate. After him, the Jew of Allschwil[18] attracted huge numbers of patients for a long time. There was also an old woman called Lülbürenen in Gerber Lane, to whom many sick people went, as also to the two municipal hangmen, the brothers Wolf and Georg Käser, whose oldest

---

16   This friend of Felix Platter was the adopted son of his father's mentor, Oswald Myconius.

17   Dorothea Helg practiced medicine in Basle until at least 1572, after the death of her husband, the humanist, physician and botanist Otto Brunfels (1488–1534), who published a respected herbal in 1530.

18   On whom see Chapter 5, this volume.

brother was renowned in Schaffhausen for his medical skills, as is their father Wolf, the hangman of Tübingen. In the meantime, I began to attract a clientele among the local citizens and nobility, who generally tested me out by sending their urine samples, from which I had to make predictions. I dealt with these so well that many were impressed and started to come to me.[19]

The young French-trained doctor was not in a position to turn away business or disappoint local expectations. He tackled routine tasks of a type delegated by more established physicians, and dealt with endless requests for uroscopy from sceptical patients who came to try out his skills. He goodhumouredly interpreted a man carrying a urine sample in his parent's street, whom he encountered on his return from France, as a positive omen for his own future career. Even so, references to this hugely popular diagnostic method such as his criticism of a rival's 'tricks with uroscopy', indicate that he followed the latest medical thinking in rejecting its medical and theatrical aspects as outmoded showmanship, inappropriate to educated physicians.[20] Within Basle, he collaborated with the surgical practice of his in-laws, the Jeckelmann family. On house calls outside the city, he frugally deployed the full range of his own medical skills. As late as 1562, he notes his extreme exhaustion, and disappointment at being rewarded with only 30 crowns, on attending his wealthy patient Dela Deschamps of Belfort virtually round the clock from 16 January to 7 February: 'not only as his physician, but also as his surgeon and his apothecary'.[21]

Felix Platter's hard work established the foundations for his brilliant career as Basle's wealthiest and most distinguished physician, with a wide network of private, religious and noble patients in and outside Basle. He was on sporadic call to many French and German courts, for example visiting the court of Lorraine at Nancy in March 1601, and accepted long-term professional responsibilities for the Bishop of Basle and Georg Friedrich, Margrave of Baden and their courts (Diagram 2).[22] In 1561, his father gave him the house next door to his own, and thereafter his career quickly gathered pace. In 1562, he was appointed Dean of Basle's medical school and in 1570 he became Vice-Chancellor. In 1571, when Basle had around 10,000 inhabitants, he accepted the chair of practical medicine, and became the city's public health officer, responsible for managing epidemics

---

[19]   *Felix Platter Tagebuch*, 335–8 (Spring 1558, Basle).

[20]   *Felix Platter Tagebuch*, 294 (9 May 1557, Basle), 414 (19 July 1563, Grächen), 449 (12 July 1566). See also Stolberg, 'The decline of uroscopy', 321, 328, 335. By the 1650s, Guarinonius is dismissing uroscopy as an unhygienic gypsy trick (Innsbruck UL, Cod.110, IV, f.496ᵛ).

[21]   *Felix Platter Tagebuch*, 383–4 (1562, Belfort).

[22]   Platter, *Obseruationum*, 574 (Plat[t]er, Culpeper and Cole, *Platerus histories*, 380: 'sent for by the Duke of *Lotharing* [Lorraine], to see the Cardinal his Son'). Baumann questions the extent to which Platter's municipal and academic commitments allowed him to take on formal long-term court engagements ('Ernst Friedrich von Baden Durlach', 336).

and overseeing autopsies, physicians, surgeons and midwives, hospitals for the poor, physically sick and mentally ill, and for training and examining medical students. He oversaw construction of a botanical garden and an anatomy theatre at the medical school, and introduced teaching practices from Montpellier, such as taking students on clinical hospital visits.[23] After the death of his father, Felix Platter moved to a larger home, the so-called Samson House. Here he established his curiosity cabinet, library, laboratory and study, considerable collections of *materia medica*, geological, botanical and zoological specimens, ethnological and artistic artefacts, and musical instruments. He also grew herbs, citrus trees and other medical simples, and bred canaries, doves, rabbits, guinea pigs, marmots and silkworms.

Exotic animals, whether live or as preserved specimens, were popular 'props' habitually displayed by itinerant quacks. Many great museums originated in curiosity cabinets, and such spectacle, commercially motivated by quacks' own medical agendas and their clients' scientific curiosity and medical anxieties, is relevant to the history of collecting, and the scientific and cultural pursuits of qualified physicians. Felix Platter confessed to 'a great enthusiasm for all sorts of living creatures'. As a young physician, he was repeatedly presented with animals of precisely the type associated with quacks, including a monkey from his patient Hannibal von Bärenfels, and, during his visit to the Valais, a marmot which died within a day.[24] Felix Platter's interests put him at the forefront of developments in academic teaching museums and research collections, while his excellent business sense allowed him to earn large sums by charging entrance fees and trading in silk, plants, animals and medical simples. The collections were eventually passed to Thomas Platter's great-granddaughter Helena and her physician husband Claudius Passavant, and dissipated as far afield as Sweden and Russia when their physician son sold it off in the late eighteenth century, after their deaths.[25] The apothecary, local politician, amateur scientist and great man of the theatre Renward Cysat visited Felix Platter repeatedly from the 1580s. He records his open-mouthed astonishment at his ethnographical exhibits, and Jacques Auguste de Thou was fascinated by Platter's live catfish and elk in 1579.[26] Montaigne, who dined with Felix Platter and his friend and colleague the humanist and physician Theodor Zwinger[27] in October 1580, was impressed by the imposing size and attractively painted exterior of Platter's house, his human skeletons and the new method for preserving the herbal specimens he had been collecting for over 20 years in

---

[23]   Trinkler, *Pathologie*, 30–1.

[24]   *Felix Platter Tagebuch*, 378, 391 (1562, Basle), 420 (22 June 1563, Visp).

[25]   For the Platter family tree, see Boos (*Thomas und Felix Platter*, 373).

[26]   Lötscher, *Felix Platter und seine Familie*, 128, 146–8; Bujok, 'Ethnographica', 17. Cysat produced Lucerne's civic Passion plays in 1583 and 1597.

[27]   1533–88. Stepson of Conrad Lycosthenes, former scholar of Platter's father, and Professor of Medical Theory at Basle's School of Medicine.

volumes.[28] Thomas Platter inventoried 18 of these volumes in his housebook after Felix's death, and eight are still in the University of Basle's botanical institute.[29]

Felix Platter's reputation was consolidated by his medical publications. His three-volume anatomy treatise of 1583 was based on the groundbreaking treatise of Andreas Vesalius, whose visit to his father's house in 1543 to discuss its publication he recalls in his journal.[30] Other treatises addressed aspects of the plague, the human eye, and gynaecology. In 1602, 1603 and 1608, Platter published his collected lectures in a three-volume so-called 'Praxis medica', summarizing his medical knowledge in generic form.[31] Rejecting the traditional 'top to toe' format of medical treatises, which commonly started with ailments of the head, working down the body to conclude with the feet, this attempt to introduce a more scientific classification of medical conditions continued to be republished until at least 1736. *Observations*, published in the final year of his life, 1614 and dedicated to his patron, the Margrave of Baden, presented 680 specific case-studies classified in similar manner.[32] Most soberly anonymize details of personal patients treated by Felix or his brother Thomas, providing symptoms and outcomes (unsuccessful as well as successful), and sometimes outlining treatments and medicines. A few concern travelling performers and others he observed and interrogated outside his own practice, or heard or read about. These latter include a wandering beggar boy who made a public show of swallowing stones for money at fairs; a comic stage-player in St Gallen whose act went horribly wrong when the large live eel he was pretending to swallow dived down his throat into his gut;[33] a country fellow whose gut was allegedly invaded by a live mole that burrowed its way up his fundament; three dwarfs and numerous other anatomically exceptional humans, and theology student Sebastian Rosæus Herbipolensis, who travelled round fairs begging, after suffering a spectacular scrotal prolapse of his guts.[34] Early modern English citations of Platter are not limited to medical publications.[35] A 1662 English translation of *Praxis medica* incorporating specific cases into the original edition's generic

---

[28]   Montaigne, *Complete works*, 1069.

[29]   Basle UL, Ms.A λ V.9 ('Hausbuch'), f.507. Guarinonius collected pressed plants in a leather-bound single-volume *Herbarium* preserved in Innsbruck (Tiroler Landesmusem Ferdinandeum, Botanik nr.01).

[30]   Platter, *De Corporis Hvmani Strvctvra*; *Felix Platter Tagebuch*, 61 (1543, Basle).

[31]   Platter, *Praxeos*.

[32]   Platter, *Obseruationum*.

[33]   Goulart attributes versions of these two stories respectively to Vesalius and Conrad Gesner (*Admirable and memorable histories*, 79, 81). The eel was ingested, digested and expelled within a day, as Platter pointed out to another patient, whom he vainly hoped to disabuse of the delusion of having hosted a live frog within his digestive system for over seven years (Platter, *Obseruationum*, 43; Midelfort, *A history of madness*, 177–8).

[34]   Platter, *Obseruationum*, 413–14, 456–8, 545–64, 709–10.

[35]   References in their publications confirm that Platter was read by medical authors such as Diemerbroeck (*The anatomy of human bodies*) or Hart (*Klinike*) and more general

text, some lifted from Platter's *Observations*, some added anachronistically by the English editors, was evidently successful enough to warrant the same team's translation and publication of *Observations* itself, in 1664.[36]

Felix Platter was born into a world in which the annual cycle of church and academic-sponsored mystery plays underpinned a lively performance culture, further enriched by amateur performances of classical and contemporary drama. Acting and music-making, important to Protestant as well as Catholic education, were integral to the pastoral and academic care provided at his father's boarding house. By his own account born to the sound of the Carnival Sunday church bells on 10 February 1499,[37] Platter the Elder was keenly interested in performance practice as a didactic aid. He employed older boarders to instruct his boarders in music, and directed and even wrote plays for them himself. The schoolboy Felix acted in some of these, and as an adult, his collections included 42 musical instruments. Unlike his brother Thomas, Felix was a precociously talented actor, dancer and musician, whose love of music started early:[38]

> I had a special interest in and inclination towards music, and specially for playing instruments [...] and for this reason, when I was only eight, my father allowed me to start studying with Peter Dorn the lutenist, whom he engaged to teach his boarders to play the lute [...] so that my lute-playing was later so well practised that in Montpellier they called me "the German with the lute", and I played at many banquets and serenades [...] I also greatly enjoyed playing the spinet and organ [...], clavichord [...] and harp.[39]

His exceptional lute-playing put him in demand as a music teacher and professional lutenist during his schoolboy and student years. Even after returning to Basle from Montpellier, he excelled at exploiting his amateur musical ability to enhance his social standing and contacts, as when he entertained the noblewomen with whom he was sharing a carriage, on the way to a court wedding of 1577, on his lute.[40] Felix Platter's journal illuminates early modern music education, and records some dozen religious and secular theatrical performances in Basle during the 1540s of

---

writers such as Burton (*The anatomy of melancholy*), Goulart (*Admirable and memorable histories*) or Jonstonus (*An history*).

[36]   Ignoring its anachronistic additions, Cranefield ('Little known English versions'), suggests that the English translation of *Praxis medica* (Plat[t]er, Cole and Culpeper, *A golden practice*) is more reliable than that of *Observations* (Plat[t]er, Culpeper and Cole, *Platerus histories*).

[37]   Platter the Elder, 'Thomas Platters Lebensbeschreibung', 18.

[38]   Staehelin, 'Felix Platter und die Musik'.

[39]   *Felix Platter Tagebuch*, 70–3 (1543–4, Basle). See also 251, 255–6 (August–October 1556, Montpellier).

[40]   *Felix Platter Tagebuch*, 459 (15 August 1577, Donaueschingen).

which he had direct on or offstage experience (Diagram 3).[41] His recollection of the raised heaven constructed for an outdoor production of *The Conversion of St Paul* by Valentin Boltz records an unexpected outcome of its special effects. He observed this from a house on the corner of the Basle Cornmarket on 6 June 1546: 'Balthasar Han[42] was God the Father, in a circular heaven, that hung up on The Peacock, out of which came the ray of light: a fiery rocket that set alight Saul's costume as he fell from his horse, [...] in the heaven thunder was produced, by turning barrels filled with stones, etc.'[43] In a production of this play staged by himself and his father's boarders, Gavin de Beaufort, as Paul, was badly wounded when Felix, as God the Father, accidentally hit him in the face with a makeshift thunderbolt improvised from a log.[44] A production of *Hamanus* could have ended disastrously if the quick thinking hangman, played by Balthasar Hummel's brother Ludwig, had not rescued his victim, played by Gamaliel Gyrenfalck, when the mechanism of the stage gallows failed and left him hanging by his neck.[45] Felix's schoolboy theatrical career was significantly motivated by a lifelong love of fine clothes. As Lycondes in a production of Plautus's *Aulularia*, he delighted in wearing 'a beautiful cloak'. Conversely, when he and Gavin de Beaufort were asked to recite extracts from Virgil's *Eclogues* at the house of Hieronymus Frobenius, the thought of wearing pastoral shepherd costumes improvised from 'our neighbour Christelin's torn clothes', repelled him to the extent that he 'feigned an illness in order to stay at home'.[46]

All the early modern Platter family life writings owe their existence to the initiative of Felix Platter. His father Platter the Elder may have used earlier journals and correspondence to compile the well-known account of his life that Felix encouraged him to write in the first weeks of 1572,[47] to which he later added a brief account of his second marriage. The journal of Felix's half-brother Thomas Platter solely covers his half-decade away from Basle, when Felix supported him in completing his medical studies and touring Europe. The scattered evidence concerning Felix and Madlen Platter's barren but far from childless marriage stands at the heart of the family's domestic interrelationships, which profoundly inform interpretation of the Platter journals. Felix Platter became an only child shortly before leaving for Montpellier. Throughout his childhood, he and his sister Ursula shared the family home with up to three dozen male boarding scholars each

---

[41]   See also Le Roy Ladurie, *The beggar and the professor*, 93–100.

[42]   This local stained-glass painter, a Platter family friend, attended Felix's wedding (*Felix Platter Tagebuch*, 318: 20 November 1557, Basle).

[43]   *Felix Platter Tagebuch*, 82–3 (1546, Basle).

[44]   *Felix Platter Tagebuch*, 85–6 (1546, Basle).

[45]   *Felix Platter Tagebuch*, 84–5 (1546, Basle).

[46]   *Felix Platter Tagebuch*, 85, 94 (1546, Basle); Lötscher, *Felix Platter und seine Familie*, 58–9; Hochlenert, 'Das "Tagebuch" des Felix Platter', 114–15.

[47]   Platter the Elder, 'Thomas Platters Lebensbeschreibung', 158, 160.

year. While Felix and Madlen took in far fewer paying boarders,[48] several children entered their household as wards. In 1560, the two-year-old orphan Abraham Bechius became the ward of Felix, who had stopped treating his father, the physician Philip, for cirrhosis of the liver, after overhearing Abraham's shrewish mother insultingly dismiss his diagnosis. Felix Platter supported Abraham throughout his short life, paying for his medical education in Basle and France.[49] In 1565, on the death of Madlen's older brother Franz Jeckelmann, she and Felix took in his nine-year-old daughter Crischona Jeckelmann.[50] Around 1572, a newborn baby, Margreth Simon, was welcomed into the household.[51] Formal adoption, with its attendant inheritance regulations, was then uncommon, particularly among wealthy couples.[52] Gredlin, as she was known, although unadopted and keeping the surname of her widowed, homeless father, was brought up as Felix and Madlen's daughter in all but name, and remembered with parental affection and generosity in their wills. Taught the customary feminine skills of running a household, sewing, embroidery and music-making, she was only reluctantly parted with in 1604, to marry the tailor Michel Rüedin. In 1580, two years after Crischona left to get married, Madlen's younger brother Daniel died, and her household was joined by his two-year-old youngest child. Also called Crischona Jeckelmann,[53] she left the household in 1602 to marry Felix's half-brother Thomas Platter.

Eight-year-old Thomas Platter and his five-year-old brother Niklaus joined Felix and Madlen's household in 1582. Following the death of their father that year, their mother Esther Gross moved out of the Platter family home next door to Felix, with her sons Thomas and Niklaus and four daughters, and remarried. *Observations* notes that during the Basle plague epidemic of 1582–3, Felix Platter 'lost three sisters, *Anne, Vrsula* and *Elizabetha*, infants, my two Brothers and eldest Sister being out of Town […] I sent all the young of my family to my country-house'.[54] Gross's second husband seems to have been the tiler Hans Lützelmann. Born in January 1561, his oldest child, Jakob, was baptized in May 1582, four months after Platter the Elder's death. A kinswoman, Barbara Lützelmann, stood godmother

---

48   Lötscher, *Felix Platter und seine Familie*, 88–9.

49   *Felix Platter Tagebuch*, 364–5 (1560, Basle).

50   1556–1629. Lötscher, *Felix Platter und seine Familie*, 161–2.

51   'Histori vom Gredlin' (*Felix Platter Tagebuch*, 451–3); Lötscher, *Felix Platter und seine Familie*, 108, 116–18, 164.

52   Davis, 'Ghosts, kin and progeny', 104–5.

53   1577–1624.

54   Platter, *Obseruationum*, 309 (this translation: Plat[t]er, Culpeper and Cole, *Platerus histories*, 199–200). He did not offer to take in his healthy nine-year-old half-sister Magdalena (1573–1651). The Platter journals appear to suggest that when death, poverty or remarriage prevented two parents from running a joint household, it was customary for their daughters to be raised in the household of the mother or her family, and sons in that of the father, or his family.

to Thomas Platter in 1574.[55] Felix Platter refers harshly to his bereaved young stepmother in two letters of October 1582. They are addressed to the physician Basilius Amerbach, whose aid he enlisted in removing Thomas and Niklaus from their mother's plague-stricken household:

> You wanted to achieve an agreement with my stepmother, that she sends me the two boys, and gives and entrusts them to me [...] two of the little girls are complaining of stomach pains, they are throwing up and running temperatures, which is increasing my concerns even more. So if it is God's will I would like to rescue the boys, provided they are still healthy [...] If she obeys and gives them to me, I will treat them as my own children. If she doesn't, she will surely suffer for it.

> [*And later that month:*] She has only sent me one boy, and is keeping the other, whom I would like to have with the other one [...] In the event that the boy is not ill apart from having fallen on his nose, she should at the very least show consideration for her own children by sending him now, so that he escapes the rabble. But in the event that he really is ill, in the name of God he should stay with the others, may God show them mercy.[56]

Felix's uncharacteristically belligerent threats proved successful. He took responsibility for raising and educating his half-brothers.[57] Thomas matriculated at Basle in 1590 and left for Montpellier on 16 September 1595.[58] Niklaus followed Thomas to Basle Medical School in 1595, where he died of bloody diarrhoea in 1597.

Thomas Platter was awarded his medical doctorate in Montpellier in March 1597.[59] After 18 months of professional practice in nearby Uzès and three months in Avignon, he made his Grand Tour through France, Spain, the Low Countries and England, returning to Basle on 15 February 1600. His detailed four-and-a-half-year travel journal is preserved as a fair-copy manuscript compiled during the period 1604–5, from earlier notes. In 1936, its 804 numbered and many unnumbered

---

[55]   Platter the Elder, 'Thomas Platters Lebensbeschreibung', 165.

[56]   Lötscher, *Felix Platter und seine Familie*, 154–5.

[57]   Le Roy Ladurie, *The beggar and the professor*, 343–5; Frenken, *Kindheit und Autobiographie*, 533–5.

[58]   The dates in Thomas Platter's journal conform to the customs of the country he is in. Swiss dates were then 10 days behind those of the Gregorian calendar (although the days of the week remained the same), presented in a Papal bull of 1582 and already adopted in Spain, Portugal, the Italian states, France and other regions. In much of Protestant Europe, the Julian calendar did not give way to the Gregorian calendar until 18 February 1700 (directly followed by 1 March 1700), or even later in England, Sweden and the Swiss Grisons. See also Blackburn and Holford-Strevens, *Year*, 683–8.

[59]   *Thomas Platter d.J*, 210 (22 March 1597, Montpellier).

folios were bound into two volumes, kept together with his friendship album in Basle's University Library.[60] The fashion for keeping these pocket-sized volumes spread across central Europe from Protestant German-speaking regions in the 1540s, creating a book-based forerunner of modern social networking websites. Tens of thousands of such albums, blank or interleaved with printed books, into which friends, teachers and acquaintances of travellers entered brief signed, dated, and occasionally illustrated inscriptions, survive in European museums, archives and libraries.[61] Felix Platter refers to his album soon after his arrival in Montpellier, noting that Oswald Myconius 'died of a stroke [...] who not long before, when I took my leave of him, wrote this saying in my little friendship album'. In March 1557, the itinerant quack Samuel Hertenstein signed Felix Platter's album in Toulouse ('and thereafter there was no further news of him, where he went, or when he died'), and he collected more than 20 entries from mainly Protestant Germans studying at the University of Orléans.[62]

Thomas published some editions of Felix's medical works but no independent writings. Although he refers to a collection of case studies from his practice in Uzès and other lost works, his only surviving manuscripts are a housebook kept from 1615, containing copies of wills and inventories, and his travel journal.[63] Some scholars have criticized what they perceive as the 'colourless mediocrity' of Thomas's life and journal, by comparison with his brother Felix. Clare Williams, whose expression this is, provides a helpful introduction to Thomas's extensive borrowings from the accounts of other early modern German travellers and their shared published sources, notably Braun and Hogenberg, and Sebastian Münster (Plates 2–3). Labelling Thomas Platter's journal a 'dull and tedious [...] patchwork of undigested information', she offers no insights into early modern enthusiasm for what would now be viewed as literary plagiarism, or why the approach and style of a journal written by an ambitious newly qualified physician specifically for the older brother who generously supported and financed his studies and travels, and covering a brief five-year period near the beginning of his adult life, might differ from a life narrative of his younger decades written by a successful man in his seventies.[64] The style of Thomas's journal is much less personal than that of Felix. He hardly mentions his mother's family, beyond briefly noting a meeting with his 'late stepfather Johannes Lützelmann' in Lyon, and arrangements for transferring money to him.[65] In stark contrast to that of Felix, his journal rarely reveals personal thoughts or feelings, or even mundane details of his everyday life. Exceptionally,

---

[60]   Basle UL, Ms.A λ V.7–8; Vischer, 'Stammbücher'.

[61]   Schnabel, *Das Stammbuch*, 244–9.

[62]   *Felix Platter Tagebuch*, 155 (January 1553, Montpellier), 269, 276–7 (March 1557, Toulouse and Orléans).

[63]   *Thomas Platter d.J*, 221 (9 May 1597, Uzès); Basle UL, Ms.A λ V.9 ('Hausbuch').

[64]   Williams, *Thomas Platter's travels in England*, 112, 117, 136–40.

[65]   *Thomas Platter d.J*, 36, 40 (30 September and 2 October 1595, Lyon).

two references to his 'maistresse', in August 1598, afford an unfamiliar glimpse into the 24-year-old's domestic set-up in France.[66]

Although both brothers inherited their father's love of theatre, Thomas, unlike Felix, inclined more to the visual arts and architecture than to music. His travels were motivated by touristic as well as educational concerns, indicating an obsessive interest in keeping up with court and municipal festivals, and visiting well-known local sights, including academic institutions.[67] Intended for circulation outside the immediate family, perhaps even for eventual publication, his journal is heavily influenced by the science of apodemics, which theorized systematic observational methods for travel-based information gathering, and historio-geographical and ethnographical approaches to travel writing. The University of Basle was then at the cutting edge of this newly emerging field of study, producing publications such as *Methodus apodemica* or *Synagoga Ivdaica*, respectively published in Basle in 1577 and 1603 by Felix Platter's university colleagues Theodor Zwinger and Johannes Buxtorf the Elder.[68] As an unusually well-educated, acute and reliable observer and an appreciative dependent, he spared no effort in writing up matters of special interest to Felix, drawing on the very latest developments in apodemics to record the routine customs and practices of people of other regions, nationality or religion. As a trained physician, he had a lively professional interest in spectacle with any sort of medical relevance. He describes general customs concerning such events as weddings, dances, royal entries and processions, and specific theatrical performances and performers he witnessed in the later 1590s. Valuable and accessible accounts of theatrical events and practice abound in early modern travel accounts, such as those of the Englishmen Thomas Coryate, Fynes Moryson or John Evelyn.[69] Thomas Platter's diary is not unusual for its period in describing itinerant professional performers and spectacle and ceremony, such as that relating to quacks or carnival, in general, and for including eyewitness set pieces describing spectacular court festivals. However, it provides exceptionally detailed information regarding professional practice, including a wide range of eyewitness descriptions of actual performances, and records with particular attention traditional carnival practices and the activities of travelling entertainers, including their promotion of medical goods and services. Some of Platter's descriptions of the actual stage routines of specific professional performers draw

---

[66]   *Thomas Platter d.J*, 283 (27–29 August 1598, Uzès).

[67]   He claimed to have visited all 10 French universities known to him (*Thomas Platter d.J*, 608: 9 August 1599, Paris).

[68]   Deutschländer, 'Allein auß begirdt', 58. On *Synagoga Ivdaica*, see Chapter 5, this volume.

[69]   Coryate, *Crudities*. Fynes Moryson (1566–1630) wrote up his extensive European travels of the 1590s in four parts. Parts I–III (London BL, MS.Harley 5133: Latin), were published in a heavily edited English translation of 1617, as *An Itinerary*. An abridged version of Part IV (Oxford CCC, MS.CCC 94: English), was first published in 1903, as *Shakespeare's Europe*.

on observations collected over a longer period. It is hardly coincidental that it took a physician to bring into such sharp focus the marketing and theatrical strategies of mountebank troupes combining commedia dell'arte performances with quack activity.

Felix himself produced the third autobiographical Platter account. In the final half-decade of his life, he drew on his own French student and travel journals, and correspondence with his parents, his French 'exchange students' Jacques and Gilbert Catelan, and numerous Basle friends, to compile the fair copy of his life writings. The student journals, and, to whatever extent they existed, childhood diaries, are lost, but some letters, including many of his father's (but not Felix's replies), survive in Basle's University Library. Lötscher edits several chronologically overlapping sections into one continuous narrative. They cover the period of his childhood, student years and early professional practice, from birth to the early 1560s, and append accounts of his informal adoption of Gredlin, and participation in festivals of 1563, 1577, 1596 and 1598. Although later sections are written in the hand of his half-brother, Thomas, Felix started writing his fair copy himself in 1609, at around the age his father had been during the 16 days or so in early 1572 in which he allegedly composed and wrote his entire life account. Commenting of a dissection he undertook in April 1558 that he still had the resulting skeleton over 53 years later allows the writing of this section of Felix's journal to be dated to around 1611. By the time it reaches the mid-1560s, it postdates the death in 1613 of his wife Madlen. Brief unfinished notes on a fifth festival of 1600 indicate that his life writings were cut short by his death in 1614.[70]

Evaluated by some as an artless chronology, more recent literary analysis points to a structured, reflected composition, in which knowing contrasts and parallels to his father's life writings, and rhetorical, thematic and other devices, support the interweaving and juxtaposition of personal reminiscences with exemplary anecdotes and biographical sketches.[71] The chosen episodes are carefully presented to articulate Felix Platter's stated ambitions and unstated opinions. He traces a self-disciplined progress from squeamish, phobia-ridden child to confident, competent and successful physician and self-constructed *pater familias*, in a narrative intended to triumphantly trump the pivotal boost to his family' social and professional rise recorded in his father's life-writings. The central role of medicine in this strategy is self-evident. Here, attention is drawn to the crucial contribution made to this process by theatrical skills, practice and interests. At a time when the significance of a holistic approach to the study of early modern theatre is receiving ever increasing recognition, Felix and Thomas Platter's journals, with their extensive descriptions of spectacle and detailed eyewitness accounts of a wide range of professional entertainers of many nationalities, offer exceptional insights into links between theatre and medicine in the age of Shakespeare.

---

[70]   *Felix Platter Tagebuch*, 353, 438 (April 1558 and January 1565, Basle).

[71]   Hochlenert, 'Das "Tagebuch" des Felix Platter', 144–54, 162, 165.

Chapter 3
Hippolytus Guarinonius (1571–1654)

The physician Hippolytus Guarinonius wrote at least 15 works in German, eight in Latin, and one in a mixture of German, Latin and Italian, of which eight were published and the rest are known only in manuscript.[1] None of his major writings are yet translated outside these languages, and unlike the Platter brothers, he is little known beyond German- or Italian-speaking Europe. The illegitimate son of north Italian Catharina Pellegrini and Bartolomeo Guarinonius,[2] he was born in Trent in the South Tirolean Alps. In the Catholic Etschtal region between Trent and Bolzano, then as now largely bilingual in German and Italian, the wealthy Guarinonius family owned extensive vineyards. Shortly after his birth on 18 November 1571, his father, the son of a physician and grandson of a goldsmith, was called to Vienna to take up an appointment as court physician to Emperor Maximilian II. Hippolytus's younger half-brother Bartolomeus Guarinonius was 'Doctor of medicine in Schwaz' to at least 1659, and another half-brother, Johann Andreas Guarinonius, was a courtier in Graz, to Emperor Ferdinand II (Diagram 2).[3] The now discredited suggestion that Hippolytus served as a pageboy at Cardinal Carlo Borromeo's court in Milan is unsupported in his publications. Their autobiographical passages do, however, refer occasionally to Vienna and Trent, and frequently to Prague and Padua. By his own account, Guarinonius spent the first 11 years of his life in Vienna, where he had a tutor, and in 1583 followed his father, by now serving as physician to Emperor Rudolf II, to Prague, where he spent 11 years as one of around 150 boarding scholars at Prague's Jesuit College in preparation for his medical studies at the University of Padua .[4]

Rhetoric and acting were essential components of the Jesuit teaching curriculum.[5] Jesuit schools and colleges were renowned for the extravagantly costly sets, costumes, and elaborate specially printed programmes known as periochs, of the didactic religious plays most staged on an annual basis. Produced and often written by Jesuit teachers, and with social standing trumping acting abilities when parts were distributed to pupils, these plays were often staged for the general public, even for high-ranking dignitaries, as well as for parents and

---

[1]   Dörrer, 'Quellen', 205–7; Neuhauser, 'Die Überlieferung der Schriften', 189.

[2]   1534–1616. See also Guarinonius, *Grewel*, 'Dedicatio', (b)iˇ.

[3]   Naupp, 'Über Bad-Curen', 175.

[4]   Guarinonius, *Grewel*, 118, 126, 153, 568, 1192, 1237.

[5]   Thomas Platter, surveying Ghent from the tower of St Bavo's Cathedral, spotted a 'delightful comedy' being rehearsed by the Jesuits and their scholars in a courtyard of the nearby Jesuit college (*Thomas Platter d.J*, 751–2, 10 September 1599, Ghent).

others directly connected to the school. Guarinonius learned to play the theorbo at school, but only rarely refers to his own participation in Jesuit school plays or music-making, although it seems likely that he continued to play music in Padua and Hall, and his accomplishments as a musician were praised in 1646 by Christoph Sätzl, choirmaster of Hall's imperial convent.[6] In contrast to Felix Platter, Guarinonius strongly disapproved of the growing trend for wealthy families to ape the nobility by teaching their daughters as well as their sons to play music, and of secular music in general.[7] However, his schoolboy enthusiasm for sport and games became a lifelong solace, informing the content and writing process of his best known work, a medical treatise published in 1610 under the biblically-influenced title *The abominations of the desolation of the human race* (Plate 6).[8] While working on *Grewel*, he would often:

> push aside pen and paper and go for a walk towards Innsbruck. Thus walking, I worked on this book more, and with much greater pleasure, and afterwards got more onto paper. And if pushed to tell the whole truth exactly how it is, I can't deny that for the most part I planned and composed this very modest and simple little work while walking or riding, then got my planned simple ideas down onto paper back at home.[9]

The 'friendly conversations and discussions' he enjoyed during some of these walks with professional colleagues such as Dr Paul Weinhart contributed materially to his treatise, and were a continuation of the longstanding habit of taking regular sociable exercise central to his approach to health.[10]

Book 6 of *Grewel*, 'On exercise', has noticeably more frequent autobiographical references to his decade in Prague than any of the treatise's other six books. The Platter brothers' journals offer numerous endearing passages. One of the few in Guarinonius's writings is an extended lyrical description, in 'On exercise', of an Alpine climb, that concludes by warmly inviting the reader to join him on the

---

[6]   Guarinonius, *Grewel*, (a)ii, 227, 1228; Senn, *Aus dem Kulturleben*, 559, 575; Drexel, 'Quelle zur Musikgeschichte', 53–5.

[7]   Guarinonius, *Grewel*, 370, 1160.

[8]   Guarinonius, *Die Grewel der Verwüstung Menschlichen Geschlechts*, here referred to throughout as '*Grewel*'. *King James Bible*: 'Matthew' 24 v.15: 'When ye therefore shall see the abomination of desolation, spoken of by Daniel the prophet, stand in the holy place'. See also Grass, 'Ein Vorkämpfer', 60–3, and on Guarinonius's use of biblical quotations: Vonach, 'Die heilige Schrift', 292, 297.

[9]   Guarinonius, *Grewel*, 1173, 1234.

[10]   Guarinonius and three fellow students at Prague's Jesuit College had undertaken a three week midwinter walking trip to Leipzig in deep snow, during which they experienced 'much strange luck, good and bad' (*Grewel*, 1234).

next expedition, planned by himself and his companions for August 1610.[11] It was undertaken by Guarinonius in August 1607 to gather medicinal plants, of which, as he notes, the best grow only on high mountains.[12] Accompanying him were a porter, a goatherd, his friend Simon Kolb, and brothers-in-law Georg Thaler and Heinrich Altherr. Kolb was Sätzl's predecessor as director of music at the imperial convent of Hall, an important centre for church music, whose choirboys studied at the neighbouring Jesuit College.[13] Thaler was Archduke (then Emperor) Ferdinand II's imperial accountant until 1638, when he entered a religious order to live out his final decade as a hermit. Altherr was married to Thaler's sister Ursula, and Guarinonius married another of his sisters, Charitas, in 1599.[14] During the first two decades of the seventeenth century, perhaps on the initiative of their brother Johann Baptist Thaler, a Capuchin monk, Guarinonius worked closely with Kolb, Georg Thaler and Altherr to revitalize Hall's Marian Congregation from a defunct group of less than a dozen, into an active spiritual focus for the town, with over 3,000 congregants.[15] The Congregation sponsored a chapel, whose account books of 1603–4 confirm Guarinonius's contribution of 'a beautiful pair of tin plates' and 'a beautiful picture of Our Lady' painted by himself. Led by the Jesuits of Hall, supported by the noblewomen of its imperial convent and guided by its prefect and officers, the Congregation took responsibility for staging Hall's civic religious plays and Good Friday and Corpus Christi processions. Guarinonius and Kolb, assistant prefects in 1605, respectively became prefect in 1606 and 1607, and in the three following years the office passed to Altherr, then back to Guarinonius, then to Thaler. Between them, the four held further office many times in the following decades.[16] In this capacity, Guarinonius, an enthusiastic supporter of Jesuit school drama, is said to have taken part in municipal stagings of religious plays in Hall, in 1606 or 1607 directing a Jesuit tragedy, Mathäus Rader's *Theophilus*.[17]

The *Vitae* of Guarinonius circulated by the Congregation on his death in 1654 confirms his participation in their processions, and his devotion to the Jesuit priest Peter Canisius (1521–97). Appointed professor of theology at the University of Ingolstadt by Duke Wilhelm IV of Bavaria in 1549, and founding head of Ingolstadt's Jesuit College by Wilhelm IV's son Albrecht V in 1555, his move to Switzerland in 1580 was possibly precipitated by a falling out with Albrecht's son

---

[11]   Guarinonius, *Grewel*, 1206–8 (for a similar invitation, see 579); Haslinger, 'Hochgebirgsbesteigung'; Breuer, 'Hippolytus Guarinonius als Erzähler', 1123–6.

[12]   Guarinonius, *Grewel*, 434.

[13]   Senn, *Aus dem Kulturleben*, 180–1, 206.

[14]   Nothegger, 'Aus Guarinonis Freundeskreis', 31–2.

[15]   These figures were estimated by Christoph Sätzl in 1646 (Drexel, 'Quelle zur Musikgeschichte', 55).

[16]   Klaar, *Dr Hippolytus Guarinoni*, 20–2, 40.

[17]   Senn, *Aus dem Kulturleben*, 498, 575; Dörrer, 'Guarinoni als Volksschriftsteller', 142, 164; Bücking, 'Hippolytus Guarinonius', 67 and *Kultur und Gesellschaft in Tirol*, 126.

Wilhelm V.[18] Innsbruck and Hall's Jesuit Colleges were founded on Canisius's initiative in 1562 and 1573:[19]

> out of deep compassion for his crucified saviour, he [Guarinonius] played the part of this suffering person praiseworthily and with great piety in the Congregation [procession] on Good Friday for several years. [...] He celebrated the feast days of Francis, the Romans Ignatius and Xavier, as also of the highly estimable P[ater] Peter Canisius, with his whole household. Proof that these devotions did not take place without awe is given by a sleeve from the vestments of the highly respected P. Canisius, which our late physician carried with him when visiting infected people, saying that it had always protected him from appreciable, actual danger of illness better than the most highly regarded medicines.[20]

A broadsheet of 1655 associated with the initiative to have Canisius canonized as a healer-saint confirms Guarinonius's use of the Jesuit leader's sleeve to treat pregnant women threatened by miscarriage, and reveals that he also used a letter from him as a personal plague amulet.[21] Guarinonius's faith in the curative powers of religious relics is well-documented with respect to his great friend and spiritual mentor, Fra Tommaso da Bergamo, a lay brother at Innsbruck's Capucin Monastery since 1619, and a successful healer whose 'Thomas spoons', small wooden spoons said to work genuine miracles in healing the sick, were much sought after.[22] While an imperial artist painted Fra Tommaso's death mask immediately after his death in 1631, Guarinonius spent two hours in prayer, supplicating his help with a serious cancer on his left palm. He rubbed the hand and fingers of Fra Tommaso's corpse on his cancerous growth: 'and in that instance the pain stopped and has not returned now for twelve years'. Before leaving, he requested hairs from Fra Tommaso's beard and a scrap of his habit as holy relics; the first of many such requests, resulting in 'such a crowd that two lay brothers couldn't keep up with cutting and distributing scraps of habit'.[23]

Guarinonius viewed universities as excellent facilitators of upward social mobility, and argued strongly in favour of fathers paying the necessary premium to enable their sons to study abroad.[24] During the mid-1590s, when Thomas Platter was at Montpellier medical school, Guarinonius studied medicine at Padua, widely celebrated, not least by Shakespeare, whose Lucenzio is drawn to: 'fair Padua,

---

[18]   Baader, *Der bayerische Renaissancehof*, 197–8; Lederer, *Madness, religion and the state*, 72–4.

[19]   Nagl and Zeidler, *Deutsch-Österreichische Literaturgeschichte*, I, 581.

[20]   *Vitae* of Guarinonius (cited in: Klaar, *Dr Hippolytus Guarinoni*, 37–8).

[21]   BHStA, Jesuitica 513/III (cited in: Lederer, *Madness, religion and the state*, 109).

[22]   Neuwirth and Witting, 'Die sprechende Architektur', 219; Guarinonius, *Thomas von Bergamo*, 69.

[23]   Guarinonius, *Thomas von Bergamo*, 80–4.

[24]   Guarinonius, *Grewel*, 260–2.

nursery of arts [...] Here let us breathe and haply institute a course of learning and ingenious studies' (Plates 4–5).[25] By all accounts, Guarinonius did just that. He matriculated in 1594, the year Girolamo Fabrici d'Acquapendente's new anatomy theatre was constructed for Padua's medical school, led a normal student life featuring diversions involving wine, secular music and theatre, within a few years being condemned in his writings, and qualified as a physician in 1597.[26]

His increasingly unforgiving attitude to man's earthly pleasures drew on devout Catholicism fundamentally shaped by his Jesuit education, fostered by the uncompromising monotheism of his adopted Tirol and several watershed experiences, notably two 'special Graces from God'.[27] In September 1598, he nearly drowned while riding to his father in Trent after staying in nearby Teutschen Mötz, the family home of his aristocratic student friend Niclaus von Firmion. Guarinonius became stranded in midstream when he and Firmion, whose exemplary mastery of all chivalric arts, including athletics, he repeatedly praises,[28] had to ford a river on horseback because recent flood waters had swept away a bridge. Unable to swim and fearing for his life, he was forced to remain up to his nose in the current, while Firmion's manservant Remigius Römisch was dispatched to fetch a sturdy 'water-experienced peasant' from the nearest village. Screaming 'misericordia', the terrified peasant stripped off and waded in, but couldn't get close. Guarinonius was eventually pulled out by Firmion's scribe Christoff, with a rope improvised from two bridles.

Drowning was a serious risk of early modern travel, and some near escapes had lasting effects. Felix Platter was impressed that after surviving an accident in which several German students at the University of Bourges, including a former boarder of his father, drowned in the River Auron, Caspar Olevianus of Trier honoured the pledge he made to God while in fear of his life, to change his course of study from law to theology, and become a preacher.[29] Guarinonius's own delivery, which he attributed to divine intervention, motivated him to become one of the first postclassical physicians to write informatively on the sport of swimming.[30] Regarding it as 'the first Grace this great and mighty God showed my deeply sinful and unworthy self', he bracketed this delivery together with a second 'Grace', his survival with an unmarked body of a dangerous sledging accident in

---

[25] Shakespeare, *Taming of the Shrew*, I.i.2–9.

[26] Guarinonius, *Grewel*, 627, 659, 1140, 1210.

[27] Guarinonius, *Grewel*, 156–9. On Guarinonius and the Jesuits, see Gemert, 'Tridentinische Geistigkeit', 61.

[28] Guarinonius, *Grewel*, 1191 (see Iazzo no.32 in Chapter 18, this volume), 1193, 1214. Firmion, who died at the age of 35 shortly before Guarinonius started writing *Grewel*, also seems to be the subject of one of the treatise's darkest accounts, concerning the bloated corpse of a young man who had been in the peak of physical health, until he embarked on an extended bout of gluttony concluded only when he choked to death (*Grewel*, 763–4).

[29] *Felix Platter Tagebuch*, 248–9 (1 August 1556, Basle).

[30] Guarinonius, *Grewel*, 1216–18.

January 1603, in which a bolting horse ripped his clothing to shreds. These two 'graces' heighten his devotion to the Catholic faith, signalling the beginning of a new life to him, and confirming his belief in an intimate interconnection between earthly health and everlasting afterlife.[31]

Among the first four novices to enter Innsbruck's new Servite monastery, founded by Archduchess Anna Katharina in 1617, were Guarinonius's son Karl, who took the name Seraphin, and his foster son Dionok O'Dale, who published a life of the physician and Servite leader St Philip Benizi and other theological tracts under his new name of Cherubin Maria O'Dale.[32] Karl was born in 1599, the year of Guarinonius's first marriage. Stillborn triplets followed in 1604, and within a year he started work on *Grewel*, whose manuscript has two portrait sketches of a plump-cheeked, curly-haired daughter born in 1605, probably Margretha Charitas, whose planned entry into the Hall convent in 1622 was delayed by serious illness.[33] Six of his children died between 1605 and 1609, and writing was also delayed by his and his wife's lengthy bouts of a debilitating *'febrem continuam Anginam'*. A temporary cure, affected in March 1608 by the physician Paul Weinhart, led Guarinonius to:

> praise, respect and thank the almighty grace of God for giving me back my life, which I again totally dedicate to him [...] and will let my gaze stray from the truth much less even than before, but proclaim it with great clarity and courage, and steadfastly speak out against the political hypocrisies of our contemporary world.[34]

He survived a serious relapse in 1609, but his wife Charitas did not. She died in early 1610, having signed her last will on 23 December 1609, eight days before Guarinonius signed off the completed first volume of *Grewel*.[35] Repeated regrets that marriage prevented him from taking holy orders, and longwinded warnings to his readers of the folly of remarriage, did not prevent Guarinonius's own remarriage in January 1611, 10 months after Charitas' death, to Helene von Spieß.[36] Guarinonius's strenuous religiously-motivated attempts at marital celibacy were unsuccessful. His second wife bore him several children who died young, a physically disabled son who died aged 22 shortly after graduating in 1637, and his two youngest children. Seraphim Ignaz (1624–89), was a qualified doctor by

---

[31]   Guarinonius, *Grewel*, 156. See also Breuer, 'Hippolytus Guarinonius als Erzähler', 1129–30 and 'Schöne des Leibs', 128; Locher, 'Beglaubigungsstrategien', 147.

[32]   Guarinonius, *Grewel*, 1206, and *Thomas von Bergamo*, 4; Klaar, *Dr Hippolytus Guarinoni*, 9, 30–1.

[33]   Innsbruck UL, Cod.110, I, f.528ʳ; Klaar, *Dr Hippolytus Guarinoni*, 32.

[34]   Guarinonius, *Grewel*, 791.

[35]   Guarinonius, *Grewel*, 969; Klaar, *Dr Hippolytus Guarinoni*, 30.

[36]   Guarinonius, *Grewel*, 1118.

1648, when he contributed one of four epistles to the frontmatter of Guarinonius's Latin treatise on fasting, and Maria Franziska married in 1654.[37]

Raised to the minor nobility by Ferdinand II, who became Holy Roman Emperor in 1619, and honoured by the Pope, Guarinonius was from 1601 the respected, pious and successful public health officer of Hall, where he spent his whole professional life. The town's lavish 1511 production of the local Easter mystery play had marked the peak of a prosperity founded on trade routes and the local salt-mining industry.[38] Guarinonius tirelessly praised the beauties and health advantages of Hall, whose well-preserved medieval centre has a street named after him.[39] His deep-seated suspicion of what he saw as the 'poisonous' politically-motivated deceitfulness promoted as essential to successful court life by Machiavelli and others was formed in the late 1590s, when his father was ousted as imperial court physician by the intrigues of a relative, Dr Christoforo Guarinoni.[40] Early in his own career, Hippolytus Guarinonius turned down the opportunity to be Ferdinand II's personal physician in Graz, but in 1605 he entered his direct employ, albeit in the relatively low profile role of court physician with responsibility for the fluctuating community of two to three dozen nuns in Hall's imperial convent. Founded in 1569 by three aunts of Ferdinand II, the Archduchesses Magdalena, Helena and Margaretha, with the support of Peter Canisius, it became an increasingly important centre for sacred music, and, from 1607, the final home of Ferdinand II's sisters Maria Christina, widow of Sigismund Battor, and the spinster Eleonore (Diagram 2).[41] Apart from pilgrimages to Rome,[42] Guarinonius's own travels were largely confined to German-speaking regions. Although he also wrote Latin medical treatises, for *Grewel* he chose the then less commonly used vernacular, repeatedly emphasizing that 'he wanted to be understood in German by the Germans', so that his recommended methods for the promotion of the healthy body, mind and soul would reach the widest possible

---

[37] Guarinonius, *Grewel*, 1142–4, *Thomas von Bergamo*, 26–31, 61–2, and *Chylosophiæ*; Klaar, *Dr Hippolytus Guarinoni*, 33; Granichstaedten-Czerva, 'Die Familie Guarinoni'.

[38] Guarinonius, *Grewel*, 428, 458; Katritzky, *Women, medicine and theatre*, 30–1.

[39] Guarinonius, *Grewel*, 456–63: Book 3, chapter 11, 'On the air and location of this our city of Hall in the Inn valley'.

[40] Guarinonius, *Grewel*, 379, 392; Grass, 'Dr Hippolytus Guarinonius', 12.

[41] Guarinonius, *Grewel*, 'Dedicatio' B^v, 189, 462, 1227; Senn, *Aus dem Kulturleben*, 134–8; Bücking, *Kultur und Gesellschaft in Tirol*, 90; Schennach, 'Der Innsbrucker Hof', 238.

[42] Manuscript accounts of his 1613 pilgrimage survive (Neuhauser, 'Die Überlieferung der Schriften', 188) and an earlier visit is noted in *Grewel* (1313–14). The source of his sporadically displayed knowledge of Madrid was almost certainly his then Madrid-based colleague Tobias Zächen (*Grewel*, 505, 1177).

readership, uneducated people and children included.[43] In practice, his writings were aimed at one distinct section of this readership, Catholic Alpine German-speakers, whom he never tired of stereotypically favourably contrasting with the predominantly Protestant lowland Germans.[44] Celebrated by cultural and literary historians for its early use of vernacular German in a professional context, and for its insights into the arts of its time, *Grewel* quickly influenced writers such as Ægidius Albertinus and Jeremias Drexel, but made little impact beyond the German-speaking regions. There are sporadic direct pre-1800 British references to Guarinonius's predominantly Latin medical treatise *Chylosophiæ* and to his vernacular plague treatise *Pestilentz Guardien*, both listed in the 1787 catalogue of British Library holdings, but those to the vernacular *Grewel* are at second hand, via Latin treatises by other authors.[45]

Guarinonius's didactic and theological works include popular hagiographies, two of which successfully argue for the addition of the peasant girl Notburga of Rottenburg and Eben, and the fictitious Andreas Oxner, to the roster of local Tirolean saints. Most specialists accept that his position regarding Italy cannot be dismissed with a formulaic 'Italian = negative, German = positive' construct.[46] He greatly admired the leading Italian counter-Reformationist Carlo Borromeo,[47] a vigorous opponent of professional and itinerant theatre, whom he followed in taking a robust stand against superstition, quackery and the secular stage, and after whom he named his firstborn in 1599. In 1618 Guarinonius published his German translation of Pietro Giussano's substantial biography of Borromeo, containing passages recording the consistently aggressive attempts of this profoundly anti-theatrical prelate to root out carnival and other festivals, itinerant performers and quacks. Borromeo's energetically ministered systematic programme to bless every building on land under his jurisdiction, in order to protect their inhabitants against the plague, excludes all those 'used for the staging of commercial public acrobatic

---

[43]   Guarinonius, *Grewel*, 4, 110, 112, 162, 866; see also 8, 173, 249. In this last, 'verständlich' (clear) replaces the 'teütsch' (German) of the manuscript version (Innsbruck UL, Cod.110, I, f.355ᵛ) a sense in which 'teutsch' is also widely used in the treatise. See also Kemp, 'Hippolytus Guarinonuis als Schriftsteller', 12; Siller, 'Die Sprache des Hippolytus Guarinonius', 42. Felix Platter, who also chose the vernacular for some medical publications, emphasized his wish to write 'non cum tanto fastu, sed simplicitate' (Hochlenert, 'Das "Tagebuch" des Felix Platter', 135).

[44]   Guarinonius, *Grewel*, 429–56; Moser, 'Deutsche und Tiroler', 182.

[45]   For example, Salmon, *Medicina practica*, 134–5, 154; James, *Pharmacopœia universalis*, 353.

[46]   *Pace* Battafarano ('Zettelkraut statt Zitronen', 146 and *L'Italia ir-reale*, 25–6). A more nuanced approach is, for example, already advanced by Bücking ('Hippolytus Guarinonius', 73–4).

[47]   1538–84.

spectacles or comic plays, ropedancing, fencing displays, foolish clowning, or similar unseemly or dangerous or dishonest plays or public diversions'.[48]

Just two years after Borromeo's posthumous canonization in 1610, Guarinonius dedicated a substantial plague treatise to 'the most highly worthy, holy Count, nobleman and master, Carolus Borromæus', declaring in it his intention of dedicating a church to 'San Carlo'.[49] Six years later, at his own expense, Guarinonius, a talented amateur architect and artist, initiated construction of the precociously exuberant baroque Karlskirche. Overlooking a bridge across the River Inn between Hall and the nearby village of Volders, where Guarinonius bought a family estate in 1618, the Karlskirche is prominently visible, some 12 kilometres before Innsbruck, to modern travellers heading south down the Austrian motorway towards the Brenner Pass. Guarinonius oversaw its building, raised funds, produced architectural designs, painted a lost altar-picture and collected holy relics from Rome. He is even said to have hurried along construction work, sometimes under the pseudonym 'Meister Pölten', sometimes, as recorded in the Hall Congregation's posthumous *Vitae*, openly greeting friends while dressed in workmen's clothes.[50] He became estranged from his son Karl, Pater Seraphin of the Servite monks, after constant financial arguments with the Servite order, for whom the Karlskirche was built, and died six weeks before its official consecration, outliving Karl by a decade.[51]

Of *Grewel*, the medical treatise containing Guarinonius's quack commedia dell'arte descriptions, only the first volume, which he wrote in his thirties, achieved publication. Addressing hygiene issues and the maintenance of human health, its surviving partial manuscript clarifies pre-publication editorial changes, for example including more autobiographical passages than the published version, where some are re-edited into the third person or dropped altogether.[52] My comparison of the published volume of *Grewel* with this manuscript, and identification of internal evidence such as dates, confirms that, in some ways not unlike a medical blog, Guarinonius wrote the contents of its 1,400 published pages almost entirely sequentially, from first to last page, during the half-decade 1604–9. Four decades after its publication in 1610, Guarinonius started the companion volume on human

---

[48]   Guarinonius, *In memoria æterna*, 340–1.

[49]   Guarinonius, *Pestilentz Guardien*, 3, 22. The copies consulted (HAB, 128.3 Med; Munich, Bayerische Staatsbibliothek, Path.513) share identical unconventional pagination. Here, I use asterisks to indicate repeat pagination, giving the full sequence as follows: pages 1–144, 81*, 85*, 83*–84*, 85**, 86*–99*, 200–12, 113*–24*, 251, 126*–9*, 230, 131*–44*, 145–78, 159*, 180–99, 200*–3*.

[50]   Klaar, *Dr Hippolytus Guarinoni*, 38; Guarinonius, *Grewel*, 1227; Trapp, 'Guarinoni als Baukünstler'; Brückle and Müller, 'Die unzimblichen *Gemåhl*', 115; Rapp, *Guarinoni, Stiftsarzt*, 39.

[51]   Koch, 'Karlskirche', 198, 200–4.

[52]   E.g. two autobiographical anecdotes dated 1583 and 1589 are excluded from publication (Innsbruck UL, Cod.110, I, f.540v; Guarinonius, *Grewel*, 373).

pathology to which it makes so many references.[53] Never published, this survives only in partial manuscript, unfinished at his death in Hall on 31 May 1654, aged 82, shortly after returning from Trent to attend the wedding of his daughter Maria Franziska.[54]

A monument to its author's pioneering contributions to healthcare and social policy, the first volume of *Grewel*, written as 'not a medical treatise but a health manual',[55] offers a comprehensive guide to the attainment and maintenance of human health, in the widest sense of physical, mental and spiritual well-being.[56] Its combined treatment of personal, public and moral hygiene champions the benefits of frugal nutrition, daily physical exercise, moderate living and due regard to spiritual health. Many of its numerous suggestions for promoting health run counter to the accepted medical wisdom of its day. Guarinonius provides measured warnings concerning the health dangers of procedures such as routine bloodletting or purging, mixed public baths, alchemy and medical astrology. He gives detailed support for practices such as thorough ventilation of living quarters, and a diet high in fish and vegetables and low in meat, alcohol or outlandish fashionable foreign foods such as turtle, chantelle mushrooms, oysters or snails (let alone the 'roast owl, good plump, well-garnished cat, or ass's head' he ironically offers sinful 'guzzle-fools'), and above all based on fresh, unadulterated bread and water.[57] The treatise makes important advances in linking occurrences of communicable diseases and epidemics with the purity of air, food and water, availability of private indoor bathrooms and sanitary facilities, and levels of personal, household and civic hygiene. The 42-page unpaginated index, directly following the list of contents in *Grewel*'s frontmatter, succinctly overviews

---

[53]   E.g. Guarinonius, *Grewel*, 4, 69, 70, 101, 114, 330, 376, 390, 520, 591, 641, 897, 909, 914, 915, 961, 962, 985, 1053, 1057, 1079, 1162, 1324, 1330. *Pace* Schadelbauer, 'Von den kranken Menschen', 91.

[54]   Koch, 'Karlskirche', 204; Dörrer, 'Quellen', 205–6. The *Grewel* manuscripts form part of the largest collection of Guarinonius's autograph manuscripts, preserved as four bound volumes in the University of Innsbruck Library. The first two volumes of this codex include the manuscript draft for the first two-thirds of the published first volume of *Grewel* (up to the third chapter of Book V), written, with many deletions, on the versos, the rectos being reserved for numerous *addenda* and *corrigenda* (Innsbruck UL, Cod.110, I, f.595ff. and II, f.672ff.; Guarinonius, *Grewel*: 'Vortrab' and I–V, 3). Its fourth volume contains the draft manuscript for Books II and III of the unpublished second volume of *Grewel*, written continuously on both sides of each folio in a frail, barely legible script (Innsbruck UL, Cod.110, IV, ff.390–531, on which see: Schadelbauer, 'Von den kranken Menschen'; Neuhauser, *Katalog*, 32–47). The penultimate folio of Book 3 refers to Book 5, but the whereabouts of any manuscripts for this, or the other missing books of this volume, or the missing final third of the published first volume of *Grewel*, are unknown.

[55]   Guarinonius, *Grewel*, 50.

[56]   Gerster, 'Diätiker', 728; Fischer, 'Hippolyt Guarinonius', 285; Grass, 'Ein Vorkämpfer', 89; Mann, 'Gesundheitswesen und Hygiene', 114–16.

[57]   Guarinonius, *Grewel*, 378, 733, 800, 814; Mayr, 'Volksnahrung', 119–20.

Guarinonius's personal and medical priorities. It flags up his engagement with issues such as the importance of friendship, female foolishness, and the superiority of highland over lowland nations, vegetarians over meat-eaters, water over wine and religious orders over married family life. Guarinonius's enthusiasm for sport and exercise is reflected in his provision of nuanced advice for those of different stamina levels and age, gender and social groups, and his informed instructions and recommendations for pursuing many specific sports and games. Noting that it was popular with noblewomen, Guarinonius describes the fashionable and still relatively recent game of pall-mall, together with real tennis and a dozen or so other games.[58] Paediatrics and pedagogy are another focus. Guarinonius notes his unrealized intention to expand on them in a 'separate brief handbook', and repeatedly emphasizes the need to treat babies and children not as miniature adults, but with specifically tailored child- and healthcare.[59]

Grewel also conveys profoundly disturbing prejudices, both within the specifics of its content, and in the choice of tones deployed to deliver them to the reader. It equates health with beauty and identifies the anatomically abnormal as expendable vermin, repeatedly denigrates women for their 'long hair, long dresses, long tongues, short wit and brains',[60] exhibits ingrained misogyny and anti-Semitism, condemns all non-Christians and every type of Protestantism, whose preachers and 'preacheress' wives think that 'they and their listeners are flying to heaven, when they are really heading for hell',[61] and warns against the dangers of performance-based earthly pleasures such as music, dance and theatre. In contrast to Felix Platter's case studies, those embedded in Grewel are judgmental of the perceived shortcomings of patients and fellow professionals.[62] Ole Grell and Andrew Cunningham's helpful reminder of the extent to which the religious beliefs of early modern physicians coloured and shaped their medical practice is particularly relevant for Guarinonius. He regarded the ultimate source of health as God, and based his medical practice and publications on the belief that 'the fundamental art of maintaining complete health cannot be initiated or undertaken without the support or acknowledgement of the Lord of all nature'.[63] His attempt to establish a specifically German Catholic medical tradition draws heavily on the teachings of Jesuits and classical physicians, and is remarkably free of contemporary non-German medical influence.[64] His acknowledged

---

[58] Guarinonius, *Grewel*, 1208–15. Thomas Platter was also a keen sportsman who enjoyed pall-mall, not yet documented by Felix Platter in the 1550s. His sport-related writings, which, unlike Guarinonius's, ignore health aspects, are better known (referred to, for example, by Behringer, 'Arena and Pall Mall', 339, 341, 343, 349).

[59] Guarinonius, *Grewel*, 310, 362.

[60] Guarinonius, *Grewel*, 1062.

[61] Guarinonius, *Grewel*, 1169, 1240.

[62] Guarinonius, *Grewel*, 778, 811, 1064, 1136.

[63] Grell and Cunningham, 'Medicine and religion', 2; Guarinonius, *Grewel*, 137.

[64] Fischer, 'Hippolyt Guarinonius', 291.

authorities are: 'for the natural world, Aristotle and for medicine, Hippocrates and Galen', and he particularly denigrates the 'poisonous, murderous cow and horse medicine' and 'bestial madness' of 'false, harmful and deceitful Paracelsus'.[65] Probably drawn from Galen's *Ars medica*, Hippocrates's 'six non-naturals', namely air, exercise and rest, sleep and wakefulness, food and drink, elimination and retention of superfluities, and the passions of the soul, provide the basis for *Grewel*'s concept and structure. Tacitly acknowledging as his main source the Christian Bible, Guarinonius adds a seventh concept, namely 'God'.[66] Following a substantial introduction, the remainder of the treatise is organized into seven 'books' reflecting this schema:

1. On God
2. On the human mind
3. On air
4. On food and drink
5. On physical elimination
6. On exercise
7. On sleep.

From these sparse and conservative sources, the treatise builds up a comprehensive interlinked consideration of physical, mental and spiritual health, to which Guarinonius vigorously anticipates antagonism:

> The goodnatured reader says: what business is it of the physician to deal with mental illnesses? Because they are not physical, but quite clearly spiritual? The trustworthy physician replies that such mental complaints are more physical than spiritual for the following genuine reason: the more spiritually a man lives, that is to say according to his reason, the less he is plagued by such complaints, from which it follows that the more physical and bestial a man is, the more he is laid low by such complaints and illnesses.[67]

Himself torn between the physical and the spiritual, Guarinonius dedicates *Grewel* to the Virgin Mary, but also, in a second dedication, to his father's eminent patron Emperor Rudolf II. Despite dismissing its 1,400 pages as his 'tiny little manual on health and healing',[68] he spares no expense or trouble to ensure that its frontispiece engraving presents his features in the best possible light, by commissioning it from

---

65   Guarinonius, *Grewel*, 4, 58, 114, 216, 1169.

66   Guarinonius, *Grewel*, 110–11; Gerster, 'Diätiker', 727; Bücking, 'Hippolytus Guarinonius', 69–70 and *Kultur und Gesellschaft in Tirol*, 11–12; Breuer, 'Hippolytus Guarinonius als Erzähler', 1118, and 'Schöne des Leibs', 126; Lederer, *Madness, religion and the state*, 68; Schiendorfer, 'Vorformen zu Guarinonis Lehre vom "Gesondt"', 244.

67   Guarinonius, *Grewel*, 163; see also Gemert, 'Medizinisches Naturverständnis', 1126.

68   Guarinonius, *Grewel*, 'Vortrab' (a)ii.

Europe's foremost portraitist, Munich-based Raphael Sadeler.[69] The treatise opens with extended discussions of factors contributing to longevity.[70] While assuring his readers that his only concern in writing *Grewel* is to encourage fellow Tiroleans to prolong their lifespans and survive into healthy old age, numerous direct appeals to 'responsible municipal authorities' reveal highly motivated political ambitions, to influence local and regional health and social policy.[71] Guarinonius identified the 40 inns supported by Hall's 6,000 or so inhabitants in 1609, as squalid hotbeds of immorality and contagion.[72] Highlighting public order and health and safety issues, such as the effect of the availability of alcohol to minors on crime rates, or of putrid and contaminated meats on outbreaks of plague and other diseases, he urges the authorities to introduce, strengthen and strictly police regulations regarding private banquets and festivities, the testing and sale of food and drink, the licensing of public inns, taverns and bathhouses, and the conduct and sphere of influence of physicians' healthcare 'inferiors'.[73] As well as extended criticisms of barber-surgeons and public bathhouse superintendents, Guarinonius includes a chapter precisely setting out the exact regulations he suggests for reforming their practice.[74] Although his guidelines had little impact beyond his own city, they did influence municipal reforms of provisions for the sick and poor of Hall in 1617.[75]

Shaped by the rigidly determined structure and mores of the society in which Guarinonius lived, *Grewel* is addressed solely to his fellow Catholics, and primarily to men. To attract and keep the interest of lay readers as well as medical professionals and policymakers, Guarinonius, in the manner of many writers of his time, deploys an impressive range of literary strategies, drawing extensively on dialogue, rhetoric, poetry and proverbs, historio-geographical and autobiographical accounts, and topical digressions based on current news broadsheets. He conceptualizes his suggestions with concrete examples drawn from diverse sources, notably the stage. The Tirolean historian Adolf Pichler's communication of the existence of *Grewel*'s theatrical episodes to the theatre historian Johannes Meissner led to recognition of their literary and cultural significance from the 1880s.[76] Guarinonius wrote at a time when the civic and religious authorities were becoming increasingly negative towards popular carnival and theatrical traditions. During the decade before he studied medicine in Padua, the authorities of neighbouring Venice systematically increased their

---

[69]   Via a painted portrait by Hieronymus van Kessel. Guarinonius, *Grewel*, 1309; Hochenegg, 'Die Bildnisse Guarinonis', 22.

[70]   Guarinonius, *Grewel*, 1–4, 12–18.

[71]   Guarinonius, *Grewel*, 5–8; Bücking, *Kultur und Gesellschaft in Tirol*, 24.

[72]   Guarinonius, *Grewel*, 819–39; Bücking, *Kultur und Gesellschaft in Tirol*, 151–3.

[73]   Guarinonius, *Grewel*, 747, 830, 832, 840–59.

[74]   Guarinonius, *Grewel*, 938–40, 958–61, 1046–7, 1062–8, 1074, 1086.

[75]   Bücking, 'Hippolytus Guarinonius', 76; Schennach, 'Der Innsbrucker Hof', 240, 242.

[76]   Meissner, *Die englischen Comoedianten*, 1–12; Meissner, 'Die englischen Komödianten', 115–17; Bücking, *Kultur und Gesellschaft in Tirol*, 95–8.

opposition to public theatres and performance, even within the carnival period.[77] Public dancing, including carnival dancing, was repeatedly restricted in sixteenth-century Hall, and a Jesuit preacher persuaded Hall's authorities to ban carnival celebrations altogether in 1586. Forty-hour prayer services, during the last days of carnival, were introduced in the churches of Hall in 1608, and of nearby Innsbruck in 1609, and Hall's annual 'Fish supper', which, by long tradition, saw out the first Sunday of Lent with all-night feasting, drinking, music, dancing and theatre, was banned in 1610.[78]

Various types of source inform Guarinonius's knowledge of performance practice. His secondary sources range from a days old report of a tournament at a Stuttgart court wedding of November 1609[79] to tired old recycled theatrical anecdotes concerning Gonella and other court fools and entertainers, some of highly dubious historical authenticity.[80] His own eyewitness accounts of Italian quack troupes are examined in Chapters 13–15. He also draws on his personal experience as spectator and participant, throughout his lengthy and varied working life, of a wide range of other spectacle in the Tirol and German-speaking Europe. As well as supporting Hall's municipal religious processions and plays through his leading role in the town's Marian Congregation, Guarinonius observed Jesuit school drama, professional travelling troupes, rope-dancers, actors and acrobats.[81] He repeatedly criticizes professional comic entertainers or stage fools who mounted trestle stages, to offer one-man shows or short dramatic entertainments based on the popular farce tradition, at private festivals, in public houses or on the street.[82] He implies that such 'entertainers, court fools, teasing jokers and the like motley rabble' look to sixteenth-century popular literature of the type of *Eulenspiegel*, a collection of satirical short stories in which a young peasant makes fools of educated citizens, or Gabriel Rollenhagen's allegorical travesties of classical epic

---

[77]   Even while actively engaging the best professional actors to perform in support of the Republic's political agenda, the ageing Doge Nicolò da Ponte presided over a Council of Ten increasingly concerned to suppress Venetian public theatre. The brief respite it enjoyed after the plague years of the mid-1570s culminated in the building of two public theatres in 1580. In 1585, they were demolished by the authorities, who in 1584 had refused the Gelosi troupe permission to perform in public at the Venetian carnival, even though, at the Doge's request, they had performed privately for prominent visiting dignitaries, including a German party brought to Venice for the 1579 carnival by Archduke Ferdinand of the Tirol. See: Johnson, 'Two Venetian theatres', 950–1, 954; Katritzky, *The art of commedia*, 93–4.

[78]   Senn, *Aus dem Kulturleben*, 461, 471; Graß, 'Der Kampf gegen Fasnachtsveran-staltungen', 221–2.

[79]   See Chapter 6, this volume.

[80]   One concerning a king and a court jester is deleted and replaced in the published version with another, involving the choice of a servant by a contemporary head of household: Guarinonius, *Grewel*, 645 (see also 140, 233, 502–3, 725, 1160, 1309); Innsbruck UL, Cod.110, II, f.344^v.

[81]   Guarinonius, *Grewel*, 214–15, 222–3, 1233, 1255.

[82]   See Guarinonius, *Grewel*, 236–8.

poetry. Guarinonius brands their comic entertainments sinful temptations to the over-inquisitive, and their 'bad, useless and wicked blood' as fair prey for daily or even hourly bloodletting, in order to cure them of their folly.[83] In one such anecdote, Guarinonius recalls: 'taking part in a festivity yesterday [...] at which the players were requested to perform songs of the most unimaginable obscenity'. This performance, in front of a mixed audience of four packed tables, was not limited to singing. Quite the reverse; Guarinonius notes that one enterprising entertainer placed his bench, specially designed for this purpose, in the middle of the room, 'so that he could be seen clearly by everyone', sprung onto it, and started to present a repertoire of songs accompanied with 'gestures of a type of which to this hour I am still ashamed to the bottom of my heart to think of, of a type of which I have never read in any heathen writings, let alone thought that they could ever be performed in the presence of such honest people'. Shocked to the core, Guarinonius voiced his concerns to a nobleman sitting next to him, who immediately interrupted the act and had the entertainer thrown out. Guarinonius records with uncompromising satisfaction his own later confrontation with this 'shameless simpleton', who 'soon after died a miserable death. And thus a due verdict was reached on his sins'.[84]

Guarinonius recommends that readers of his treatise turn from the entertainments of such 'indecent' professional fools or street quacks, to performances sponsored by the Catholic Church. He identifies Catholic church music as the highest form of music, a 'medication and cleanser of the soul' whose therapeutic powers are favourably contrasted with the negative, unhealthy effects of, for example, secular dance music.[85] Similarly, one type of theatre is praised above all others, the 'spiritual, seemly, modest, virtuous, Godly' amateur, all-male, religious, Jesuit school drama.[86] According to Guarinonius, its powerful use of the most beautiful and advanced machines and scenery to present Christian themes offers its Catholic spectators 'physical and spiritual health', and non-Catholics the possibility of salvation.[87] He urges his educated readers to forgo in its favour the coarse diversions and shameless lewdness of the mixed-gender professional players, the Italian commedia dell'arte quack troupes whose 'tricks, laughter, and worldly scenes [...] whoring and villainy' are designed to appeal to the base instincts

---

[83] Guarinonius, *Grewel*, 217, 234, 369, 986.

[84] Guarinonius, *Grewel*, 187.

[85] Guarinonius, *Grewel*, 190–1. Without distinguishing between secular and church music, Bodin pronounces music 'one of the things with the greatest power against evil spirits [...] music is divine, and because the Devil loves only discords [...] it heals the body through the soul, just as medicine heals the soul through the body' (*Demonomanie*, sig.159ʳ).

[86] Guarinonius, *Grewel*, 222.

[87] Guarinonius, *Grewel*, 215.

of servants and other simple people, and teach nothing but 'lust, unseemliness, ungodliness and dishonour'.[88]

As an established and respected court and civic physician, Guarinonius often attended festivals of a type at which it was traditional for hosts to provide music and entertainment in keeping with their standing. For him: 'one virtue is seldom without other virtues, one depravity, sin or vice seldom unaccompanied by many other related depravities and related sins', and his treatise draws on his own experiences to mine festivals and their associated spectacle primarily not as enjoyable earthly pleasures, but as a rich and varied resource of dangerous hazards gravely threatening his patients' spiritual and bodily health.[89] Of the numerous health dangers he directly associates with festivals, one of those emphasized most in his treatise is overindulgence in food and alcohol at festival banquets, from which: 'many return home with cut and ripped skin, whose skin was whole when they left, and most ill and unhealthy, who were healthy and strong, not a few are even carried away dead, who were alive and healthy and raised at great expense. The sole cause of all this is over-eating and over-drinking'.[90] Even by the standards of his own community, this ambitious and respected physician was unusually ascetic and devout. *Grewel*'s detailed descriptions of scatological and other theatrical routines have to be viewed in the light of his deep religious beliefs. All Guarinonius's writings were profoundly motivated by his conviction that earthly life: 'is purely and wholly a comedy and brief play. Soon and unexpectedly, the winds of truth and justice blow away the curtain and the masks [...] revealing who should have been more respected and better rewarded, and who, by contrast, cursed and expelled'.[91]

---

[88]   Guarinonius, *Grewel*, 214–15, 222–3, 1256.

[89]   Guarinonius, *Grewel*, 795.

[90]   Guarinonius, *Grewel*, 791.

[91]   Guarinonius, *Pestilentz Guardien*, 201*–2*.

PART II
Ceremony and Festival

Chapter 4
'Christian fools with varnish'd faces'

Court-, community-, and above all Church-controlled feasts and fasts, of diverse length and type, punctuated and defined the early modern festive year, regulating and restricting the activities of both amateur and professional performers to specific dates and seasons. François Laroque highlights some challenges in identifying and interpreting informative evidence relating to festivals in early modern Protestant England.[1] He potently explores the fundamental theatre-historical importance of the 'matrix of time' established by the annual cycle of the Christian festive year. Previous festival-based literary studies tended to concentrate on carnivalesque aspects of festival, particularly revealing from a theatre-historical perspective. By setting carnival enquiries within a holistic consideration of their accompanying year-round manifestations, Laroque encouraged a welcome widening of focus in a fertile field of enquiry. Some of the most substantial of all accounts of early modern carnival festivities, those in the journals of Felix and Thomas Platter, remain little-known to non-German scholars. Their documentary value is further enhanced by their contextualization within these informative journals. Recognizing the value of Laroque's approach, this chapter identifies numerous references to European sacred, civic and court ceremonies and festivals in the Platter brothers' and Hippolytus Guarinonius's writings, many not previously available in English translation, and draws on them to piece together the three physicians' experience of carnival and the festive year within which it is set, and insights into their healing dimensions.

Saints' days and other feast and fast days acquired diverse local and Confessional significance. Diagram 4 indicates some of the fixed feasts, whose calendar dates remain unchanged from year to year, and the two major cycles of movable feasts, whose dates are calculated with respect to the day of the week of any particular year's Christmas, and the date of its Easter. The longest Christian fast is the 40-day period of Lent from Ash Wednesday to Holy Saturday. Lent separates Easter from the Christian year's most theatrical festival, carnival. By the sixteenth century, courtesy of complicated date shifts precipitated by repeated calendar reforms, many regions celebrated carnival for weeks, or even months. Typically it started on Twelfth Night and culminated on Shrove Tuesday, although certain festivities related to carnival started in November or intruded into Lent itself.[2]

---

[1]   Laroque, *Shakespeare's festive world*, 15, 77, 179, 197.

[2]   According to the modern Gregorian calendar, depending on when Easter Sunday falls, between its earliest and latest possible dates of 22 March and 25 April, Shrove Tuesday falls between 3 February and 9 March (or 8 March in a leap year). Blackburn and

Local festivals powerfully bonded early modern communities, but also alienated and excluded nonconformists (see Chapter 5). As Shylock reminds us, in a play performed before King James VI/I on Shrove Tuesday 1605,[3] carnival was for Christians:

> What, are there masques? Hear you me, Jessica:
> Lock up my doors, and when you hear the drum
> And the vile squealing of the wry-neck'd fife,
> Clamber not you up to the casements then,
> Nor thrust your head into the public street
> To gaze on Christian fools with varnish'd faces.[4]

Although the fast periods of the festive year prevented professional performers and quacks from earning a year-round income within their own communities, it supported their itinerant practice through a rich network of annual fairs (Plates 4, 31), around which safe seasonal trade routes developed, until calendar reforms disrupted their traditional itineraries. Rooted in annual church consecration celebrations, many took place on saints' days that came to represent their local communities' most significant economic and festive highlight. The Platter journals richly reflect the diverse number, type, length and dates of annual fairs, and their contrasting potentials for attracting itinerant healers and performers. Antwerp's two annual fairs lasted six weeks from the Eves of St Ivo and Nicholas; Bourges had six (marked by the saints' days of Laurence, Lazarus, Martin, Ursino, Oûtrille and Ambrose); Niort three.[5] His mind concentrated by the almost continual tolling of the funeral bells for the victims of the city's deadly dysentery epidemic, Thomas Platter left Lyon without experiencing any of its four annual fairs (held at Twelfth Night, Easter, August and All Hallows'), whose 'exceptional privileges attract many skilled people, and more publishers than any other city'.[6] Some fairs, like Montpellier's St Bartholomew Day onion fair, were modest one-day single-produce markets.[7] The St Firmin's fair of Uzès, held for a fortnight from the equinox, 25 September, was the largest of any Languedoc city without a port, attracting numerous French and Italian merchants, but trading only two main commodities, the local serge fabric and sweet chestnuts.[8]

Holford-Strevens overview Catholic and Orthodox computations for dating Easter (*Year*, 68, 602, 791–9.).

[3]   Kernan, *Shakespeare, the king's playwright*, 70.

[4]   Shakespeare, *Merchant of Venice*, II.v.28–33.

[5]   *Thomas Platter d.J*, 461 (14 May 1599, Niort), 522, 674–5 (14 July and 24 August 1599, Bourges and Antwerp).

[6]   *Thomas Platter d.J*, 40 (2 October 1595, Lyon).

[7]   *Felix Platter Tagebuch*, 175–6 (24 August 1553, Montpellier); *Thomas Platter d.J*, 172 (24 August 1596, Montpellier).

[8]   *Thomas Platter d.J*, 233 (25 September 1597, Uzès).

Basle's annual fair attracted a profusion of merchants, traders, performers and healers from far beyond the region for the fortnight from 27 October (St Simon and St Jude's Eve), to St Martin's Eve (10 November). Felix Platter knew that his birthday was in late October, because his father recalled bringing the 1536 fairings to his mother's lying-in chamber.[9] He also recalls some memorable rages of his mother during Basle fairs of the 1540s. One was triggered when instead of buying a useful dagger, he squandered a coin from his cousin on dolls and other foolish trinkets, another after he was assaulted by an aggressive stall-holder:

> At the Basle Fair, someone was selling patterns of the type used for pressing out gingerbread biscuits, on a stall on the Cornmarket. Being eager to examine these works of art, I stood there and touched one, at which the old wretch ripped the wooden pattern from my hand and threw it so hard at my face that I thought he had knocked my teeth out, grabbed back the pattern and threw it high over all the stalls that had been set up. He chased after me as I ran away, returning home with a thick lip. My mother was angry with the trader, went down in the morning, reprimanded him as an old degenerate. He replied with insults, wanted to be paid for his pattern, which broke when he threw it.[10]

Felix Platter finally married 23-year-old Madlen Jeckelmann on 18 November 1557, a month after qualifying as a physician and turning 21, and one week after the Basle fair ended. Madlen kept house for her widowed barber-surgeon father, one of whose interminable excuses for postponing the couple's wedding was that it should postdate the Basle fair. On 27 October 1557, Felix hid for three hours in the Jeckelmanns' bitterly cold attic, in order to be the first to greet Madlen with the traditional Basle cry of 'kromen mir' ('Give me a fairing!') when the city's bells announced the fair's official opening at midday. They exchanged gifts when she emerged from her hiding place. She accepted the Bible Felix brought her from Paris, but fear of pre-wedding gossip made her refuse the gold chain he had also bought her there, at the Pont au Change workshop of the Basle-born goldsmith Hans Jakob David.[11]

Thomas Platter illuminates the commercial attractions of Languedoc's fairs for travelling healers and performers:

> Villeneuve is divided into three separate parts [...] One of these is situated at the foot of the hill, and is a fairly large walled city, in which every year, on St Andrew's Day, an excellent annual fair is held, which I will describe in the proper sequence, because I was there in 1598. [...] Outside the time of the

---

[9]   *Felix Platter Tagebuch*, 49 (October 1536, Basle).

[10]   *Felix Platter Tagebuch*, 78–9 (c.1545), 105–6 (c.1546–7). These are among several imprecisely datable episodes woven together into a single coherent narrative by Lötscher's editorial rearrangements of Felix Platter's childhood memories.

[11]   *Felix Platter Tagebuch*, 280, 312–13 (April and 27 October 1557, Paris, Basle).

annual fair there is nothing special to be seen there. During the annual fair, huge numbers of foreign merchants come there, and all sorts of rare goods are to be found there. After that of Beaucaire it is the largest fair in the whole region. It lasts for several consecutive days, and not only does the trading take place in both the cities of Villeneuve, but many stalls are set up outside the city, and all the inns are so full that a considerable number of people have to go to Avignon to find lodgings, and I saw all this repeatedly when I was in Avignon in 1598. [...] The annual fair [of Pézenas] on 8 September is held only in the suburbs, and many merchants travel there from Lyon and Toulouse [...] there are hot baths in the town. In conclusion, nothing is missing from this city by way of diversions. Tennis courts and *jeux de ballon* are common there,as this city has a huge number of distinguished, wealthy citizens who spend their lives solely in such diverting pursuits [Plate 3].[12]

Platter's lively impression of Beaucaire's renowned annual fair, particularly noted for its healers and showpeople, singles out two shows, performing fleas and a civet cat, for detailed description:

We landed at Beaucaire [...] a city renowned throughout France, Italy and Spain because of its annual fair, held here every year on 22 July, St Magdalen's Day. It is the most famous fair in the whole of Languedoc, because the city lies on the western banks of the Rhône, so that seagoing vessels from Marseille and elsewhere can easily reach it by navigating up the Rhône by sail or by haulage, while those from Lyon or Burgundy can come down the Rhône [...] Now I want to describe what I experienced at the fair, because as previously noted, it is the most important fair in Languedoc. Within and outside the city there is such a multitude of all manner of merchants' stalls that it is impossible to describe it. On every road into the city, special huts are constructed in which goods are offered for sale, and these roads are many and long. Inside the city itself, not just is almost every house used for this purpose, but a huge number of new stalls are also built for this purpose. There you can see all sorts of beautiful foreign wares, notably pearls, precious stones, coral, and *naturalia*. Talented performers, entertainers and other wondrous acts come here all the time. There I saw a Burgundian (who constantly wore glasses on his nose, in order to improve his sight, as he said, or more likely, so that one would notice him and ask who he was), exhibit several extremely skilfully fettered live fleas, which he was allowing to feed on the arm of a young girl. On one sat a mannikin of silver, completely covered in armour, he had a little spear on his shoulder. He put the fleas in a glass electuary jar and tipped the same over the fleas. Thereafter, he lifted a light to the glass, at which the fleas jumped against the glass, because it was warm, so that it could be heard ringing. He had several similar fleas, each of

---

[12]   *Thomas Platter d.J*, 113–14 (24 February 1596, Villeneuve), 310–11 (14 January 1599, Pézenas).

which dragged after itself a little silver chain as long as a finger, and sprang with it. But these chains weighed only one gram.

Thomas Platter appends his eyewitness account with references to even more astonishing performing fleas he heard about but did not see, which apparently pulled, and even jumped with, a four-wheeled silver coach. He recorded in detail the method of producing musk, then a prized and costly medicinal ingredient, from the live civet cat he examined in another booth. Shortly after its showman refused 1,500 francs for it, it died in a heat wave at the end of the fair, while being returned to Avignon. Platter concludes his account of Beaucaire fair by noting that:

> Numerous other actors, acrobats, comedians and similar adventurers of every type are also there, as is customary at such widely-renowned fairs. Apart from that, there is such a crowd of people in the city of Beaucaire during the fair, that not all of them can stay there overnight. Instead, many of them stay at the town across [the river], Tarascon [...] We too stayed overnight in that city.[13]

As many working people's only chance of three consecutive holidays, Christmas and St Stephen's Day (26 December), Easter, and Corpus Christi, the longest festivals of the Christian year, were much used for bloodletting, a medical procedure associated with prodigious over-eating.[14] The English traveller Francis Mortoft vividly describes Romans on the final day of Carnival stuffing 'their paunches full of flesh, in regard they could eat noe more flesh after this night for 45 dayes together, unlesse they had license from the Doctors of Physicke, and those licences signed by A general of An order', and Felix Platter presents the cautionary case of a gluttonous noblewoman who died immediately after rushing back from the Easter service to gorge herself on her first taste of meat since the start of Lent.[15] Guarinonius warns his readers against gluttonous Christmas temptations: 'through alcoholic excess, a vigorous miner fell down the stairs of a tavern in Schwaz during the Christmas holidays, at 4pm on St John the Evangelist's Eve in the year 1604, and died there instantly', and identifies another high holiday health hazard, 'the abomination of female unnecessary sweeping, cleaning, bleaching and washing'.[16] In *Grewel*'s manuscript, he interrupts a discussion of the sin of envy with an autobiographical incident that 'happened to me in my youth, to my very great sorrow'. Its first-person narration is edited out of the published version:

> A long time ago, the following happened to a schoolboy who brought a beautiful new outfit to his boarding school in Prague on Christmas Eve. In his happiness,

---

[13]   *Thomas Platter d.J*, 129, 229–30 (29 February 1596 and 25 July 1597, Beaucaire).

[14]   Guarinonius, *Grewel*, 999–1000, 1017. 1069–70, 1072.

[15]   Mortoft, *His book*, 141; Platter, *Obseruationum*, 409–10. See also Diagram 4.

[16]   Guarinonius, *Grewel*, 100. This latter the title of Book 3, Chapter 18 (494–9). For other cases of deaths following alcohol abuse, see 701–2.

he showed it to a lot of people [...] At night he placed it next to his bedside on a box or chest when he went to sleep. When he reached out for it the following morning, he unfortunately found nothing. He jumped out of bed greatly shocked, but had to spend the holidays miserably crying and complaining, and the new outfit stayed forever with whoever had taken it and never again came to light.[17]

The first-person relation of another of his boyhood memories of Christmas in Prague is retained in the published version. One Holy Innocent's Day, when Bohemian custom permitted young bachelors to playfully bare and strike the legs or buttocks of unmarried women, Guarinonius's father was disturbed by his screaming female cook beating off his manservant. He entered his kitchen, thrashed his servant with his iron-studded belt, sacked him and threw him out:

> I still remember this story all the more clearly because I was there during the battle, laughing and heartily supporting the subjugation of this servant. That is why, during this entertainment, I came so close to my dear father's velvet belt that if I hadn't rushed up the next flight of stairs in three leaps, his residual anger would have broken out over me and I would have received a lame, blind and dumb holiday from my dear father. Above all, it behoves the authorities to vigorously ban this common public nuisance.[18]

Felix Platter reminisces more cheerfully on Advent and the Christmas period. He delighted in childhood St Nicholas' Eve gifts.[19] On his first Christmas Eve in Montpellier, having admired the traditional coloured Christmas candles hanging in every corner shop, the 16-year-old Lutheran was excluded from accompanying his Catholic fellow lodgers to Midnight Mass. Afraid to go to bed alone, he locked himself into his attic study with a lamp and read an old edition of Plautus's *Amphytrion* until their return just before dawn.[20]

By the 1590s, Montpellier was Protestant. Thomas Platter dismisses his youthful interest in 'Popish ceremonies, relics and all that pertains to their religion', claiming that his descriptions of them are not included to express:

---

[17]   Guarinonius, *Grewel*, 357 (manuscript version: Innsbruck UL, Cod.110, I, f.515^v).

[18]   *Grewel*, 1257. Guarinonius bore lifelong scars, from brutal schoolboy beatings received from the age of six (*Grewel*, 246).

[19]   *Felix Platter Tagebuch*, 56 (5 December 1540, Basle).

[20]   *Felix Platter Tagebuch*, 152 (24 December 1552, Montpellier). It was an octavo Plautus given him by Andreas Cratander, hidden under a hank of hemp, that his father had illictly read while working as a rope-maker's apprentice (Platter the Elder, 'Thomas Platters Lebensbeschreibung', 83–4). Plautus was also on the Jesuit school curriculum, and Guarinonius quotes a misogynous passage from the *Poenulus* and a warning against the dangers of wine from Act 5 of the *Pseudolus* (*Grewel*, 494, 1190).

praise, approval or respect, rather, because nothing else was shown to me in those places, and to offer educated Protestant readers an impression of the extent to which they replace the eternal with the transient, and matters permitted to and necessary for the soul with those that are superfluous and forbidden.[21]

He watched 'the Papists', now the vulnerable persecuted minority, walk to Christmas Mass through a city whose defences were on high alert, with night watchmen and soldiers with torches posted at every door of the Catholic church.[22] On 24 December 1598, passing through Nîmes, he registered at an inn, and 'as it was Christmas Eve we went to the Catholic Church at midnight, where we listened to excellent music and all sorts of Christmas carols'.[23]

On Christmas Day 1599, Thomas Platter witnessed one of the great sights of Paris, the healing ritual of the Royal Touch at the Palais du Louvre. Attended by huge crowds shouting 'vive le roy', Henri IV, accompanied by his guest of honour, Charles-Emmanuel, duc de Savoie, joined over 100 male and female French and Spanish tuberculosis sufferers in the Louvre's courtyard and hall. Through miraculous healing gifts transmitted by the holy oil used during the coronation ceremony, the touch of the ruling monarch was said to cure scrofula, or the King's evil, swollen nodes or crops on the neck and face caused by a bacterial complication of tuberculosis. As the son of the King of Navarre, Henri IV's claim to the French succession was highly controversial, and public enactment of the Royal Touch validated the legitimacy of his claim to the throne more visibly than any diplomatic successes.[24] Platter had anticipated the ceremony when he visited the Louvre that July, less than a week after seeing Henri IV in person, dining in Orléans with his five-year-old son César, duc de Vendôme, closely attended by courtiers and Scotch bodyguards, before playing dice and taking a carriage to the tennis court:[25]

> in this great hall at Christmas the King touches the people suffering from scrofula. [...] Of the King of France [Michael] Villanovanus relates two miraculous things. Firstly, that in the church at Rheims at the king's coronation a dish of holy oil came down from heaven that never gets used up or less full. Secondly

---

21 *Thomas Platter d.J*, 6 ('Vorred an dem Leser').
22 *Thomas Platter d.J*, 84 (1595, Montpellier).
23 *Thomas Platter d.J*, 308 (24 December 1598, Nîmes).
24 Clark, *Thinking with demons*, 657–8.
25 César's mother Gabrielle d'Estrées had died suddenly that April at the age of 28, and in August Thomas Platter saw her embalmed body lying in state in a coffin surrounded by candles, in the Cistercian Convent of Maubuisson near Pontoise, whose Abbess was Gabrielle's sister. *Thomas Platter d.J*, 536–9 (22 July 1599, Orléans), 617–18 (10 August 1599, Pontoise).

that the king, solely with his bare touch, can heal the crops (les escruelles) that grow on peoples' necks.[26]

Even though Henri IV favoured Scotch rather than Swiss guards, Platter managed to talk one of them into letting him past the crowds that Christmas:

> When the king himself entered the hall, the patients all kneeled down all around the hall. The king went from one to another in sequence, raising his right hand and touching one after another with his thumb and index finger on their chin and nose, then with the same fingers in the form of a cross, on both cheeks. At the first touch, he said (le roy te touche) the king touches you, at the second, on the cheeks (dieu te guerit) God is healing you. He made the same cross for every face, and followed this by (ausmonier) giving alms, always, as far as I could see, 5 steuber, that is around one franc, counting it into his hand. Everyone had high hopes of being healed through these touches. [...] I was told several times in England that the queen also had the same power to cure this affliction through touch, she too is said to present each person with a small coin after touching them. Others say that every seventh son, if no daughters are born between them, has the same power. But I think that the exercise of travelling, and moderation in eating and drinking, as well as secret cures arranged by royalty, give them the ability to have and strengthen such powers.[27]

During his 1599 visit to London, Thomas Platter evidently informed himself of an English variant of this Europe-wide custom, in which the reigning monarch washed the feet of paupers and distributed alms to them at court on Maundy Thursday.[28]

Tuberculosis was rife in mountainous regions, because of the low iodine content of Alpine drinking water. In January 1607, Guarinonius, who ascribed the disease to the ice-cold temperature at which Alpine water was drunk:

---

[26]   *Thomas Platter d.J*, 579, 611 (28 July and 9 August 1599, Paris). Platter's source for Villanovus is Abraham Ortelius. Dulieu reproduces a print of 1628 illustrating Henri IV touching for the king's evil (*La médecine a Montpellier: La Renaissance*, 159).

[27]   *Thomas Platter d.J*, 899–900 (25 December 1599, Paris).

[28]   Shakespeare's allusions to the English ceremony accord closely with Platter's observation in Paris (*Macbeth*, IV.iii.140–59: 'a crew of wretched Souls that stay his cure'). See also Blackburn and Holford-Strevens, *Year*, 617. Recognizing its powerful placebo effect, the sceptical James VI/I carried on the practice (Wilson, *The history of Great Britain*, 289). Samuel Johnson received the Royal Touch from Queen Anne as a child, in 1702 (Wright, 'Quacks', 163). Moryson witnessed Emperor Rudolf II distributing maundy money at his Prague court in 1592 (Oxford CCC, MS.CCC94, 328; Holeton, 'Fynes Moryson's "Itinerary"', 399).

had seven boys with scrofula under my care all at the same time. They were all lodging and studying here [in Hall] together in one house, which was over-heated throughout the winter, and drinking a great deal of cold water, and all became scrofulous together. They were also all cured of it together, within three weeks.[29]

Dismissing 'the actual efficacy or inefficacy of the Royal Touch (its "reality") as an interpretative red herring', Stuart Clark accepts as genuine the belief in the authenticity of its miraculous healing powers published in print by many early modern medical professionals.[30] Thomas Platter's robust privately expressed misgivings, and astute intimations that the Royal Touch exploited proactive and reactive patient response, were informed less by his observations of the actual ceremony in Paris than by his own medical practice in Uzès, where tuberculosis was endemic. Even with the Royal Touch, he reports, local sufferers 'are seldom properly and fully healed, and it generally breaks out again before long'. They were often also resistant to the waters of the 'Fontaine du Maine', a healing spring between Uzès and Beaucaire that drew many French and Spanish sufferers uncured by the Royal Touch.[31]

Christmas and St John the Baptist's Eve approximate the winter and summer solstices. For each, Thomas Platter records traditional ritual practices involving fires producing ash with perceived medicinal benefits. On Christmas Eve 1597, he joined the 'cachefioc [cover the fire]' ceremony at the house of a former patient with whom he had lodged in Uzès,[32] the wealthy landowner M. Carsan. He and his son, whom he bought into the nobility, remained Catholic, his wife and daughter were Protestant converts:

> That same evening, a large wooden log was laid on the grate in the fireplace over the fire. When it caught fire, the whole household assembled by the fire, and the youngest in the house, unless too young, in which case the father or mother make proxy arrangements, has to hold a glass full of wine, some breadcrumbs and a little salt in their right hand and a burning wax or tallow candle in their left. Then the boys and men all bare their heads and this same youngest person, or their father in their name, speaks thus in their mother tongue:

> Ou Monsieur (le maistre de la maison)
> S'en va et vent
> Dious donne prou de ben,
> Et de mau ne ren.
> Et Diou donne des fennes enfantans,

[29] Guarinonius, *Grewel*, 446.
[30] Clark, *Thinking with demons*, 656–8.
[31] *Thomas Platter d.J*, 215, 232 (21 April and 26 July 1597, Uzès and Beaucaire).
[32] *Thomas Platter d.J*, 232 (7 August 1597, Uzès).

Et des capres caprettans,
Et des fedes agnolans,
Et vacques vedelans,
Et des saumes poulinans,
Et de cattes cattonans,
Et de rattes rattonans,
Et de mal non ren,
Si non force ben.

[…] After pronouncing this, the same child throws a little salt on one end of the log in the name of God the Father, then on the other end in the name of the Son, and lastly in the middle, in the name of the Holy Spirit. When this has been done, they all shout together "Allegre, diou nous allegre", that is: "happy, God make us happy". The same is done with the bread, and then with the wine, and finally the candle is allowed to drip in all three places in the name of God the Father, Son and Holy Spirit, and every time they shout, as described above: "happy". They say that a glowing ember from such a log will not burn through any table on which it is placed. They diligently save the ashes right through the year and believe that if they draw around the growth of any human or animal with a swelling with these same ashes, it can't grow any bigger and will soon disappear. Once this was completed, an impressive banquet was held, without fish or meat, but with excellent wine, sweets and fruit. The table was left laid all night with a glass half full of wine, bread, salt and a knife. And I saw all this myself.[33]

Platter's German translation of the Occitan monologue confirms it as a fertility incantation, wishing fertile women, fertile domestic animals, even fertile vermin, upon the head of the household. His account is the earliest of the French version of this transregional ritual, now known as the 'bûche de Noël', and still commemorated in many parts of Europe with the traditional Christmas yule-log cake.

The medicinal ash associated with midsummer's day or St John the Baptist's Day came from the fires of a saint's day also associated with many other traditions. In the medical context, St John the Baptist, who immersed Christ in the waters of the River Jordan, is revered as the patron saint of spas. Some communities, not least Basle, marked St John's Day with the appointment of councillors or other officials, or with purely local legends; for others, such as Saint-Denis near Paris or the Loire Valley village of Soings, it marked their annual fair.[34] Thomas Platter relates one

---

[33]   *Thomas Platter d.J*, 233–4 (24 December 1597, Uzès). Jennett translates the original Occitan as follows: 'Our master comes and goes, God give him many blessings, and guard him from harm, and God give his wife children, and his goats kids, and his sheep lambs, and his cows calves, and his hens chickens, and his cats kittens, and his rats young, and nothing ill be done, but many blessing come' (*Journal of a younger brother*, 268).

[34]   *Thomas Platter d.J*, 514 (24 June 1599, Soings), 892 (30 November 1599, Saint-Denis), 927 (15 February 1600, Basle).

legend about a small nut tree his landlord, the apothecary Antoine Régis, showed him in a field outside Uzès, said to flower and immediately bear fruit on St John's Eve: 'of which many people in Uzès afterwards also assured me; everyone has the freedom to believe this', and another about a tower in the fortifications of Remolins, from which a 'devilish' swarm of beetles was said to fly each St John's Eve.[35] Montaigne, unimpressed by the procession staged in Florence in 1581 for the city's patron, St John, notes the fireworks on the roof of Florence Cathedral, even though, unlike many parts of France, St John's Midsummer bonfires were not customary in Italy. In 1596, Thomas Platter took part in the traditional St John's Eve parrot shooting festival in the deserted village of Lattes, where he often collected medicinal herbs.[36] That evening, in nearby Pérols, locals danced round and through St John's fires burning in front of every farmhouse, in similar fashion to a carnival custom he knew from Basle. Eventually everyone helped themselves to the ash, whose medicinal qualities Platter hints at: 'they hold it in high regard, as being good and useful for a lot of purposes'. Next morning, he joined the male and female bathers who swim in the sea on St John's Eve and Day, 'in the hope that this will protect them from numerous illnesses with which they feel they would otherwise have a high chance of being afflicted'.[37] Following his close escape from drowning in a Rhine tributary in 1552, Felix Platter's father had forbidden him from swimming in the Mediterranean.[38] Thomas Platter got out of his depth during his 1596 St John's Day swim, and was saved from drowning only by a fortuitous tide.

St Theobald's festival, which Felix and Madlen Platter experienced in 1558, is also celebrated with bonfires, albeit only in Thann. This 'very beautiful' town, which Montaigne briefly passed through in September 1580, is built around the Collégiale Saint-Thiébaut, an ornate gothic church consecrated to St Theobald, patron saint of the 'holy' or falling sickness.[39] Specialists disagree on whether Thann's saint is the Italian Bishop Ubaldus, the eleventh-century St Theobald of Provins, or conflates them. According to legend, a traveller founded Thann in 1160, when his walking stick, concealing an inherited ring prised from his recently deceased master, Bishop Ubaldus of Gubbio, took root against a pine tree. Witnessing this and three burning pines, an Alsatian ruler vowed to honour the Bishop's relics with a church. In 1976, tests confirmed that skin fragments formerly attached to the now lost ring match those of Ubaldus's relics in Gubbio's Basilica of Monte Ingino.[40]

---

[35]   *Thomas Platter d.J*, 207 (27 February 1597, Remolins); 277–9 (11 August 1598, Uzès).

[36]   *Thomas Platter d.J*, 151–2 (23–24 June 1596, Lattes and Pérols).

[37]   Montaigne, *Complete works*, 1226–7.

[38]   *Felix Platter Tagebuch*, 124, 185 (August 1552, Basle; September 1553, Montpellier).

[39]   Epilepsy. Montaigne, *Complete works*, 1067; Pinkus, *St Theobald in Thann*.

[40]   On Ubaldus, see Blackburn and Holford-Strevens, *Year*, 209.

Impressed by the recently qualified 22-year-old's medical expertise during a visit to Basle earlier that year, where two of his sons were boarding with Felix Platter's father, Dr Theobald Surgant called him to Thann in 1558.[41] A councillor of Thann and graduate of Basle medical school, Surgant had been experiencing increasingly painful angina and swelling in his legs since falling from his horse on a return journey from Speyer that May.[42] His lackey and carriage arrived in Basle on 29 June. After dinner on Friday 1 July, both couples went to Thann's town square to watch crowds of boys descend the hills with torches, carry the civic flag around the fire with a delegation of local dignitaries, and set alight a pine tree near the church. On Sunday 3 July, the Platters departed after Felix medicated his patient's swellings, which he diagnosed as dropsy. He published the case in anonymized form.[43] Surgant, whose symptoms worsened, called Platter to Thann seven more times. He attended him at his death on 25 September 1558, and continued to treat many patients in the town, including, until her death in 1566, Surgant's widow.[44]

St Magdalen's Day 1556 brought varied expectations in Montpellier. Courtesy of Felix Platter, who bought its German medical students pies in honour of his future wife Madlen, they celebrated the German custom whereby someone romantically linked with a girl treated his friends on her saint's day.[45] Felix Platter also relates that certain terrified locals interpreted weather conditions in Montpellier, with winds hot enough to scorch the crops, hailstones the size of hens' eggs, and flash flooding that drowned people and left streets knee-deep in water, as an apocalyptic sign of the approaching ending of the world, and Day of Final Judgment, on 22 July, St Magdalen's Day 1556.[46] The thunderstorm that toppled the church tower of Saint-Hilaire that summer was a foretaste of the bitter French religious wars that converted the region's elite classes to Protestantism during the following decades. According to Thomas Platter, by 1595 hardly a local church tower, or even a single stone of a single monastery, was left unrazed: 'in short, nothing that belonged to those of the church remains standing'.[47]

Proof of successful completion of the demanding annual pilgrimage of the Triumph of the Cross on 14 September, to La Chapelle de la Sainte Croix on Mont Ventoux near Carpentras, was a coniferous twig or branch from the otherwise rare larches and cedars proliferating on the lower slopes of Provence's iconic mountain. The pilgrimage dated at least to the time of Petrarch's ascent in 1336,

---

[41]　Lötscher, *Felix Platter und seine Familie*, 87; early examples of some 700 horseback journeys Platter made on house-calls outside Basle (Koelbing, 'Felix Platters Patienten', 61).

[42]　*Felix Platter Tagebuch*, 334–5, 344–5 (Spring 1558, Basle; July 1558, Thann).

[43]　Platter, *Obseruationum*, 610.

[44]　*Felix Platter Tagebuch*, 449.

[45]　*Felix Platter Tagebuch*, 252 (August 1556, Montpellier). See also Diagram 4.

[46]　*Felix Platter Tagebuch*, 221, 245–7 (August 1555 and May–July 1556, Montpellier).

[47]　*Thomas Platter d.J*, 63 (October 1595, Montpellier).

and locals rarely ventured onto Mont Ventoux outside high summer. Thomas Platter scheduled an expedition for May 1598, in order to gather rare medicinal plants to send back in bulk to his brother Felix in Basle. Chosen for his excellent local knowledge, his guide, the local surgeon Master Adolff, accompanied Platter's group from nearby Caromb, stopping off to tend his patients. With a porter for their provisions, they started the strenuous 10-hour ascent from Bédoin at 2am, Adolff pointing out numerous crosses commemorating pilgrims who had died during the climb.[48] At the top, where cold winds had blown 10 feet of snow into the chapel, Platter energetically stripped off to dry himself and his clothes out in the sun, but the cold affected Lucas Just so badly that he barely managed the descent. Thomas Platter lacked his brother's rare gift for characterizing people of all social groups as individuals in his journal. He reveals little more about Just, a younger relative of the Lucas Just (1535–95) who had been Felix Platter's school fellow, and a longstanding friend who had been among the group who bade him farewell when he left Basle in 1595, followed him to Montpellier's medical school in 1597, and was his travelling companion throughout this 44-day expedition.[49]

The costumes, ceremony and spectators of religious processions gave them an obvious theatrical dimension. In March or April 1557, Felix Platter was impressed to see so many clerics and monks in a Parisian religious procession organized by the Eglise des Innocents in the rue Saint-Denis, that they took nearly an hour to file past him.[50] Thomas Platter records numerous diverse processions. In early 1599, he watched a procession in honour of Narbonne's patron saint, on St Sebastian's Day, and religious and secular participants 'carrying many strangely shaped and coloured lights around and back into the church again' in honour of the Purification of the Virgin in Barcelona.[51] That May, he watched local bakers accompanied by pipers, drummers and bagpipers, carry blessed bread loaves around Poitiers' Augustine Church, in a Rogation Sunday procession.[52] In Blois, he joined 'almost all the citizens and womenfolk of the town, all very magnificently dressed' to observe costumed local fishermen and sailors compete in their boats on the Loire in the traditional Whitsun water tournament.[53] That July, in Paris, he viewed treasures and reliquaries of Saint-Chapelle annually processed around the city on Easter Sunday.[54] He saw the two great religious treasures of Arras, shown annually to the public in separate public processions, the holy manna in its reliquary in the Church of Nôtre Dame on Quasimodo, and the holy candle in the

---

48 Now joined by memorials to Tom Simpson (1967) and other cyclists claimed by the Tour de France's defining stage.

49 *Thomas Platter d.J*, 246–8 (28 May 1598, Mont Ventoux).

50 *Felix Platter Tagebuch*, 280 (1557, Paris).

51 *Thomas Platter d.J*, 318 (20 January 1599, Narbonne); 350 (2 February 1599, Barcelona).

52 *Thomas Platter d.J*, 467 (16 May 1599, Poitiers).

53 *Thomas Platter d.J*, 508 (May 1599, Blois).

54 *Thomas Platter d.J*, 561–2 (28 July 1599, Paris).

chapel of Nôtre-Dame des Ardents (destroyed during the French revolution), on the Petit Marché on Corpus Christi. The holy candle, now in a nineteenth-century church, was venerated after the minstrels Norman and Itier successfully cured 149 local people of St Anthony's Fire, or ergotism, with it in 1105. They obeyed instructions received in a vision from the Virgin Mary, to treat patients with water into which its wax had been dripped. Platter, who retells this legend at length, observed numerous visitors take such water for medicinal use for a wide range of ailments in addition to ergotism.[55] In the Cathedral of St Mauritius, he viewed the treasures and relics paraded annually in the Angers Corpus Christi festival, said to be the most impressive in France.[56]

Platter did not experience the Arras or Angers processions themselves. However, his eyewitness account of the 1598 Avignon feste Dieu conveys the immense importance, prestige and expense associated with Corpus Christi festivals.[57] Hippolytus Guarinonius indicates the distances pilgrims were prepared to travel to witness this most important of all early modern church festivals. His references to personal pilgrimages to Munich to the Jesuit Corpus Christi procession that annually attracted over 17,000 visitors to the city, include one of c.1604 undertaken on horseback and one of 1607 with his brother-in-law Georg Thaler and three further companions, via various Bavarian monasteries, in traditional pilgrims' costume. He also relates a cautionary tale about a Protestant wine merchant from Ulm who was said to have been struck dead by God on 2 October 1609, as a direct result of insulting Günzburg's Catholics by labelling their Corpus Christi procession a 'work of folly'.[58]

In 1305, Pope Clement V had relocated the papal court to Avignon (Plate 3). After it officially returned to Rome in 1378, a parallel papacy held court in Avignon until Benedict XIII fled the city in 1403. Thereafter, Roman papal legates and vice-legates oversaw the garrison that supplied the Italian soldiers and Swiss guards who respectively guarded the city gates and the Palais de Papes, and ensured that Avignon, not re-annexed to France until 1791, remained firmly under Vatican jurisdiction. Avignon's high religious status was reflected in its prolific Catholic hierarchy, displayed to the full in a magnificent procession lasting from 8am until midnight. An eyewitness account of the 1581 Roman Corpus Christi procession[59] suggests that the Avignon procession's sumptuous decoration of house façades along its route with carpets, or protection of streets from rain with linen sheets suspended along their middle at first floor level, were only two of many customs whose blueprint was provided by the Roman procession. Until midday, Platter

[55]   *Thomas Platter d.J*, 642–8 (16 August 1599, Arras).

[56]   *Thomas Platter d.J*, 481 (21 May 1599, Angers).

[57]   *Thomas Platter d.J*, 238–9 (21 and 24 May 1598, Avignon). Corpus Christi festivals were suppressed in Reformation England in 1547 (Laroque, *Shakespeare's festive world*, 56).

[58]   Guarinonius, *Grewel*, 615, 841–2, 1224–5, 1277–8.

[59]   Gregory Martin, quoted by Blackburn and Holford-Strevens (*Year*, 634).

watched the procession file through Avignon's Place du Change. The priests and secular male participants, dressed according to rank and carrying diverse holy relics, were followed by nuns and local women, and accompanied by excellent groups of musicians. Meanwhile, on a raised stage in one corner of the square, actors performed a tragic religious play concerning the destruction of Jerusalem. Various plays and masquerades were staged on raised stages on other street corners. In other streets and squares, beautifully decorated flowing fountains were set up, or beautiful hills or other artistic creations were placed in front of the houses:[60]

> In conclusion, everything was so richly decorated, covered and embellished, that it is almost impossible to describe, and of course everyone can imagine for themselves that on this most important of festival days, there will have been no penny-pinching in a city in which the popes lived for so long.[61]

Three days later, on the morning of Sunday 24 May, again in the Place du Change, Platter witnessed the very different procession of 'des battus'. Fully clothed under their costumes, they theatricalized a brutally physical religious ritual originating with devout mid fourteenth-century Christians desperate to harness magical salvation to placate the divine wrath they believed was causing the plague.[62] This remained a genuine threat in the 1590s, and Thomas Platter's travel plans were repeatedly affected by stringent quarantine regulations. Just a month later, he was to write: 'in Marseille and Aix, deaths are very numerous [...] and if the plague takes hold in a town, it does far more damage than at home. If they didn't have and enforce such regulations, whole cities would die out, perhaps because of the great heat'.[63] Like over 4,000 he saw in a religious procession in Marseille in February 1597,[64] Avignon's flagellators filed past, intermittently beating themselves, in four companies distinguished by white, black, blue or grey painted shirts. These covered them:

> from the crown of their heads to their ankles and were open only at the eyes, mouth and at the back where they beat themselves, although they wore their everyday clothes underneath. The white and black companies were each accompanied by very excellent musicians, including some locals, and some sent from Toulouse. And each company had around 60 singers, some in front, some behind and some in the middle, going two by two, and holding up round sticks with which they beat out the rhythm. Each group of musicians included several cornet and trumpet players, as well as shawm players, all playing very sweetly

---

[60]   *Pace* Jennett (*Journal of a younger brother*, 150–1), the fountains and hills were independent of the theatrical performances on the raised stages.

[61]   *Thomas Platter d.J*, 239 (21 May 1599, Avignon).

[62]   Kreuder, 'Divine flagellation', 181, 186.

[63]   *Thomas Platter d.J*, 263–4 (14 June 1598, Montpellier).

[64]   *Thomas Platter d.J*, 192 (16 February 1597, Marseille).

in tune with each other. When they reached the Place du Change, they stood still and sung one or two impressive motets. This procession also lasted until nearly midday.[65]

Montaigne confirms that by no means all 'battus', even at this late date, were play-acting: 'Do we not vpon every good-friday, in sundrie places, see a great number of men and women, scourge and beate themselves so long till they bruse and teare their flesh, even to the bones; I have often seene it my self, and that without enchantment'.[66]

Carnival was a festival of contained social anarchy. In many regions, restrictions on public music, dancing and plays were relaxed, and strict dietary and sumptuary regulations were suspended. Particularly during the last days before Ash Wednesday, participants from every social group were encouraged to celebrate together to the point of excess. They routinely indulged in foolish behaviour involving sins such as gluttony, sloth or lechery, disguised in face-masks and costumes deliberately chosen for their inappropriateness to their trade, their social standing, even their gender. Such mummers and masqueraders populate Felix Platter's earliest childhood memories. He recalls his extreme fear when, aged four, he saw fools running amongst a masked parade of pipers and carnival mummers in Basle in early 1541, hitting boys with their folly sticks.[67] He was deeply impressed by the lute-playing at carnival time by a boarder of his father: 'how very much I enjoyed it, and how I wished that I could learn to play like that, thinking I couldn't possibly play any better', and by his participation in Shrovetide carnival masquerading in Neuenburg a few years later, cross-dressed as a girl.[68] He first documents the Montpellier carnival in January 1553, two months after arriving: 'At the start of the new year', he reports, 'all sorts of diversions immediately began'. While the plague raged in Basle, night-time serenading and dancing continued in Montpellier's most affluent streets and houses until Fat Monday and Shrove Tuesday. Then groups of masqueraders with musicians and costumes performed all sorts of diverse dances.[69] Around New Year 1555, Platter was sought after at dances and mummeries, for his skills in lute-playing and dancing in the French fashion.[70] That March, his exchange student Gilbert Catelan got into trouble with his professors over a carnival masquerade at a Basle wedding. At New Year 1556 Felix, under pressure to return home, reports to his father that while he studied late into the night, Gilbert, now back in Montpellier, went to dances and slept in.[71]

---

[65]   *Thomas Platter d.J*, 239 (24 May 1598, Avignon).

[66]   Montaigne, *Essayes*, 133.

[67]   *Felix Platter Tagebuch*, 57 (1541, Basle).

[68]   *Felix Platter Tagebuch*, 71, 88 (c.1544, Basle and c.1547, Neuenburg).

[69]   *Felix Platter Tagebuch*, 153, 158 (January and 8–12 February 1553, Montpellier).

[70]   *Felix Platter Tagebuch*, 211 (January 1555, Montpellier).

[71]   *Felix Platter Tagebuch*, 216, 240–1 (April 1555 and 14 January 1556, Montpellier).

Felix Platter records several pre-Christmas carnival-like maskings and disguisings. Entering Montpellier for the first time on 30 October 1552, the homesick teenager was cheered by the city's All Souls' Procession, held in annual commemoration of the dead.[72] Numerous citizens disguised in white shirts, including aristocrats, paraded with musicians and banners, dispensing sweets from silver bowls with silver spoons to the magnificently dressed young women in the streets. Arriving at his boarding house, Platter found his hosts Laurent Catelan and Eléonore Depuech watching outside the door of their apothecary, the renowned 'Pharmacie de la Licorne', closed for business because it was a Sunday.[73] Aristocratic students sometimes organized runnings at the ring in Montpellier. Felix Platter watched one in the terrible hot June of 1556,[74] and Thomas Platter another on All Souls' Day 1595:

> On 2 [12] November, All Souls' Day, the wealthy young citizens of the town, all daintily disguised in women's clothes, ran at the ring at a tournament in the city, not far from the Saunerie, in a narrow alley near the Couple Inn. They were all masked, and some costumes were covered with thin yellow sheet-metal, which made a loud noise as they ran.[75]

In late November 1554, Felix Platter danced and played the lute with a masked group who performed at several masquerades and balls.[76] In early November 1556, while taking part in masked 'cherubin' mumming, he entered the house of his personal tutor, Antoine Saporta. Here, he joined in the dancing and, because he knew and liked her, revealed his identity to Saporta's new young wife, Jhane de Sos.[77] On 2 December 1562, returning to Basle from a house-call, Felix danced until daybreak with a group of masked girls who came to his inn after visiting local houses, spending two crowns on food and drink.[78]

In some regions, the Festival of the Three Kings marked the official start of the carnival period. In 1553, the German-speaking students of Montpellier celebrated

---

[72]   Two days earlier, he had been so overwhelmed with homesickness that (before gaining some relief through church music), in an episode recalling his father's account of his youthful visit to Munich around the year 1518, he had wept, then collected his thoughts at a vantage point overlooking the nearest river (*Felix Platter Tagebuch*, 142: 28 October 1552, Avignon; Platter the Elder, 'Thomas Platters Lebensbeschreibung', 52).

[73]   *Felix Platter Tagebuch*, 144–5 (30 October 1552, Montpellier). On the Catelan family, see Dulieu, *La médecine a Montpellier du XIIe au Xxe siècle*, 315, 341–3.

[74]   *Felix Platter Tagebuch*, 246 (7 June 1556, Montpellier).

[75]   *Thomas Platter d.J*, 91 (2/12 November 1595, Montpellier).

[76]   *Felix Platter Tagebuch*, 208 (21 November 1554, Montpellier).

[77]   *Felix Platter Tagebuch*, 257 (4 and 8 November 1556, Montpellier).

[78]   *Felix Platter Tagebuch*, 390 (December 1562, Dannemarie).

the Three Kings with a banquet at which Felix Platter was the lutenist.[79] On Twelfth Night 1554 itself, in the College of Medicine, a student from Constance, Andreas von Croaria, drew the bean and was crowned as their king. Their celebratory meal was cooked by the elderly beadle, who had spent many years in Greece, and whose his son was publicly executed as a highwayman in Montpellier weeks later. Two days later, the students celebrated Twelfth Night again, in the home of the medical professor, ichthyologist, and respected author of numerous treatises on botany and anatomy, Guillaume Rondelet. Here Felix, lute teacher to Rondelet's daughter Catherine, first gained the confidence to dance in the French manner.[80] Possibly because travelling showmen performed in Montpellier on 6 January 1556, the German medical students celebrated that year's Three Kings only on 13 January. After the meal, two students newly arrived in Montpellier that December, Melchior Rotmundt of Swabia and Johann Ludwig Höchstetter of Augsburg, argued drunkenly over Rotmundt's beardlessness.[81] Höchstetter, who had continued to correspond with Felix after boarding with his father in Basle in the 1540s, was a great joker.[82] The argument was resolved by Rotmundt paying a barber to cut off Höchstetter's mighty beard, disguising him in a coat and hat, and introducing him in the morning as a new arrival with letters from home for the German students. Taken in, they treated Höchstetter to an expensive meal at the Salamander Inn before recognizing him, with much laughter.[83]

On Saturday 27 February 1557, having finished his studies in Montpellier, Felix Platter exchanged emotional last farewells with Laurent Catelan and Eléonore Depuech, and left as the carnival celebrations reached their peak. Accompanying

---

[79] *Felix Platter Tagebuch*, 154 (January 1553, Montpellier). Related customs were then still current in France and England (Blackburn and Holford-Strevens, *Year*, 23–4).

[80] *Felix Platter Tagebuch*, 192, 194–5 (January and March 1554, Montpellier). As the founder of one of the world's first botanical gardens, Rondelet, son of a perfumer, brother of an apothecary and Chancellor of Montpellier University, has secured a significant place in the history of collecting and museums. Rabelais commemorates him as 'the Physitian our honest Master *Rondibilis* […] married now, who before was not' and presents his 'cure of cuckoldry' in terms suggesting amorous student adventures (*Gargantua and Pantagruel*, 414–15, 429–33; Oppenheimer, 'Rondelet', 822; Le Roy Ladurie, *The beggar and the professor*, 169–70). Rondelet's nephew Pierre evidently inherited these extra-curricular preoccupations. He 'personally confided' to Thomas Platter that he transferred his law studies from Toulouse to Montpellier after escaping execution for seducing the daughter of a high Toulouse official only by being cross-dressed in women's clothes and hidden in a local convent by several hundred masked, armed fellow law students, who literally snatched him from the gallows (*Thomas Platter d.J*, 414: 27 April 1599, Toulouse).

[81] *Felix Platter Tagebuch*, 239–40 (13 January 1556, Montpellier); see also Chapter 9.

[82] Höchstetter, *Ein Brief*, 2–5.

[83] Earlier that year, the still beardless Felix Platter had stayed up a whole night copying out medical recipes. Rondelet's leaving present to two fellow students, they included a 'secret' for making hair grow (*Felix Platter Tagebuch*, 248, 257: 14 July and 22 November 1556, Montpellier).

him were his dog Pocles, Theodor Birkmann, a talented amateur wind and string musician who had studied medicine in Montpellier with Felix since May 1555 and whose family were publishers in Cologne, the Catelans' son Gilbert, and two of the German students who saw them off, Sigismund Rot and Johann Wachtel of Strasbourg, who later visited Felix in Basle.[84] Reaching Béziers the following day, the last Sunday of carnival, they were eating their midday meal at an inn when a masked group of young carnival masqueraders entered with their musicians.[85] They unmasked, revealing the merchant who had married Gilbert's sister Isabelle, his sisters, and other relatives, all, as were the Catelans, conversos. While they feasted and danced, Platter, aware that his future wife impatiently awaited his return to Basle, resisted the flirtations of a converso girl in yellow silk knitted stockings. Then Gilbert's relatives invited his group to stay with Isabelle's father-in-law.

The following morning, Monday 1 March, the Germans left without Gilbert. Gaining extra privileges by all four claiming to be Swiss, they entered Narbonne, registered at a hostel and ordered the midday meal. Here, a nobleman among the 'masqueraders who come to every meal, because it is carnival time' addressed them in German. Removing his carnival mask, he spent that afternoon showing them the city.[86] On Shrove Tuesday, 2 March 1557, Rot and Wachtel returned to Montpellier. Felix Platter, who travelled on to Paris with Birkmann, notes that from the next day, Ash Wednesday, he ate no more meat before reaching Basle.[87] Just as the German medical students of Montpellier fêted their German-speaking visitors, Platter and Birkmann were welcomed with special food and entertainment in March 1557 in Orléans, whose university had the largest community of German students in France. In deference to Lenten food regulations, a fish banquet with local wine and various rich deserts was organized in their honour by Sigmund von Andlau, who had provided Felix and other fellow pupils with much amusement as a reluctant child actor, while boarding with Thomas Platter the Elder (Diagram 3). Felix ate and drank prodigiously, becoming extremely ill during the night. Rumoured to be dying, by midday he had recovered sufficiently to attend festivities in the house of another German, impressing fellow guests with his French dancing, and harp and lute-playing.[88] Sigmund had not outgrown a messy habit of poking his fingers into

---

[84]   *Felix Platter Tagebuch*, 218–19, 263, 338 (May 1555 and February 1557, Montpellier; 20 January 1558, Basle).

[85]   *Felix Platter Tagebuch*, 264 (28 February 1557, Béziers).

[86]   *Felix Platter Tagebuch*, 265 (1 March 1557, Narbonne). Excluding the Archbishop's Palace. Michelangelo's statue then adorned the fountain in Narbonne's market square. Thomas, who admired the Palace's chief treasure (Sebastiano del Piombino's *The raising of Lazarus*, since 1824 in London's National Gallery), during carnival 1599, provides an embroidered version of Vasari's account of the sculptor's involvement as co-painter (*Thomas Platter d.J*, 316, 318: 18–19 January 1599, Narbonne).

[87]   *Felix Platter Tagebuch*, 265–6 (2–3 March 1557, Narbonne, Carcassonne).

[88]   *Felix Platter Tagebuch*, 275 (23–25 March 1557, Orléans).

inappropriate places when with Felix. Some dubious physical experimentation they had got up to as young children ended only when 'Sigmund's reward was that he had to wash his hands'.[89] In Orléans, the now 20-year-old injured himself by fingering Felix's new Parisian gun until it accidentally backfired, causing him to bleed profusely.[90] Thomas Platter, who rarely let Lenten dietary regulations get in the way of a hearty meal, was surprised that the traditional Lenten fast, and year-round weekly two-day abstention from meat were observed in Protestant England.[91] He ordered duck at Saint-Cannat's White Horse Inn during Lent 1597 (albeit in a private dining room to decrease the risk of being caught and punished), and meat for himself and eggs for his young lackey Daniel Olivier during Lent 1599.[92]

Of the 1558 Basle carnival, his first since returning, Felix Platter notes that a group of masqueraders entered an inn one evening as he was dancing and playing music with friends. They left swiftly, on seeing Ursel Wachter, the girl their leader, the iron merchant Isaac Liechtenhan, was interested in impressing, seated on the knees of the fiancée she married days later, Jacob Myconius.[93] In the 1560s, Felix Platter experienced contrasting carnivals while attending patients in religious orders. From November 1561, the Bishop of Basle, Melchior von Lichtenfels, repeatedly called him to his court at Pruntrut to treat his chancellor, Esaias Dankwart, for serious symptoms of colic and gout. On 7 February 1562, the last Saturday of carnival, Felix Platter attended the delirious Dankwart all night while he suffered seven seizures, the last, at dawn, fatal: 'which greatly saddened the Bishop. And although the Bishop had always taken pains to observe carnival with great magnificence, he cancelled everything and had many parts of the castle covered with black cloth'.[94] In 1564 Felix and Madlen Platter enjoyed carnival with Katharina von Hersberg, abbess of the Cistercian convent Kloster Olsberg, 'a cheerful woman' who allowed at least two men to become 'almost too familiar' with her. A regular patient since at least 1560, she was not above staging playful tricks, such as convincing Madlen that a painted wooden carving

---

[89] *Felix Platter Tagebuch*, 92 (c.1546, Basle).

[90] *Felix Platter Tagebuch*, 287 (24–25 April 1557, Orléans).

[91] *Thomas Platter d.J*, 824 (25 September 1599, London).

[92] Whereupon Olivier surprised Platter by announcing that he would prefer meat, and had lied to him about being Catholic while in Spain, to make himself appear more employable: 'which I more readily believed, as he had been unable to cross himself properly when asked to do so in Spain'. *Thomas Platter d.J*, 201 (20 February 1597, Saint-Cannat), 395 (13 March 1599, Mèze).

[93] Myconius's intemperate lifestyle, his fellow physician Platter notes, widowed Wachter within the year (*Felix Platter Tagebuch*, 339, 348: March 1558 and February 1559, Basle).

[94] *Felix Platter Tagebuch*, 372, 384–6 (November 1561; 31 January and 7 February 1562, Pruntrut). Dankwart's wife Euphrosyna was the daughter of von Gundelsheim, the bishop of Basle whose personal physician, Epiphanius, had mentored Platter the Elder.

of a naked child lying in a cot in her private rooms was a live baby. This made the others laugh, and Felix comment: 'I thought that in some convents that could be a way of hiding real children'. Her nuns and visitors were encouraged to stage 'all sorts of diversions during carnival, when we played the lute and had mummings and other performances'.[95]

Thomas Platter describes carnivals of the 1590s in Avignon, Marseille and Barcelona, at which he joined the masked and costumed carnival masqueraders who danced, ran or rode through the streets far into the night, accompanied by torch-bearers. Some, in uniformly costumed groups he interchangeably calls masqueraders or mummers, stopped regularly at houses and inns, where they removed their masks to perform chosen dances to the music of their instrumentalists before being offered seasonal refreshments, perhaps in the manner depicted in Plate 21. A passage in John Marston's *Histrio-Mastix* describes a related English custom of the 1590s. Here, a nobleman's servant announces that 'a Morrice-daunce of neighbours crave admittance'. They are referred to as players, enter with their poet, and are expected to entertain the assembled company by singing and performing plays, in exchange for 'beefe and beere, and beds'. The noblemen dismiss their puffed up repertoire as 'home-spun country stuffe [...] lame stuffe indeed'.[96] The *branles* and other street dancing Thomas Platter saw performed by 'fishermen, sailors and vintners' of Villeneuve-lès-Maguelonne on Sunday 18 February 1596, in the company of his fellow student Rudolff Meiß of Zurich and landlord Jacques Catelan, were modest rustic examples of this carnival practice, celebrated with competitive lavishness in urban centres.[97] His description of the following Sunday and Monday's Avignon carnival festivities identifies typical examples of masquerade costume as those of pilgrims, peasants, Netherlandish sailors; Swiss, Italian, Spanish or Alsatian national costume, or the dress of women; or 'other unusual types'. It was customary for each uniformly-costumed group to replace their outfits for each year's carnival celebrations. The masqueraders were all masked, each group accompanied by its own musicians, generally including some who played steel or bronze cymbals shape like flat horse-brasses with handles. Their mighty noise when clashed together could be heard above the playing of the other instruments, of which there were usually many, including violas, violins, lutes, bagpipes, pipes. Each group ran and danced around the town, removing their masks when they entered houses, to dance with each other, and sometimes also with those in the houses. These visits were kept brief so that each group could get around the whole town.[98]

Platter names the typical dances of the masqueraders as the '*branle, gagliarda, corrente, volta* and others', and describes a particularly attractive hoop dance

---

[95]   *Felix Platter Tagebuch*, 358, 373, 431 (1560, 1561 and 13–15 February 1564, Kloster Olsberg).

[96]   Marston, *Histrio-mastix* II.i (sigs.C2ᵛ–4ʳ).

[97]   *Thomas Platter d.J*, 99 (18 February 1596, Villeneuve).

[98]   *Thomas Platter d.J*, 120–1 (25 February 1596, Avignon).

performed by four aristocratic young couples. Dressed in white trimmed with gold, they visited the inn where he eaten that evening in order to ensure a good seat for viewing the masqueraders. Each pair held a white half hoop trimmed with gold upright in their hands, and stayed in perfect time with the beat of their musicians as they wove under and over each other's hoops, dancing first in the street, then in the inn. They danced the hoop dance right through, then took off their masks and danced a *volte*, accepted a drink, replaced their masks, and returned to the streets. A friendship album depiction of the 1590s shows costumed males performing an elaborate hoop dance of this type (Plate 8). The masqueraders visited local inns and public houses, but also grand mansions and palaces, including one to which a nobleman from Tarascon took Thomas Platter and his companion, in which many women sat in a large hall. Platter watched one group of masqueraders after another enter, many dancing with the women, others sitting down and socializing with them. They always left on the arrival of another group, although sometimes one or another took his mistress with him. The master of the house played cards with other noblemen, while others played at dice, for high stakes of gold or coin. It was after midnight before each went home with the woman of his choice.

The following morning, Monday 26 February 1596, Platter again saw various masqueraders running and dancing through the streets with their musicians, less than on the previous day, and all costumed differently. After breakfast, he watched a religious procession from the Palais des Papes to the Church of Nôtre-Dame and other Avignon churches. Its purpose was to pray for God's pardon for the follies of the carnival masqueraders, some of whom were running about in the same streets, giving way to the religious paraders when they met. These walked in rows of three. Each priest, carrying a cross or reliquary and the symbols of the Apostle, saint or Evangelist they represented, was flanked by two girls or boys under the age of 21, dressed in white and carrying books.[99] That evening, he again accompanied the nobleman from Tarascon to several grand private houses, leaving only after midnight. He was particularly impressed by a group he watched arriving in a coach lined, covered and hung about with silk, preceded by several riders on stately horses, and surrounded on all sides by so many white wax torchbearers that they shone as brightly as daylight, and the jewels inside the coach glittered astonishingly. In the coach were four unmasked noblemen in matching outfits of golden velvet, trimmed with gold, silver and jewels. At their sides sat the four most beautiful noble girls in Avignon, unmasked and in matching outfits of golden taffeta, embroidered with pearls and gold and silver thread, their breasts and necks uncovered according to local custom. 'In short', he comments:

> they rode towards us with their stately chief ornaments on display, as one paints goddesses [...] As soon as they came to a house at which they were expected, they got out, and the doors were immediately closed again behind them. When I too had entered, the hall was already filled with people to every last corner,

---

[99]   *Thomas Platter d.J*, 121–2 (26 February 1596, Avignon).

and with such thick smoke from the torches and nightlights that I was not really able to see them dance. But I was well aware that they danced a stately *ballet*. Afterwards, they drove to other houses until after midnight, it was said that their expenses for this *ballet* had been above 1000 crowns.[100]

On Shrove Tuesday, Platter, who went to a wedding and a play in the morning, then registered at the city hall before going to the pall-mall alley in the afternoon, 'still passed masqueraders in the streets, running with their musicians, but no longer as many as on the day before'.[101]

Platter spent the following carnival in Marseille. On 11 February, he detailed the miserable on-board life of Mediterranean galley-slaves.[102] The following Sunday morning, he watched a gang of them, chained together, working at speed to prepare the narrow road stretching from the city hall to the ducal palace for the carnival. They lifted the paving, covered the surface with sand, and erected a long raised platform along one side for seating, to accommodate the maximum possible audience, although Platter notes that wealthy spectators preferred to watch from inside houses along the road. In the afternoon, Charles de Lorraine, fourth duc de Guise arrived at the cleared square, with many gentlemen and noblemen on good Berbers or other racehorses, all impressively costumed, and unidentifiable because of their daintily masked features. Here they skilfully ran to the ring for several hours, after which the Duke's favourite mistress, Mme de Castellane, presented the prizes. Platter was highly impressed by the expense to which the Marseille womenfolk went regarding their appearance. Contrasting their luxury with the proverbial austerity of the dowry expected by earlier generations, he noticed with surprise that strings of pearls to the value of 500 or 1,000 crowns are commonplace, but finds the bright colours and bold combinations of the women's clothes unfeminine, making them 'look like parrots'.[103] All day, he saw groups of masqueraders and mummers, each accompanied by their musicians, parade the streets, but does not describe them individually, instead referring back to his descriptions of the 1596 carnival.

In Charles de Lorraine's palace, Platter watched the nobility dance the *volta*, pavane, *branle* and *gagliarda*, and after supper he put on a carnival mask and visited public carnival dances with a Nürnberg bell-founder until 2am. At one, he saw a graceful ballet performed by Charles de Lorraine and several women, including Mme de Castellane and her sister. Despite masks and costumes, their identity did not remain secret, because the spectators recognized the Duke's excellent musicians, who accompanied the dance and (as Guarinonius confirms):

---

[100] *Thomas Platter d.J*, 122 (26 February 1596, Avignon).

[101] *Thomas Platter d.J*, 123 (27 February 1596, Avignon).

[102] *Thomas Platter d.J*, 181–3 (11 February 1597, Marseille). Evelyn describes a similar set-up in 1644 (*The diary*, 89).

[103] *Thomas Platter d.J*, 186–8 (16 February 1597, Marseille).

It is quite clear and certain that even when someone's face is hidden, it is easy to recognize them from their outer gestures, as is clearly demonstrated by the mummers during the carnival period, who because of their disguise can be recognized by nothing apart from their gestures, and that is enough to identify them.[104]

Thomas Platter found the 1597 Marseille festivities similar to those of Avignon in 1596. Carnival gaming during a visit by masqueraders is a popular subject for depiction (Plate 10), although he was surprised to note a woman, the wife of the mayor, among those whiling away the time between masqueraders' visits by gaming for high stakes with cards or dice.[105] Later that month, he travelled to Pont de Sorgue near Orange, to watch the locals perform the drowning of 'The Old Carnival'.[106] Represented by a straw man, Carnival is paraded joyfully around the whole town on a donkey, and finally taken to a bridge from which he is drowned, by being thrown into the water. This ritual, still considered noteworthy in the nineteenth century, is comparable to the Easter Sunday burning of the English Jack-a-Lent.[107]

Thomas Platter describes the carnival of 1598 not at all, and that of 1600 only briefly. He returned to Dijon in late January 1600 at the height of carnival, and saw many beautiful ballets, masquerades and dances by day and by night, extending his visit to include 'the great festival day of Candlemass, when I saw the magnificence and expense of the inhabitants' costumes'.[108] His planned participation in further carnival festivities that year was cut short when he left Besançon to avoid taking up the sinister comte de Cantecroy's invitation to see out the carnival with him.[109] His account of the 1599 Barcelona carnival again refers readers to his descriptions of the 1596 Avignon carnival, for details of the activities of individual groups of masqueraders. The carnival activities peaked between 18 and 22 February 1599, when, as in Marseille in 1597, he saw one masked group of mummers after another parade through the city, day and night, those on foot running in and out of houses with their musicians, those on horseback riding slowly through the streets and around the large squares near Barcelona's School of Medicine. Platter remarks on their small riding boots, sometimes decoratively gilded, with a single spur one span in length, like a spindle, at the side of which is a small round wheel with which they spurred the horses, because if they were to use the spur itself,

---

[104]   Guarinonius, *Grewel*, 71.

[105]   *Thomas Platter d.J*, 194–6 (17 February 1597, Marseille).

[106]   *Thomas Platter d.J*, 206 (24 February 1597, Pont de Sorgue).

[107]   Frédéric Rivarés describes the annual Ash Wednesday 'trial and condemnation of the Carnival' of Pau of the 1840s (Eyre, *A lady's walks*, 218–19, in translation). On Jack-a-Lent, see Laroque, *Shakespeare's festive world*, 103–4.

[108]   *Thomas Platter d.J*, 912 (21/31 January to 23 January/2 February 1600, Dijon).

[109]   *Thomas Platter d.J*, 921–2 (30 January / 9 February 1600 Besançon). See Chapter 10, this volume.

they would pierce their horses to the gut.[110] He considered the dancing and riding skills of the Spanish less cultivated than those of the French, and noted that a favourite dance was the sarabande, which they danced in groups of up to 50 mixed pairs, each couple always facing each other. He describes their strange, grotesque gestures and movements and use of castanets in this dance. Large numbers of masqueraders, on foot, on horseback (sometimes two to a horse), or travelling by coach, each group masked, and differently costumed, rode and drove up and down the squares, slowly enough to get a good look at the richly-dressed women watching from their windows, and allow the women to observe them at leisure.

These French and Spanish carnivals featured many customs Thomas Platter was unfamiliar with from his native Basle. One frequently depicted is the throwing of citrus fruit or eggs (Plate 9). Felix Platter observed this custom at the Montpellier carnivals on Shrove Tuesday. In 1553, he saw local young people with cheap bags of rotting grapefruit hanging round their necks. Using baskets as shields, they threw so many at each other in the Place Nôtre-Dame, that the whole square was littered with split fruit.[111] On Shrove Tuesday 1554, the Montpellier law students went around in a masquerade group while the locals pelted each other with grapefruits.[112] Thomas Platter notes that by February 1597, the oranges in Marseille are yellowing, soft and beginning to rot. Shiploads continue to be delivered and sold for almost nothing, so that many thousands are thrown by boys at every carnival, at each other, and sometimes at passersby. Those in the Place Neuve on 16 February 1597 reminded him of snowballing Basle boys.[113] In 1599, in the suburbs of Barcelona, he saw 'many beautiful gardens in which grapefruit, lemon and orange trees, together with pomegranate trees, grew as naturally as apple or pear trees in our country [...] and many fruits had been left on the trees, mostly so that people could use them to throw at each other during the carnival'. Every Barcelona masquerader was armed with sacks of rotting citrus fruit, sometimes filled with perfumed water or powder, or strange written messages, carried by themselves or their servants, or even eggshells filled with perfume, for throwing at the exquisitely dressed women who watched them from every window of the city's houses. These caught them in their hands, or simply let them fall through their windows, so that they could then use them again, to toss down to masqueraders who took their fancy. It was considered a sign of popularity to be targeted by these missiles, and any that fell on the road were picked up and thrown again by small boys. Platter estimated that many thousands were thrown in this way each day, and considered them far less dangerous than the hollow eggs which were also traditional: 'with which one can cause great offence to women, by refilling them with acidic liquids that can bruise or swell their faces'.[114]

---

[110] *Thomas Platter d.J*, 372–5 (18–22 February 1599, Barcelona).

[111] *Felix Platter Tagebuch*, 158 (12 February 1553, Montpellier).

[112] *Felix Platter Tagebuch*, 193 (February 1554, Montpellier).

[113] *Thomas Platter d.J*, 189 (16 February 1597, Marseille).

[114] *Thomas Platter d.J*, 353 (2 February 1599, Barcelona).

Given the severe restrictions regulating Spanish women's daily dealings with men outside the carnival period, Platter is surprised to see masked and costumed women as well as men among the Barcelona masqueraders. He remarks drily that the menfolk had to tolerate women's free participation in the carnival as a traditional custom, even though it creates numerous cuckolds even before the proper arrival of spring.[115] Platter ends his account of the 1599 Barcelona carnival by describing the Catholic ritual from which Ash Wednesday takes its name, in which, after Morning Mass, each reveller had a little ash wiped across his forehead: to prepare them for a seven-week abstention from meat, cure them of carnival foolishness and return them to their senses. The physician Platter notes that to achieve this it must indeed be a powerful powder.[116] James Howell's letter of Ash Wednesday 1654, digressing on Lenten fasting, ascribes a laboured variant on this aside to the Turkish ambassador to Venice:

> the Christians hath a kind of Ashes, which thrown upon the Head, doth presently cure Madness; for in Venice I saw the People go up and down the Streets (said he) in ugly and antick strange Disguises, as being in the eye of human Reason stark mad; but the next Day (meaning Ashwednesday) they are suddenly cur'd of that madness, by a sort of Ashes which they cast upon their Heads.[117]

If Howell and Shakespeare's Shylock remind us of non-Christian disapproval of carnival, Guarinonius confirms that neither were its excesses by any means favourably regarded by all Christians. He highly praises the anti-carnival initiatives of Tolosa, a 25-year-old Paduan monk. While Guarinonius studied in Padua in the 1590s, Tolosa invited those preparing the main square for the carnival Sunday tournaments to a sermon, calling on them to joust for the Church. This inspired numerous Paduans to dedicate the final two days of carnival not to the customary festivities but to Confession, Communion and 40-hour prayers.[118] Guarinonius himself refused all his patients, regardless of social standing, meat certificates allowing them to prolong 'bestial' carnival gluttony by excusing them from the Lenten dietary requirements whose health benefits he so highly rates.[119] He condemns a 'frivolous' carnival-related Bohemian custom in which girls and bachelors lash anyone holding Easter eggs with the long brightly-coloured plaited rods sold on every Prague street corner and square during the Easter holidays, 'like fools with their folly sticks'.[120] He criticizes slack municipal officials for 'wandering around in masks during the Carnival' instead of enforcing regulations;

---

[115]   *Thomas Platter d.J*, 373–4 (18–22 February 1599, Barcelona).
[116]   *Thomas Platter d.J*, 374 (24 February 1599, Barcelona).
[117]   Howell, *Familiar letters*, 439.
[118]   Guarinonius, *Grewel*, 1229–30.
[119]   Guarinonius, *Grewel*, 756–7.
[120]   Guarinonius, *Grewel*, 1257.

'gross fools' who scare young children with 'voices, masks and other means',[121] and the sinful inquisitiveness of thoughtless adolescents drawn towards:

> dangerous matters [...] through which they are often shamefully injured or die in a dreadful manner, such as a type of masquerade known as the *Chiusen* often performed in Italy. Even though they are completely practiced and well-rehearsed for this, as well as being specially costumed, now and again someone slips up and loses a leg or an arm, or even falls down dead.[122]

Guarinonius's manuscript confirms this as the *mattacino*, a dangerous armed *moresco* danced with swords or hammers by professional entertainers, and increasingly imitated by carnival masqueraders.[123] Moreover, for Guarinonius, the darker side of carnival represented a genuine threat to life as well as limb:

> On the fifth day of last month, February of this year of 1606, on the Sunday before Shrove Tuesday, at a dance in a hall in Trent, most of the nobility of both sexes were assembled and present and the masquerade groups were coming and going, when without warning a terrible quarrel began in that same hall. Several people had encountered their enemies there whereupon, despite all the crowds, they had shot at them several times. Those for whom the shots were meant luckily got away. But instead of them, two innocent manservants were each hit by a single shot. Previously of sound body, both died within 30 hours. One of them was Mattheus N, one of my father's servants. He was in his forties and left a wife and child.[124]

In the journals of the Protestant Platter brothers, the essentially Catholic carnival emerges as the joyous culmination of the festive Christian year, a theatrical celebration with the healing power to unite disparate communities and social strata. In *Grewel*, the devoutly Catholic Guarinonius relentlessly emphasizes the health-, even life-threatening, aspects of 'carnal, bestial Carnival'.

---

[121]   Guarinonius, *Grewel*, 310, 794.

[122]   Guarinonius, *Grewel*, 373.

[123]   Innsbruck UL, Cod.110, I, f.540ᵛ. The six dancers in the left foreground of Plate 20 are a *moresco* troupe.

[124]   Guarinonius, *Grewel*, 136.

Chapter 5

Jewish Traditions and Ceremonies in Montpellier and Avignon

The European festive year is based on the feasts and fasts of the Christian faith. Christianity's profound roots in Judaism had complex early modern cultural and social repercussions. Jews, the most significant religious group represented within Christian festivals, were also their largest non-participating group. This chapter focuses on the Platter brothers' accounts of the reception, impact and diffusion of Jewish culture in western Mediterranean France in the 1550s and 1590s, when they lived with and were taught medicine and pharmacy by conversos: baptized Iberian Jews and their 'New Christian' descendants. It concludes by considering some Jewish representations and misrepresentations in the writings of Hippolytus Guarinonius. For over a decade until 1594, while studying at Prague's Jesuit College, he came into unhappy daily contact with the Jews of the Prague ghetto, and one of his hagiographies initiated a persistent anti-Jewish legend commemorated in drama and other literature.

Officially, Languedoc was one of many French regions with no Jews. Alluding to King Philip IV's systematic early fourteenth-century persecution of French Jews, Thomas Platter describes the 'Collibus Judaicis' district of Bordeaux as: 'the hill where the Jews continued to live long after they were expelled by Philip'.[1] The reign of Philip IV's son Louis X (1314–16) provided only a brief respite, and subsequent French persecutions include a royal edict of 17 September 1394 expelling all Jews from Montpellier. They were allowed back, under severe restrictions, only in the seventeenth century. Jews arriving from Iberia in the wake of Ferdinand and Isabella's 1492 expulsion settled in Languedoc not as Jews, but as conversos. Christian from the point of view of canon law, conversos' continuing participation, to whatever extent, in their Jewish heritage, placed them on the cultural threshold between Europe's normative Jewish communities, whose spiritual leaders regarded conversos as at best potential Jews, and its 'Old Christians', whose profound suspicions of heresy received their most sinister expression in the Inquisition of the conversos' ancestral Iberian homelands.[2] In allusion to their North African origins, during the early modern period conversos descended from Sephardic Jews were commonly referred to as Marranos, a term they themselves regarded as highly pejorative. As Thomas Platter explains:

---

[1] *Thomas Platter d.J*, 441–2 (3 May 1599, Bordeaux).

[2] Graizbord, *Souls in dispute*, 1–3.

Huge numbers of people in this country are descended from the Jews. Because they emigrated to France from Mauritania via Spain, they have settled in cities close to the border, such as Montpellier, Béziers, Narbonne, etc. And although they behave just like other Christians, because of their origins they are still called Marranos. They regard this as the most profound libel, and if they can prove that someone has slandered them in this way, they exact a high financial compensation from their slanderer. Yet hardly a carnival takes place at which the most prominent of them, represented by clothes stuffed with straw and well-garnished with bacon fat, are not hung up, sometimes with dainty verses, in public squares and alleys. Afterwards, the hangman has them taken down and carried to the city hall, where large numbers of such effigies lie. These days, their clothes are given to the poor.

In a city known to use effigies of this type for proxy enactment of public corporal or capital punishment, this theatrical custom was aggressively threatening, as well as degrading. In 1554, for example, Felix Platter had been in the crowd watching the masked and clothed effigy of a fellow medical student, the escaped murderer Jacques de Marchetti, brought out on a sledge, for Montpellier's municipal executioners to place it on a cross and hack off its limbs.[3] Thomas Platter continues:

And even though the principal regulations at the city hall are recorded in the Catalan language, from where the Marranos originate, and the Languedoc language is not dissimilar to Catalan, from which it may be surmised that the Marranos have lived here for many years, no Marranos or their children are permitted to hold the rank of mayor or city councillor, despite the fact that they include many eminent people. It is said that they continue to observe their ceremonies like the Jews, and there are indeed some among them who eat no pork and still observe their Sabbath, for whom the rest have to suffer. Both faiths include Marranos, although more are Protestant than Catholic.[4]

In 1599 he refers directly back to this passage, confirming that it describes Montpellier's conversos, when he notes of Béziers: 'the inhabitants are extremely Catholic, no Protestant people live there that are known of. But there are a great many Marranos there, on whom even more indignities are inflicted than on those of Montpellier, who are described above in folio 39'.[5]

Mid sixteenth-century Languedoc also had several ghettos, within which Jewish ceremonies were tolerated. Their inhabitants, like any women regardless

---

[3]   *Felix Platter Tagebuch*, 205 (29 September 1554, Montpellier). Marchetti's continuing misadventures outside France ended when his occupation of the throne of Moldavia was cut short after two years by his assassination in a popular uprising (Dulieu, *La médecine a Montpellier: La Renaissance*, 398).

[4]   *Thomas Platter d.J*, 77–8 (October 1595, Montpellier).

[5]   *Thomas Platter d.J*, 312 (15 January 1599, Béziers).

of their faith, and like all non-Christian men, were barred from university study, and consequently from professional practice. In early modern Europe, Jews could only practice medicine as unlicensed healers. One such was Dr Joseph. From at least the late 1550s (when Felix Platter records him in his list of medical rivals as 'the Jew of Allschwil'), until his death in 1610, he ran a thriving practice in Allschwil, the only community in the Basle region with a significant number of Jewish inhabitants.[6] In 1530, the convert to Christianity Anthonius Margaritha dismissed German Jewish medical practitioners as quacks, weak in Latin, with little or no preliminary training apart from knowledge informally handed down through the generations, and experience of working with livestock and as ritual slaughterers. He contrasted their lack of learning sharply with the excellence of Italian and Spanish Jewish physicians, whose mastery of Hebrew, Latin and Greek enabled them to study all the best works.[7] Sephardic Jewish expertise was a vital cornerstone of Montpellier's school of medicine, and Languedoc's converso population contributed leading members of its academic and healthcare communities. Notable among these were the Saporta and Catelan dynasties.

Felix Platter's tutor Professor Antoine Saporta presided at his successful baccalaureate disputation in May 1556; his son Jean Saporta awarded Thomas Platter his medical doctorate in March 1597.[8] Antoine Saporta, who succeeded as chancellor on Guillaume Rondelet's death in 1566, also served for three months of each year at the Spanish court of Antoine of Bourbon, King of Navarre. He had close professional connections to Platter's host family, the Catelans and, with his colleague Laurent Joubert, supported cooperation between physicians and apothecaries. As Montpellier medical students in the 1530s, Saporta, Rondelet, François Rabelais and several other 'ancient friends' had acted together in 'The Moral Comedy of him who had espoused and married a *Dumb Wife*', a farce affectionately recalled by Rabelais: 'I never in my Life-time laughed so much, as at the acting of that Buffoonry'.[9] His father Louis III Saporta had preceded him as a celebrated professor of medicine at Montpellier, and his grandfather Louis II Saporta, a Sephardic Jew from Catalonia, became a court physician after fleeing Spain with his parents.

Felix lodged with Montpellier's leading apothecaries, the Catelan family, throughout his four-and-a-half years in Languedoc. Thomas lodged with them only for his first year, but maintained close social contact, as when he and other Germans were joined on a Sunday outing in June 1598 by Jacques Catelan and his daughters, or he visited Catelan's married sister Constance in Béziers in January

---

[6] *Felix Platter Tagebuch*, 337 (1558, Basle); Burnett, *From Christian Hebraism to Jewish studies*, 42.

[7] Walton, 'Anthonius Margaritha', 132.

[8] *Felix Platter Tagebuch*, 245 (28 May 1556, Montpellier); *Thomas Platter d.J*, 210 (22 March 1597, Montpellier).

[9] Rabelais, *Gargantua and Pantagruel*, 435. On Rondelet and the Saporta family, see also Dulieu (*La médecine a Montpellier: La Renaissance*, 345–9, 420).

1599.[10] In March 1599 he returned from a two-month tour of Spain to spend his last month in Languedoc in a rented room in the house of M. Gauseran, next door to the apothecary of Jacques Catelan, who was at his farewell lunch in April 1599.[11] From mid-1553, Felix roomed in a magnificent house left to Laurent Catelan by the Spanish-born converso physician Jean Falcon, on his death in the 1530s. One locked room still contained Falcon's medical papers, which Felix secretly broke into 'not without danger, using a ladder' and copied for his own use, in an episode reminiscent of one in his father's journal.[12] Catelan had fled Spain as a Jew, and founded the family apothecary in Montpellier. His wife Eléonore Depuech, whose sister had married Jhan de la Sala, a Spanish converso doctor who practiced in Lyon, was also a converso.[13] In the 1590s, when Thomas Platter was in Montpellier, the Catelan's studious younger son Jacques took over the family apothecary. He was followed by his son, Laurent III, who qualified as a master apothecary in 1595, and later founded a curiosity cabinet and wrote many publications.[14]

Jacques Catelan and his older brother Gilbert studied medicine at the University of Basle, where Gilbert resisted repeated paternal attempts to call him home. According to Felix, 'he thought his father might fear he would become a Lutheran', although it was in fact Jacques who converted to Protestantism. The brothers lodged from April 1553 for two-and-a-half and nearly four years with Felix's father, according to whom Gilbert 'got up to endless follies with his sweetheart', the Swiss girl who motivated his prolonged stay in Basle.[15] In a letter of 1555, Felix clarifies converso expectations to his father, namely that:

> Gilbert would be required to attend Mass and Confession again when he returned home, because in addition to the Jewish ceremonies that they observe, Marranos hold Mass in high regard, and the Virgin Mary more than Christ. Catelan had many Masses sung for his sons to ensure their continuing safety. My master asked me once whether Lutherans believe in Christ, and when I explained our

---

[10]   *Thomas Platter d.J*, 266, 312 (21 June 1598, Sellaneuve; 16 January 1599, Béziers). In October 1596 Thomas moved from the Catelans to the widowed Mme de Gras's lodgings: 'where many French lived, in order that I might learn the French language better', a few months later to the powder merchant François Rossonat, and in April 1597, now as a newly qualified physician, from Montpellier to Uzès (*Thomas Platter d.J*, 172–3: 1 October 1596 and 1 February 1597, Montpellier; 220: 21 April 1597, Uzès).

[11]   *Thomas Platter d.J*, 395, 397 (17 March and 18 April 1599, Montpellier).

[12]   Recording that Platter the Elder rose early every morning to secretly copy Theodor Bibliander's Hebrew grammar, during Bibliander's visit to Oswald Myconius (*Felix Platter Tagebuch*, 173, 202: June 1553 and 2 August 1554, Montpellier; Platter the Elder, 'Thomas Platters Lebensbeschreibung', 78).

[13]   *Felix Platter Tagebuch*, 163, 231 (22 April 1553 and 6 October 1555, Montpellier).

[14]   *Thomas Platter d.J*, 72 (October 1595, Montpellier).

[15]   *Felix Platter Tagebuch*, 171, 186, 331–2 (May and October 1553, Montpellier; December 1557, Basle).

religion to him, he said "If I get enough money, I would like to take care of my salvation. If I can leave enough for my children that they can have Masses sung for me after my death, I will be at peace." Item, how he always says "noli foenerari fratri tuo sed alieno", which is still strictly observed by the Marranos between themselves. All in all, he was a good man, who treated me with love.[16]

Because Felix Platter arrived knowing neither the 'langue d'oc' (Occitan) of Montpellier's locals, nor the 'langue d'oïl' (French) of its educated elite, Laurent Catelan got into the habit of speaking to him in Latin, 'in his way, badly', according to Felix. Sometimes they discussed religion. The literal meaning of Laurent Catelan's Latin phrase here is 'rather lend to a stranger than to your own brother'. Swiss-Germans would have recognized this as a Deuteronomic law vehemently rejected by Jean Calvin. Felix heard him in 1541, conversing with his father when they stopped off at The Keys, the inn opposite the townhall of Liestal at which Calvin was staying en route from Strasbourg to Geneva, and in 1552, delivering a French sermon he could not understand, in Geneva, where he delivered a letter from his father to him, receiving in exchange an approving comment that he was travelling on to Montpellier in the company of the Protestant surgeon Michel Héroard.[17] One evening, Catelan handed the Lutheran student:

> an old Latin Bible, in which there was no New Testament, from which I read to him, occasionally commenting on a few verses, especially when I read to him from the Prophet Baruch, how he wrote against images and idols, which pleased him greatly. Because, being a Marrano, he, like the Jews, did not think much of them, and although he could not speak openly about this, he often said "ergo nostri sacerdotes?" That is: then why do our priests allow them? Then I talked to him about how they were doing wrong, and how they were not tolerated in our religion, and cited many passages demonstrating that they are forbidden by God. This pleased Catelan very much, and he asked how it could be that I understood such things while still so young, and had come so far with my studies that he already considered me exceptionally learned.[18]

On Sunday 11 November 1554, less than a month after the Catelan's daughter Anna was born, their eldest daughter Isabelle married the converso son of a Béziers merchant in the large hall of Felix's lodging house. Here they hosted a banquet and dance for their mainly converso guests, and Felix was smitten by Jhane de Sos. This 'very friendly girl, who behaved in such a friendly way to me while dancing and conversing that I could easily have made a complete fool of myself over her',

---

[16] *Felix Platter Tagebuch*, 221 (14 August 1555, Montpellier).

[17] Father of Jean Héroard (1551–1628). *King James Bible*: 'Deuteronomy' 23, v.20: 'Unto a stranger thou mayest lend upon usury; but unto thy brother thou shalt not lend upon usury'. *Felix Platter Tagebuch*, 93, 135 (1541 Liestal; 15 October 1552, Geneva).

[18] *Felix Platter Tagebuch*, 156–7 (12 January 1553, Montpellier).

was to marry his professor, Antoine Saporta, in May 1555, a year after the death of Saporta's first wife.[19]

During the 1550s, the Catelans served a broadly Spanish cuisine modified according to the custom of the conversos, 'who do not eat any of the foods avoided by the Jews'.[20] Lent was strictly observed in their household and Felix Platter suffered considerably, as recorded for his first, 1553, Lenten fast under Catholic Montpellier's dietary regime. From Ash Wednesday, it was the custom to discard the earthenware pots in which meat had been cooked, and replace them with new ones for the fish, and the diet revolved around cabbage, onions, salad, sweet chestnuts and numerous varieties of fish.[21] There was no cheese or fruit, and lodgers were expected to abstain completely from meat or eggs. This capital offence was nevertheless transgressed by some German students, who taught Felix to fry eggs in butter melted in sheets of paper held over the open fire. Even outside the fasting period, the Catelans ate modestly, although good bread and watered red wine were always plentiful. They cooked in oil, used no butter, and Felix sometimes ordered pork when he joined fellow students for breakfast at the Three Kings Inn, 'because I ate none in the house of my master'.[22] Thomas Platter found Montpellier's Lenten fish diet and year-round lack of dairy foods even more challenging. During Lent 1596, while still lodging with Jacques Catelan, he 'took a liquid purgative, out of fear that I would become ill through the fish and foreign foods I had eaten on my travels. It worked seven times, and I felt really fit and well afterwards'. A few weeks later, on an excursion with Jacques Catelan, he and other German medical students 'almost drank themselves sick on creamy cows' milk, because it is not possible to obtain butter or good milk in Montpellier'.[23]

While Thomas Platter's comments on Montpellier's converso traditions cannot compare with Felix's informed insights, his journal offers the most detailed surviving record of Jewish life in early modern Avignon (Plate 3). With Carpentras, Cavaillon and L'Isle-sur-la-Sorgue, Avignon was one of four communities in the southern French district of Venaissin whose Jewish residents were under direct papal protection until the French Revolution. As such, rather than being expelled according to the prevailing French model, many of the region's Jews inhabited centrally located, highly taxed, largely self-contained ghettos, according to the

---

[19]   *Felix Platter Tagebuch*, 206, 219, 247 (11 November 1554, 17 May and 19 June 1555, Montpellier).

[20]   *Felix Platter Tagebuch*, 159 (15 February 1553, Montpellier).

[21]   Such Lenten foods provided the blueprint for Guarinonius's health-conscious dietary guidelines. He valued water above wine, bread over meat and for him 'among all foods, pickled cabbage is the theriac' (*Grewel*, 570; James Hart's discussion of German pickled cabbage ('sauerkraut') indirectly acknowledges Guarinonius (*Klinike*, 52). See also Mayr, 'Volksnahrung', 121; Battafarano, 'Zettelkraut statt Zitronen', 141–2).

[22]   *Felix Platter Tagebuch*, 158, 162 (February–April 1553, Montpellier).

[23]   *Thomas Platter d.J*, 145, 148 (21 March and 30 April 1596, Montpellier and Sellaneuve).

Italian system.[24] On 26 May 1598 Thomas Platter left Avignon for two small towns on the River Sorgue, Le Thor and neighbouring L'Isle-sur-la-Sorgue:

> because it [Le Thor] lies within papal territory, it is inhabited by many Jews, with the same customs and freedoms as those of Avignon. [...] The German for Lisle is island, because this town [L'Isle-sur-la-Sorgue] is surrounded like an island on all sides by the Sorgue. It is quite populous, and also inhabited by many Jews, who as far as I can tell are also permitted to buy landed property, apart from that they share the freedoms and restrictions of those of Avignon.[25]

The following day, Platter was in Pernes-les-Fontaines, a small town whose Jews, unlike those of nearby L'Isle-sur-la-Sorgue and Carpentras, had been officially expelled from their ghetto in 1569 (Diagram 1). Even so, he noted that: 'some Jews also live there, as in Avignon but not as many'.[26] A few days later, his host in Carpentras took him to the city's crowded Jewish ghetto, whose synagogue, founded in 1367, is the oldest now surviving in France: 'Dr [Guillaume] Albert also showed us around the Jewish street, in which a great many live. It is thought that more live there than in Avignon. In any case, they are treated in the same way as them'.[27]

Thomas Platter's many visits to Avignon include 10 weeks at the end of 1598, when he lodged in the Petit Paris Inn with Christoph and Wolf Dietrich Lasser von Lasseregg of Salzburg, aristocratic brothers he met in Lyon in 1595.[28] In Avignon, they taught him Spanish, and 'practiced many unusual skills' with him, 'on which they spared no expense'.[29] His longest description of the city's Jews dates to this period. Presented not as an account of normative Sephardic Judaism in general, but as a specific description of the Jews of Avignon's ghetto, it lightly modifies, in the light of his own eyewitness experiences during visits to their ghetto in February 1596 and late 1598, information Platter lifted from secondary sources.[30] Emphasizing his personal discussions with Avignon's Jews and his familiarity with the many unfamiliar customs he observed them practicing both within and outside their synagogue in its introduction, its concluding paragraph explicitly acknowledges his reliance on published sources. Twenty-three thematic sections[31] cover Jewish law, circumcision, the Mikvah or women's baths, religious education, rituals and prayer, the synagogue, Sabbath preparations, fasting and

---

[24]   Iancu, 'The Pope's Jews'; Calabi, 'Les quartiers juifs', 794.

[25]   *Thomas Platter d.J*, 240 (26 May 1598, L'Isle-sur-la-Sorgue).

[26]   *Thomas Platter d.J*, 245 (27 May 1598, Pernes).

[27]   *Thomas Platter d.J*, 251 (30 May 1598, Carpentras).

[28]   *Thomas Platter d.J*, 41 (2 October 1595, Lyon).

[29]   *Thomas Platter d.J*, 287 (27 October 1598, Avignon).

[30]   For the full account (compressed by Jennett into a few lines: *Journal of a younger brother*, 181), see *Thomas Platter d.J*, 289–305 (27 October – 24 December 1598, Avignon).

[31]   For English translations of 10 of these 23 sections, see Chapter 17, this volume.

food, weddings and divorce, illness, punishment, death and the Coming of the Messiah. Holy days discussed include the five major annual feasts and fasts of the Torah: Rosh Hashanah (Head of the Year), Yom Kippur (Day of Atonement), Sukkot (Feast of Tabernacles), Pesach (Passover) and Shavuot (Pentecost), as well as the monthly Rosh Chodesh, celebrating the new moon that ushers in each month of the lunar Jewish calendar.

Platter's sections closely follow the 37 chapters of *Synagoga Ivdaica*, first published in 1603.[32] The author of this substantial vernacular manual on Jewish rites was the successor to Sebastian Münster's chair of Hebrew Studies, the Christian Hebraist Johannes Buxtorf the Elder.[33] It was the definitive representative of an approach to Hebrew and Jewish culture that widened the mainstream academic perspective to include contemporary Jewish life and practices. By supplementing philological and theological techniques with ethnographical methods heavily influenced by new developments in travel writing, it facilitated 'a new era for the study of Judaism'.[34] Converted Jews made a significant, under-recognized contribution to the eventual standardization of the rich conglomerate of overlapping regional and social dialects representing medieval German. At a time when serious writers in the German-speaking regions routinely wrote in Latin or Hebrew, they represented a permeable boundary for increasingly intense transfers between Jewish and Christian culture, whose medium of choice was vernacular literature.[35] One German vernacular sub-genre unknown in pre-sixteenth-century Christian Hebraica and first pioneered by Jewish converts to Christianity, was systematic descriptions of Jewish ceremony and ritual. Its most notable early publication, and Buxtorf's main literary model, was *Der gantz Jüdisch glaub* (1530), a resolutely anti-Jewish ethnographical compendium of Jewish ceremonies and customs by Anthonius Margaritha, son and grandson of Rabbis Samuel and Jakob Margoles of Regensburg.[36] Buxtorf's *Synagoga Ivdaica*, the earliest example of this genre whose author was Christian from birth, was first published in 1603, two years before Thomas Platter finished writing up the fair copy of his journal.

While relying on Buxtorf's methodology and content, Platter significantly neutralized the Basle professor's anti-Jewish tone. Foregrounding a spirit of enquiry rather than sectarian recrimination, he in effect compresses much of the factual information in Buxtorf's lengthy treatise into a succinct 7,000 word

---

[32]   1564–1629. Buxtorf, *Synagoga Ivdaica* (anonymous English translation published in 1663 as *The Jewish Synagogue*); Burnett, *From Christian Hebraism to Jewish studies*, 85.

[33]   Buxtorf, *The Jewish Synagogue*, 13.

[34]   Stroumsa, *A new science*, 26, 41; see also Burnett, 'Distorted mirrors', 276; Hsia, 'Christian ethnographies of Jews', 44. My thanks to Asaph Ben-Tov for bringing this point, and much relevant secondary literature, to my attention.

[35]   Przybilski, *Kulturtransfer zwischen Juden und Christen*, 1–2, 103–4, 139.

[36]   Burnett, 'Distorted mirrors', 276; Walton, 'Anthonius Margaritha', 129; Diemling, 'Anthonius Margaritha', 303–4; Deutsch, 'Von der Iuden Ceremonien', 343–5.

account. Undeniably derivative, and more telling for what it discards from Buxtorf than for any factual additions, Thomas Platter's account of 1604–5 deserves recognition for its previously unnoted methodological innovation. More usefully viewed as an attempt to align himself with the forefront of the new trend in contemporary ethnographic approaches to Jewish studies, led by Buxtorf, than as a sterile exercise in derivative plagiarism, it precociously and systematically applies ethnographical approaches already informing accounts of peoples on the margins of and outside Europe, to travel writing recording Jewish life within mainstream Europe. Felix Platter did not formally record his scattered recollections of Jewish and converso life in the 1550s until shortly before his death in 1614. Montaigne set a distinguished, if brief and unpublished, precedent to the approach taken by Thomas Platter, which became commonplace in seventeenth-century European travel accounts, influencing writers such as the English travellers Fynes Moryson, Thomas Coryate, John Taylor, James Howell, John Evelyn and Francis Mortoft.

The extreme brevity with which Platter treats Jewish illnesses suggests that, at a time when many Christian church schools taught Hebrew as one of the three ancient languages,[37] Platter, unlike his father, had little or none: 'Like Christians, they too have all sorts of illnesses. They use many letters and cabalistic arts, also supernatural and magical arts against serious illnesses. All their books are filled with these matters.' However, his whole account is coloured by his keen professional interest in the daily customs, in this era of plagues and other highly contagious epidemics, of a separately housed group in uniquely high-density living quarters. Personal observation is apparent in his accounts of circumcision, morning prayers, the ritual baths, and a wedding he attended. Here, as the bridal couple drank the blessed wine:

> the mother of the bride, who was standing behind her, wiped her [daughter's] mouth with a handkerchief. And because she tried to wipe it too soon, the bride was rushed, and spilled wine onto herself. She was completely dressed in white satin and her mother chastized her severely in front of everyone. Even though it was really her own fault, no-one was allowed to blame her.[38]

Platter viewed the Avignon Mikvah, consisting of 'several tanks of water constructed under their synagogue', empty. His brief account of its use relies heavily on Buxtorf, as does his account of circumcision, observed from the dual perspective of solemn religious rite and significant medical operation, based on seeing 'two little boys being circumcised in their temple'.

As the world's oldest continuously observed religious ceremony, and the cornerstone of Judaism, the reaffirmation of God's covenant with Abraham through male circumcision attracted the increasing attention of non-Jews. Felix Platter, who customarily ate with the Catelan family while lodging with them

---

[37]   *Thomas Platter d.J*, 21 (September 1595, Lausanne).

[38]   *Thomas Platter d.J*, 303 (see also Chapter 17, this volume).

in Montpellier, records without further detail that Laurent II Catelan, to whom Eléonore Depuech gave birth on 22 April 1553 behind a curtain in the family's dining room, was secretly circumcised and named, 'according to their custom'.[39] According to Montaigne's eyewitness account of a Roman circumcision ceremony in 1580, having dressed the child's wound and been given a glass of wine, the ritual circumciser:

> takes a swallow of it, and then dipping his finger in it he three times takes a drop of it with his finger to the boy's mouth to be sucked; and afterward they send this glass, in the same state, to the mother and the women, who are in some other part of the house, to drink what wine is left.[40]

In a Prague circumcision witnessed by Fynes Moryson, the Rabbi, father and godfather drank from the chalice of wine in which the child's prepuce had been placed.[41] At the end of a Roman circumcision of 1645, John Evelyn watched the chalice of wine being shared between two of the women, the child's godfather, and the ritual circumciser himself.[42] The physician Thomas Platter was aware of the then widely attributed medical powers of human blood, routinely noted in medical treatises such as his brother's *Praxis medica*,[43] and his account of the 1598 Avignon circumcision ceremony carefully notes this aspect of the ceremony. However, the closeness with which his wording here follows Buxtorf considerably undermines his account's eyewitness reliability.

Less derivative is Thomas Platter's briefer record of February 1596, of daily life in Avignon's ghetto. At a time when the Jesuits too had been all but expelled from France, following Jean Châtel's attempted assassination of Henri IV,[44] one Avignon sight pointed out to Platter on leaving the Palais des Papes was:

> a church opposite the palace on the great, broad square, in which every Saturday a Jesuit preaches a penitential sermon to the Jews, which on pain of severe punishment, a third of the Jews, in rotation, are forced to attend. As I myself later observed; but one can't possibly imagine that this has been instrumental in converting a single Jew.[45]

---

[39]   *Felix Platter Tagebuch*, 163 (22 April 1553, Montpellier).

[40]   Montaigne, *Complete works*, 1154.

[41]   Moryson, *Shakespeare's Europe*, 495.

[42]   Evelyn, *The diary*, 142.

[43]   Plat[t]er, Cole and Culpeper, *A golden practice*, 23–4.

[44]   *Thomas Platter d.J*, 573, 580 (28 July, Paris). Platter thought the Jesuit College he visited at Agen in May 1599 was one of their last, then saw another in Saint Macaire a day later (431, 435: 1–2 May 1599, Agen and Saint Macaire).

[45]   *Thomas Platter d.J*, 118–119 (25 February 1596, Avignon).

Italian Jewish communities were widely subjected to compulsory sermons. Although the hostility with which John Evelyn dismissed a sermon of this type he attended on 7 January 1645 in Rome contrasts with Platter's measured tone, his conclusion is similar:

> A Sermon was preach'd to the Jewes at Ponte Sisto, who are constrain'd to sit, till the houre is don; but it is with so much malice in their countenances, spitting, humming, coughing & motion, that it is almost impossible they should heare a word, nor are there any converted except it be very rarely.[46]

Guarinonius too concludes an account of witnessing a court servant whipping an eight or 10-year-old Turkish girl almost daily for several weeks in summer 1598, by remarking: 'This is no way to make believers out of unbelievers. Such tyranny will rather convert some Christians to Turks'.[47]

The following day, Thomas Platter reports on a visit to Avignon's ghetto. Its Jews, barred from owning land, buying property, or training for medical or other professions, earned their living almost exclusively through trade and craft:

> After dinner we went to the street of the Jews, which can be locked at two points. They all live in the same district, there are always around 500 of them. They all trade in clothes, gems, cloth, armour, arms or linen and bedding. In short, everything that belongs on and in contact with the human body is to be found with all of them in great quantities, either for sale or for exchange, as preferred. And if they are lacking in anything, they arc in such credit with all the merchants that they immediately secretly obtain it from them. What they use, they pay for, the rest they return again, and they know the price. Apart from that, they are not permitted to purchase any other houses, gardens, fields or meadows, neither within nor outside the city, nor to follow any other trades than those noted and the exchange of money. They will pay a good price for old clothes, valuing them more highly than one would have thought of getting for them, but on the other hand, they also overprice their goods, considering that after taking into account what they pay, they still make a great profit just for mending and altering. Because almost all of them are skilled tailors as well as traders, they can sell them at the price of new ones. Their shops are on the ground floor of their houses. Because they have no daylight other than from small roof windows it is so dark that it isn't really possible to judge their wares properly, even if you carry them out to the streets. They are also dark, because the houses are high and built so close to each other, so that it is difficult to get away from them without being cheated. Of course it does happen from time to time that someone buys advantageously from them, because they deal in a lot of lost property and

---

[46]   Evelyn, *The diary*, 141.

[47]   Guarinonius, *Grewel*, 270; Breuer, 'Hippolytus Guarinonius als Erzähler', 1126–9 and 'Schöne des Leibs', 127–8.

pawned items that they get for a low price, and are able to sell on all the more cheaply. Nearly all the women are seamstresses, they sell and exchange linens, collars, caps, handkerchiefs, shirts, all beautifully quilted or embroidered. Every time, they try to sell their worst items first, overprice everything; you will get it if you offer half or less for it; only after you have bought the bad goods do they bring out such good ones that you can't resist not leaving them behind, so that some people immediately exchange yet again the ones they have just bought, but always at a loss. The Jews and their wives are always walking around the city, from one inn into another, showing the foreign travellers cloaks, clothes, linens, collars and suchlike. These they will sell or exchange, as you will, and they not only have to pay a large tax to the Pope, but also pay a certain amount of their takings to the innkeepers in whose houses or inns they sell or exchange anything. That is why you can always get a better price if you buy in the street of the Jews than in the inns. Except that it is so difficult, because they all but tear you apart when you enter their street. Everyone wants you to enter their house, and it is so dark.[48]

Thomas Platter clearly considered these trading strategies specific neither to Avignon's ghetto, nor to Jews. He recalled them in Paris: with respect to the enticing patter of the market wives on the Île de la Cité, in their booths lining the arcades of the great chamber of the Palais de Justice, and also the clothes traders of la Fripperie, near the Hôtel de Bourgogne in Les Halles, who:

> sold and exchanged them like the Jews of Avignon, there is such a screaming when someone enters their street that it is quite pitiful, everyone there wants to be the first. If someone enters their shop, they show them clothes and other goods and try to sell or exchange them, according to their preference. Because they know how to repair old clothes very skilfully, as if they were new. They also have dark houses and shops, in short their manner of trading is in every way like that of the Jews that I have described above.[49]

Felix Platter, who stayed in Avignon on his way back to Montpellier from Marseille with a group of German medical students in September 1555, confirms the longevity of its Jews' trading traditions:

> We had magnificent music in our guest-house, and the Jews came to us there, as is their custom, sold us all sorts of goods, whatever we wanted they brought, and they especially know how to repair linens and other clothes as if they were new, that's how they cheated people. In the afternoon we went around the town in order to see all the sights. [...] We went into the dark street of the Jews, where

---

48   *Thomas Platter d.J*, 127–8 (26 February 1596, Avignon).
49   *Thomas Platter d.J*, 562, 588 (28 July 1599, Paris).

you could not imagine anything that someone or other didn't have, and everyone
is at work, young and old.[50]

Since 1215, when the Fourth Lateran Council decreed that the clothing of Jews
and Christians had to be clearly distinguishable, Jews were increasingly required
to identify themselves within certain communities by wearing special signs.[51]
Thomas Platter's 1596 account next notes the Avignon Jews' mandatory costume
identifiers:

> Jewish men and boys all have to wear high yellow hats or yellow berets, while
> the women and girls have a special headgear with a high wooden ring over
> which the cloth is stretched, with a yellow silk ribbon or tape fixed or sewn to
> the top, so that they can be distinguished from the Christians.[52]

Here, his journal offers a little sketch of a Jewish woman in characteristic headgear.
Jewish dress fascinated early modern travellers. In 1641, John Evelyn describes
women in the Amsterdam synagogue as 'having their heads mabbl'd with linnen,
after a fantasticall & somewhat extraordinary fashion', almost certainly worn
voluntarily, as James Howell, writing in 1622, confirms that Amsterdam Jews wear
no compulsory 'outward Mark of Distinction'. In September 1644, Evelyn was in
Avignon 'in the Synagogue of the Jewes, who are in this town distinguish'd by their
red hats'.[53] However, Mortoft, agrees on colour with Platter, noting of his visit to
Avignon on 10 November 1658 that: 'there are abundance of Jewes inhabiting in
this Citty, and to distinguish them from other People they ware yellow hatts. They
are most of them very poore and much slighted by the Inhabitants. They have here
their Synagogue and observe the Ceremonyes of the old Testament.'[54] Evelyn and
Mortoft, neither of whom comments further on Avignon's Jews, also disagree on
the colour of Jew's hats in the Roman ghetto, Evelyn in 1645 describing them as

---

[50] *Felix Platter Tagebuch*, 229–30 (24 September 1555, Avignon).

[51] In declaring the dogma of transubstantiation, the Fourth Lateran Council also
confirmed the consecrated host as the body of Christ (Schöner, 'Visual representations of
Jews', 360, 376).

[52] *Thomas Platter d.J*, 128 (26 February 1596, Avignon). With reference to gold,
Guarinonius notes that 'no-one likes the colour yellow more than the avaricious' (*Grewel*,
182).

[53] Evelyn, *The diary*, 27, 88; Howell, *Familiar letters*, 86.

[54] Mortoft, *His book*, 29. According to the Londoner Francis Mortoft (b.1636), by
1658 there was 'not one Protestant being suffered to dwell in the Towne, or to remaine
there more then 8 dayes' (28). Grandson of the haberdasher Sir Hugh Hamersley (1565–
1636, Lord Mayor 1627–8), he had a particular eye for costume, completing his seven
year drapers' apprenticeship on 30 November 1659, before marrying Abigail Nettleship
in 1661 (http://histfam.familysearch.org/getperson.php?personID=141882&tree=London
[accessed 7 December 2011]).

yellow, Mortoft in 1659 as red.[55] Noting that most Italian Jews 'are tyed to weare a Redd or Yellowe Capp, or more commonly a litle bonett or hatt', Moryson marvels at the privileges of Mantuan Jews:

> keeping the cheefe shops in the very markett places, and hardly to be knowne from Christians, being only tyed to weare a litle snipp of yellowe lace vpon the left syde of theire Clokes, which some weare on the insyde of their Clockes, or so (they being foulded vnder the left arme), the marke cannot be discerned.[56]

Coryate reports of his 1594 visit to the Venetian ghetto that it housed up to 6,000 Jews, those of European descent in red hats, Levantine Jews in yellow turbans.[57]

In 1597, while staying at the Petit Paris in Avignon, Thomas Platter spent the day exchanging his coat with unspecified, probably Jewish, traders. He upgraded his clothes and cloak in Avignon again on 22 May 1598, in the ghetto,[58] as he had done in 1596:

> I also exchanged my clothes with them, which were not made to the style of those worn in this country. Gave them a little tip. Then they took me into their temple, which is in the basement, like a cellar. Daylight comes in only from an iron grill above. In this, a blind rabbi was preaching to the women in the Hebrew language, which is however said to be very corrupted, as they use their own dialect version, in which some Languedoc words are mixed in with the Hebrew.[59] In the upper hall, however, where the Prophets are read to the men in good Hebrew, it is light, and there is the place that is called holy. It is behind a locked grating, into which nobody apart from the Head Priest may go. Above it hangs an instrument containing 100 oil-filled glass lamps, all of which they light for their festivals. I also saw the upper stage, up to which the Holy is carried, which I afterwards, together with much else, observed taking place, and will describe at the appropriate place, when I saw it, because this time I did not stay long with them, because I had to get ready to leave.[60]

Thomas Platter recalls this characteristic synagogue architecture when describing the chapel at Woodstock Manor, where Queen Elizabeth I was imprisoned before her coronation, as 'constructed in a semi-circle in the Jewish manner. The women always stand on one side, there is a window into the men's chapel'.[61] Guarinonius compares the churches of Protestants who banish all lights, altars and pictures

---

[55]　Evelyn, *The diary*, 142; Mortoft, *His book*, 116.
[56]　Moryson, *Shakespeare's Europe*, 489.
[57]　Coryate, *Crudities*, 230–1.
[58]　*Thomas Platter d.J*, 207, 239 (26 February 1597 and 22 May 1598, Avignon).
[59]　The Shouadit dialect mixes Provençal and Hebrew (Iancu, 'The Pope's Jews').
[60]　*Thomas Platter d.J*, 128 (26 February 1596, Avignon).
[61]　*Thomas Platter d.J*, 860 (29 September 1599, Woodstock).

unfavourably to 'Jewish synagogues, which are far brighter and more laudable than these poor damnable churches, because at least the Jews have many lights in their altars and tabernacles, as I observed during my 11 years in Prague in all five Jewish synagogues there, and elsewhere'.[62]

Thomas Platter's account of late 1598 spells out why Avignon's Jews were tolerated in the papal city: 'they are staunchly protected by the authorities, who ensure that nobody does them any harm, because they have to pay a high tax to the Pope.'[63] Fynes Moryson makes a comparable point about the Prague ghetto before the Thirty Years War:

> Prague [...] hath a newe, and an olde Citty, besydes a thirde of the Jewes [...] At Prage vnder the Emperour of Germany they are allowed a little Citty to dwell in, with gates whereof they keepe the keyes, and walled rounde about for theire safety [...] free liberty of all Religions being permitted, I had oportunity (without Communicating with them so much as in the least outward reverence of standing bareheaded) not only to beholde the diuers Ceremonyes, of the Hussites, the Lutherans, the Papists, and the singular Jesuites, but also to haue free speech with the Jewes, and to enter their Synogogues at the tyme of diuine seruice. Some 500 Jewes dwelt in this litle Citty [...] they haue the priuilege of Cittizens, but they buye it and continue it with great payments of mony, as well imposed on them by the Pope, as by free guift of large sommes to the Emperour, and firnishing him with mony vpon all occasions.[64]

John Taylor, according to whom there were upwards of 50,000 Jews in Prague in September 1620, comments on their way of life ('they doe all liue by brocage and vsury'), and on the city's freedom of worship: 'I was there at foure seuerall sorts of diuine exercises; viz. at good sermons with the Protestants, at Masse with the Papists, at a Lutherans preaching, and at the Iewes Synagog.'[65] Religious freedom was rare and short-lived in early modern Europe. Despite the restrictions, oppressions and casual cruelties imposed on ghetto inmates by fellow citizens, papal Avignon offered Jews as stable and secure an environment as any available to them at the time.

Anti-Jewish repercussions of one of Guarinonius's hagiographic initiatives highlight the extreme vulnerability, in the absence of powerful protectors, of religious minority communities. Having being expelled from the central European Habsburg lands by Emperor Ferdinand I in 1543, Jews maintained a precarious presence in Innsbruck, where all Jews, local or visiting, were heavily taxed.[66] While Rudolf II was supporting Prague's Jewish presence, which represented a

---

[62]   Guarinonius, *Grewel*, 153.

[63]   *Thomas Platter d.J*, 305.

[64]   Oxford CCC, MS.CCC94, 664–6; Moryson, *Shakespeare's Europe*, 277, 487–90.

[65]   Taylor, *Trauels*, sig.C4^r.

[66]   Bücking, *Kultur und Gesellschaft in Tirol*, 51.

significant source of tax income, Ferdinand II, then still an archduke, enforced compulsory Catholicism in the Tirol, by closing down all Protestant schools and banishing Protestant preachers and teachers on 13 September 1598. In 1600 he had Lutheran books burned, and threatened with loss of property and life all Tiroleans who refused to observe Catholic Confession and Communion.[67] During this time, Guarinonius moved to Hall and entered Ferdinand II's service, and his energetic promotion to biographical hagiography of the alleged ritual murder victim Andreas Oxner of Rinn initiated continuing sectarian reverberations. Accusations of ritual murder ('blood libel') were a factor in the expulsion of Jews (only officially allowed back in 1656) from medieval England, as reflected in 'The Prioress's tale' of Geoffrey Chaucer's *Canterbury tales*. Presented as fiction and set in Arabia, its conclusion directly refers to the historically documented death of Hugh of Lincoln in 1255, then widely viewed as a victim of Jewish ritual murder. Jews were also routinely accused of attacks on the body of Christ, through the crime of host desecration, as in a fourteenth-century legend related by Thomas Platter. Three consecrated hosts he was shown in the Chapelle du Saint-Sacrement du Miracle of the church of Sainte-Gudule in Brussels were said to have been recovered from Jews who allegedly stole 16 such hosts and pierced them through with a knife in their synagogue on Good Friday 1370, until they flowed freely with blood.[68]

Two of Guarinonius's hagiographies, an unpublished prose account and a 73-verse poem published in 1642, founded the persistent folk 'legend' of a previously undocumented Tirolean saint, Andreas Oxner of Rinn.[69] They initiated dramatizations which continued to attract large Tirolean audiences well into the 1950s. Guests of honour at an early version, performed by the scholars of Hall's Jesuit College in 1621, were Emperor Ferdinand II's younger brother Archduke Leopold, and Prince Radziwill of Poland. In order to protect the community and its domestic livestock from 'veterinary diseases, contagious epidemics and extreme weather conditions', another version was performed at least eight times at Castle Ambras between 1648 and 1699.[70] Repeatedly republished and

---

[67]   Nagl and Zeidler, *Deutsch-Österreichische Literaturgeschichte*, I, 615–16. For the Habsburgs, see Diagram 2, this volume.

[68]   *Thomas Platter d.J*, 661 (20 August 1599, Brussels). Witches were said to murder infants and drink their blood (Bodin, *Demonomanie*, sig.198ᵛ; Bailey, 'From sorcery to witchcraft', 980).

[69]   The unpublished manuscript of Guarinonius's prose account (*Histori des Marter deß Haillig-Vnschuldigen Khindtß Andreae von Rinn*) is at Kloster Wilten (Stiftsarchiv, Lade 38, A/1–3); Guarinonius's poem is set to music (*Triumph Cron Marter Und Grabschrifft deß Heilig-Unschuldigen Kindts, Andreae Von Rinn*, Innsbruck 1642). Neuhauser, 'Die Überlieferung der Schriften', 198–9, 213; Frey, 'Hippolytus Guarinonius', 74.

[70]   Senn, *Aus dem Kulturleben*, 370, 394; Dörrer, 'Guarinoni als Volksschriftsteller', 143, 161–6; Hastaba, 'Vom Lied zum Spiel', 283; Tilg publishes a transcription of the 1621 perioch ('Ritualmordlegende', 633–40). The Tiroler Landesmuseum Ferdinandeum has the 1766 perioch (printed programme) of a version performed in Rinn itself and the

restaged, Guarinonius's hagiography led directly to the establishment of a local cult which gained official Vatican recognition for over two centuries from 1753. Miraculous healing powers were attributed to Andreas, the child at its centre.[71] Despite wide acceptance as a historical figure, his existence, his birth in 1459, let alone alleged ritual murder in 1462 at the hands of an unidentified group of Jewish merchants travelling through Rinn on their way to and from Bolzano's annual fair, are all unsupported by any known historically valid evidence. On the contrary. By Guarinonius's own frank admission, the 'historical' research methods underlying his account involved establishing 'facts' and dates through vague conjecture from unspecified sources, and through 'revelatory' dreams of whose accuracy and reliability he was assured by Fra Tommaso da Bergamo and Jesuit friends.[72] Scholars have long known that Guarinonius was significantly influenced by accounts of a child murder in his own birth city, that of Simon of Trent in 1475, on which he left a manuscript.[73] He retells the story of a mother in Günzburg who died of joy when her firstborn child was found alive and healthy with a group of local Jews to whom he had been sold by his father, and may have known of a case of the 1440s, in which a Christian woman and several Jewish men and women were publicly executed for allegedly murdering the three or four year old Ursula Pöck of Lienz. The oldest documentary evidence, a municipal protocol of 1475, found its way into the Hall imperial convent after his time, but he may have been aware of the 1619 restoration of a memorial to the girl.[74] Winfried Frey's scholarly investigations suggest that 'the Andreas-cult with all its elements – and that makes it a special case in the history of ritual murder accusations – is the invention of one single man, namely Hippolytus Guarinonius'.[75] His close study of Guarinonius's unpublished prose account identifies it as the source of later accounts, dismisses the damaged inscription Guarinonius allegedly copied off an undated marble tombstone in the graveyard at Rinn in March 1620 as an invention, and convincingly confirms that none of the known evidence concerning any such legend or cult in or around the village of Rinn near Innsbruck predates Guarinonius's own assertions.[76]

---

titlepage of Leopold Pirkl's 1835 playtext *Andrae von Rinn. Ein Trauerspiel in vier Ackten* (Hastaba, 'Theater in Tirol', 289, 327). Another Anderl-von-Rinn playtext is in Volders (Konventsarchiv der Serviten, J VI I–23).

[71]   Also referred to as Anderl or Anderle (little Andy).

[72]   Guarinonius, *Thomas von Bergamo*, 22–6; Marrone, 'Tommaso da Bergamo'.

[73]   Hastaba, 'Vom Lied zum Spiel', 278; Neuhauser, 'Die Überlieferung der Schriften', 187.

[74]   Guarinonius, *Grewel*, 241; Pizzinini, 'Ritualmordlegende aus Lienz', 219–20, 228.

[75]   Frey, 'Hippolytus Guarinonius', 62.

[76]   Frey, 'Hippolytus Guarinonius', 64–5. Although substantially supported by Guarinonius's own admissions (*Thomas von Bergamo*, 22–6), this reading of the evidence is not universally accepted (Kuefler, 'Anderl of Rinn', 13).

Historical uncertainties inhibited neither villagers nor pilgrims. Eagerly embracing this opportunity to enhance their community's religious and economic status, Rinn's Catholic inhabitants built an imposing seventeenth-century shrine to their Anderle, in the woodland district between Rinn and neighbouring Hall still known as Judenstein, site of the alleged martyrdom. Despite never achieving official beatification, locals called on Anderle's divine healing powers, revering him as 'their' saint. Having forbidden all such cults in the 1960s,[77] and this particular cult already in 1953,[78] the Vatican enforced its official suppression in 1994, in an iconoclastic episode mobilizing cultural, religious and political factions, and fundamentally dividing the congregation. Those who blockaded the church at Judenstein could not prevent Anderle's alleged bones, previously openly displayed in a reliquary on the main altar, from being bricked up within a church wall, or the supervised destruction of several historic works of art inside the church, graphically depicting controversial episodes from the legend. Numerous legend-related images survived these activities, but rather than deconsecrating the church and preserving it as a historical monument, it was renamed 'The Visitation of Mary', and its status as an official pilgrimage destination was revoked. It continues to serve its regular congregation, and provide a popular venue for weddings, christenings and year-round 'family pilgrimages' openly publicized by influential local community sectors.[79] Rinn's central village church remains dedicated to St Andrew. A stone memorial in its cemetery commemorates Anderl and provides cult-related information and images, as does a local farmhouse identified as 'Anderl's birthplace'. Guarinonius's writings are little known outside Austria, and his role in the Rinn cult is increasingly forgotten even within the Tirol. However, as author of the source material for this enduring Tirolean 'legend', variously depicted, staged and retold by internationally published writers such as Jakob Grimm and Karl Immermann, he initiated a cult that persists at many levels, providing a covert anti-Semitic rallying-point and troubling contributions to mainstream literature and culture.[80]

---

[77]   Second Vatican Council, 1962–5 (Wenzel, 'The representations of Jews', 412).

[78]   Kümper, 'Das Anderl von Rinn', 42.

[79]   'Veranstaltungs-Kalendar [...] Mai 2009 [...] 17. VB Imst: IV. Familienwallfahrt in der Kirche beim Anderl von Rinn/Judenstein, Beginn um 11.00 Uhr, umrahmt vom IPA-Chor mit Streichquartett, zelebriert vom Ehrenkurat Pater Clemens und organisiert von der LG Tirol mit der VB Ibk-Land' (quoted from: 'Termine.ipa.at: Veranstaltungs-Kalender', *International Police Association: I P A Panorama, Österreichische Sektion* 222, February 2009, 9 (www.ipa.at [accessed 28 September 2009]).

[80]   Grimm and Grimm, 'Der Judenstein' (*Deutsche Sagen*, I, 455–6, nr.352); Immermann, 'Das Anderl von Rinn – Tirolische Locallegende' (*Werke*, X, 255–6. This, the final episode of 'Blick ins Tirol', Immermann's travel journal of his 1833 tour of the Tirol, concludes by confirming the cult's association with medical miracles: 'The worship of this child is widespread. It stretches deep into the lower valley of the River Inn, and along this route manifests itself in numerous depictions of cases with which he helped'.)

Guarinonius's stance concerning Judaism and the Jews is extreme even by the standards of his era.[81] *Grewel*'s scathing attacks on non-Catholics, typically summarized as 'all heathens, Turks, heretics, Jews, devils and all sinful people', attracted heavy criticism from shocked contemporaries he dismissed as sycophants and dishonest Catholics.[82] Together with 'our hereditary arch-enemy the Turks', any Catholics who fall short of his standards, and above all every type of Protestant and 'godless', 'avaricious' Jews, feature prominently in these attacks, as when he notes of inorganic synthesized medicines of the type popular with Paracelsian quacks: 'they are not for humans, but for horses, heathens, Turks, Jews and the sworn enemies of Christianity', or denigrates non-Catholic fasting:

> despite ferociously punishing themselves with their uncouth fasting, Jews and Turks remain full of sins and lack of virtue. But being humble and obedient and going against their own interests is impossible for heathens, Jews or Turks, or for many immoderately excessive fasters, which is why such fasting is more of a sin than a virtue.[83]

Also in *Grewel*, Guarinonius compares the Jews' wait for the Messiah to the alchemists' futile search for a chemical means of manufacturing gold; their music to 'cats on the rooftops at night, or dogs howling at each other'; labels their synagogues 'wail and shout houses'; criticizes their banks for charging too much interest; uses 'Jewish' and 'devilish' interchangeably; relates in repugnant detail the barbaric punishment of a Jewish rapist in Prague in 1603;[84] and heightens the repellence of a schoolboy memory by publishing it as an educated adult in a medical treatise elsewhere specifically warning of the hygiene risks of precisely the actions it records:

> Dice are a Jewish game, [...] which is why, during my boyhood in Prague, whenever I encountered Jews on the [Charles] Bridge or elsewhere, I never let them alone until they had given me a pair of dice or they chased me, or I them. But mostly they me, in front of my tutor, who afforded me a good shield against the Jews. But he couldn't always protect me because though he walked behind me when taking me across the long bridge to school every day and diligently watched me, especially whenever he saw a Jew coming towards me, he was unable to guard against my inner love of dice and the Jewish nation. From the front, I would attack them nice and quietly, in the manner of naughty boys, by collecting a massive gob on the tip of my tongue as best I could and [...] spitting

---

[81] *Pace* Bücking, for whom 'the attitude of Guarinonius to the Jews is obviously that of most of his contemporaries' (*Kultur und Gesellschaft in Tirol*, 50).

[82] Guarinonius, *Grewel*, 1325 and *Pestilentz Guardien*, 189–90.

[83] Guarinonius, *Grewel*, 6, 112, 328, 706, 912, 975.

[84] Guarinonius, *Grewel*, 43, 189, 190, 262, 833, 1130 (here, 1630 is evidently an *erratum* for 1603).

it at them. When the Jews complained about this to my tutor he would rebuke them, because he had seen me walking politely in front of him and not noticed anything unacceptable, because my face, eyes and hands were at the front, not at the back.[85]

The nineteenth chapter of *Grewel*'s unpublished sequel presents a sustained, scathing attack on Jewish medical practitioners, betraying considerable resentment at their popularity with Christian patients, who are warned off with tales of alleged professional negligences and ritual murders. Guarinonius urges municipal authorities to rethink the traditional 'abuse' of tolerating Jewish communities within their jurisdictions, and accuses Christians willing to trust Jewish physicians of Moslem tendencies.[86]

Unlike Guarinonius, the Platter brothers reflect an enquiring, open attitude to Jewish ceremony, culture and traditions. Where their tone is less than respectful, as for example in their accounts of ghetto traders, it does not differ materially from that of their accounts of comparable non-Jews, such as the traders of Paris. Their journals testify to longstanding mutual support between the Platter brothers and successive generations of their converso apothecary hosts in Montpellier, the Catelans. They offer exceptional insights into Jewish and Jewish-influenced traditions practiced by normative Jews and Christian conversos in early modern Mediterranean France, and the routine daily challenges of those within, or on the cultural boundaries of, minority communities whose beliefs for many generations inhibited them from full participation in mainstream educational, social and professional networking systems profoundly supported by the Christian festive year.

---

[85]   Guarinonius, *Grewel*, 1260. See also 511 and 884–6 (Book 5, Chapter 8: 'On elimination through spitting, sneezing, coughing, throat-clearing and nose-blowing').

[86]   Innsbruck UL, Cod.110, IV, ff.522^r–5^r. His word is 'Mämäluck'.

Chapter 6
Physicians at Court Festivals

Early modern court festivals certified and celebrated the recognized high points of rulers' dynastic and territorial achievements, such as birth, coming of age, marriage, diplomatic or military acquisition, death and succession. Their characteristic union of religious ceremony, cultural performance and martial arts put court physicians right at their centre. Helen Watanabe-O'Kelly distinguishes between two types of court festival: ceremony and spectacle.[1] Ceremonies – such as baptisms, coronations, formal entries, progresses and weddings, or the Royal Touch – are actual enactments by unique protagonists, of legally binding building blocks in the creation of political power structures, formally witnessed by their spectators. Spectacles stage repeatable plays, operas, firework displays, dances or other theatrical events, acted by interchangeable performers. They can manipulate but not create power structures, and their audience has no legal witnessing role. Whether staging spectacle with or without ceremony, court festivals are typically an expression of political power and a celebration of sovereignty, often enhanced by showcasing their ruler's quasi-ceremonial victory over supernatural forces of demonic enchantment, in plots of the type that received their highest literary expression in the works of Ludovico Ariosto, Torquato Tasso and Edmund Spenser.[2] Their scope for uniting cultural and martial arts, in displays based on the values, skills and literature of classical imperialism and medieval chivalry, made tournaments the early modern court festival spectacle of first choice. Ever more elaborate and showy tournament variations took advantage of sophisticated advances in theatrical technology, but could not eliminate the inherent physical danger of their defining feature, the deployment of the weapons and skills of warfare.

The scope of court festivals ranged from modest one-day events to ceremonies celebrated with a series of spectacles, sometimes at more than one location, spread over several days or even weeks, of the type of the influential Munich wedding of 1568. The publication of the first comprehensive bibliography of printed festival books and other surviving sources for early modern European festival, in 2000, reinvigorated festival study.[3] Researchers are now casting their net over a wider geographic area. Unpicking of the often complex and conflicting aims and funding streams underpinning elaborate and expensive festivals and their printed records is being progressed. Each ruler and civic authority had their own personal agenda

---

[1] Watanabe-O'Kelly, 'Early modern European festivals', 15–16.

[2] Clark, *Thinking with demons*, 646–9. See also Chapter 10, this volume.

[3] Watanabe-O'Kelly and Simon, *Festivals and ceremonies*.

for using the festivals themselves, the publicity and propaganda they generated, and the festival books published to commemorate them, as vehicles for boosting their own self-esteem, their local and international standing, and their family and political alliances; for attracting economically and politically significant visitors, and for influencing local courtiers and citizens. Some of these shifting, conflicting agendas were ostentatiously showcased, others were deliberately hidden. As these factors become better understood, informal festival descriptions, such as those in the Platter journals, are achieving increasing recognition not just as information sources for otherwise undocumented festivals, but for their provision of alternative perspectives to polemically biased official festival records.

Early modern court festivals were unique, ephemeral events, necessarily experienced differently by every participant. They are no more reliably documented by informal descriptions than by official festival books, and the accounts of Felix Platter, Thomas Platter and Hippolytus Guarinonius all have their own agenda-driven biases. Some of the festivals they describe or refer to are also known from printed accounts (Diagram 5). Several are otherwise unknown, excluded from official permanence through the expense of specially commissioned festival books or because they were abandoned or relocated; or in the light of immediately following developments such as the infant death of a christened child, or a re-alignment of relevant political or religious concerns. This chapter considers the varying perspectives on court festival available to the three physicians. Then some ways in which their accounts augment those of officially sanctioned festival chroniclers are highlighted, taking the reporting of journeys to festivals and festival weather conditions as case studies. The focus then turns to each of the three physicians' festival descriptions in turn: firstly those of Thomas Platter as medically-qualified Grand Tourist, secondly Felix Platter's as court physician, and thirdly Hippolytus Guarinonius's, as a physician whose medical writings first and foremost served his spiritual agenda.

Felix Platter, and to a lesser extent his brother Thomas, wrote for private enjoyment rather than official publication. Their accounts acknowledge the exceptional status of court life in ways that those of some courtiers do not. In the penultimate paragraph of his account of the 1598 Hohenzollern wedding, Felix Platter quotes the farewell verse he inscribed on the wall at Hochburg Castle on 18 October, on taking his leave of Georg Friedrich, Margrave of Baden: 'Eventually, you can have enough of court life, even though it's a good life for those who enjoy it.'[4] Having served continuously as court physician for the duration of a three-week festival, he was evidently more than ready to leave the court for the city. Not tied to reflecting what the host court had planned or wanted readers to think had happened, or to disseminating or supporting court-related propaganda, the Platter journals reflect different biases and perspectives than those of official chroniclers. They are not constrained to include lengthy genealogical digressions

---

[4]   See p.301, this volume. Guarinonius is even blunter, warning his patients 'if you wish to live a pious life, stay away from courts' (Innsbruck UL, Cod.110, IV, f.436ʳ).

or sycophantic eulogies, or to assume knowledge of specialized conventions taken for granted in accounts written primarily for courtiers. Their private accounts offer fresh insights into areas of festival procedure whose official description, if included at all, is often influenced by political and polemical agendas. Sometimes, as with Felix's account of commedia dell'arte costumes at the 1598 Hohenzollern wedding tournament,[5] the Platter brothers offer new insights into significant aspects of well-documented festivals. They are at liberty to reveal information suppressed or ignored by official chroniclers: background anecdotes and rumour; deviations from the scripted 'performance' of court festivals such as disruptive weather conditions, mishaps and accidents; and details of journeys to and from festivals. And whether in the capacity of established court physician, like Felix Platter, or newly qualified, independently financed traveller, like Thomas Platter, they offer professionally informed insights into an aspect of court festival routine greatly played down by most official accounts: their health risks, notably the high rate of personal injury sustained in tournaments and other spectacular martial exercises.

Despite their similar background and training, Felix and Thomas Platter's perspectives on court festival contrast with each other as well as with those of official festival books. Felix Platter's life writings reflect participation in festivals in many different capacities during his long life, as a guest, physician and performer. An unhappy early experience as a guest at a private masked carnival ball in Montpellier in January 1557, when a deceitful noblewoman falsely accused him of stealing a valuable rosary, only temporarily put him off participating in grand festivals.[6] Long before officiating at festivals in a professional capacity through long-term engagements as a court physician, Felix Platter's exceptional ability as a musician and dancer put him in great demand as a performer at festivities. In April 1554, Simon de Sandre, a neighbour and future First Consul of Montpellier, invited the 17-year-old student, then known as 'l'Alemandt du lut', to join a group serenading a young woman he was courting:

> We arrived at midnight, and first beat the drums to wake up the neighbours in the street. That was followed by trumpets, then hautboys, then flutes, after them violas, and finally three lutes. Altogether it lasted a good one and a half hours. Afterwards we were led to the bakery, where we were treated to delicious food and drank Muscat and sweet "Hippocras" wine, and thus spent the rest of the night.[7]

---

[5]   On Platter's account of this wedding, see Chapters 7 and 16 (translation), this volume.

[6]   *Felix Platter Tagebuch*, 261 (12 January 1557, Montpellier).

[7]   *Felix Platter Tagebuch*, 72, 195–6 (1544, Basle and 16 April 1554, Montpellier).

In June 1555, Felix was one of three serenading lutenists.[8] Ten days later, he played his lute hidden with the musicians 'behind the tapestry' at a grand banquet hosted by Honoré Castellan, the professor who had matriculated him into Montpellier's medical school.[9] Castellan, who had himself only matriculated in 1544, was establishing an outstanding career as an academic, court and military physician. Felix often accepted invitations to accompany him on visits to the sick, write his prescriptions, or dine at his house, next door to the wealthy, elderly Dr Antoine Griffi.[10] When Castellan asked Felix to accompany him next door to serenade, on his lute, Griffi's beautiful young wife in her husband's absence, while he felt the temporarily bedridden woman's pulse, Platter: 'noticed quite clearly that, exactly as gossip would have it, Honoré was preferred by the woman to her husband'.[11] Castellan left Montpellier to become personal physician to Catherina de' Medici. In naming him as one of two physicians who enjoyed such success with the Valois court women that 'the noblest courtiers would have sold their souls to the Devil to keep up with them', Brantôme confirms both Castellan's reputation as a womanizer, and Felix Platter's reliability as an eyewitness.[12]

Felix Platter's multiple viewpoints were largely inaccessible to Thomas. Neither musically gifted nor a court physician, during the late 1590s, the period recorded in his journal, he completed his medical studies and started practicing. Fascinated by the routines and displays of court life, he visited academies that trained young French noblemen in courtly skills in Paris, Orléans and the now depopulated fortified port of Brouage,[13] and habitually modified his itinerary to experience court festivals. Occasionally, he gained privileged access. In England, in 1599, it was via his medical skills and family connections. More often, he befriended guards, as in 1596, when Caspar, one of 12 Swiss guards, gave Platter an extended unauthorized guided tour of all the rooms of Avignon's Papal Palace, informing him that the Pope's Italian representative, who spent most of his time playing dice, had turned one of its halls into a casino (Plate 3).[14] During the following carnival, the Swiss guard at the Palace of Marseille permitted his fellow countryman Thomas Platter to gatecrash a private carnival dance hosted by

---

8   *Felix Platter Tagebuch*, 219 (14 June 1555, Montpellier).

9   *Felix Platter Tagebuch*, 220 (24 June 1555, Montpellier).

10   Another of Felix Platter's professors, whose daughter Platter had accidentally splashed all over with mud while escorting her to a dance (*Felix Platter Tagebuch*, 154). Lötscher's single seamless narrative interpolates this undated extract from the 'Biographica' (f.14) into f.36ʳ of the 'Lebensbeschreibung', or main chronological account. On Griffi and Castellan, also known as Du Chastel or Duchateau, see also Dulieu (*La médecine a Montpellier: La Renaissance*, 329–30, 386).

11   *Felix Platter Tagebuch*, 220 (Lötscher interpolates this undated extract from the 'Biographica' (f.14) into f.71ʳ of the 'Lebensbeschreibung').

12   Brantôme, *Recueil des Dames*, 480.

13   *Thomas Platter d.J*, 452–3 (5 May 1599, Brouage), 581 (July 1599, Paris).

14   *Thomas Platter d.J*, 117, 126 (25–27 February 1596, Avignon).

Charles de Lorraine, fourth duc de Guise. He appreciated the delicious malmsey wine and silver-gilt dishes of confectionery, sugared almonds, hazelnuts and cinnamon served at the end of the dance, and the Duke's costly garments, but was repulsed by his snub-nosed host's ugliness.[15] These are exceptions, and Thomas Platter's eyewitness court festival accounts are predominantly of public formal entries. Despite more limited access to festivals, his descriptions of them, like those of Felix, are informed by the personal viewpoint of a sharply observant, highly educated, eyewitness participant with an excellent memory for events, albeit without his older brother's empathy or exceptional memory for names.

Although he claims to have attended hundreds of weddings and festivals in the decade after qualifying as a physician, Guarinonius rarely goes beyond reporting on isolated verbal exchanges of his own, such as altercations with alchemists or quacks at banquets.[16] A lengthy poem, in a chapter on festivals in *Grewel*'s second volume, criticizes an unidentified, undated formal entry for providing a convenient path to hell, and court festivals, banquets and carnival festivities reap further stern criticism in the following folios.[17] His few published references to court festivals are mostly brief autobiographical passages or second-hand reports in *Grewel*'s first volume. No less didactically motivated than any of his theatrical references, they are selected and presented to support specific health-related points in his treatise. Less comprehensive and more public than the festival commentaries of the Platter brothers, they reflect his standing as a respected public health officer, court physician, and devout Catholic.

The Platter brothers' status at court festivals informed every aspect of their accounts of them, including their reporting of journeys to festivals, and of weather conditions. Journeys, although rarely described in official accounts, were integral to the festival experience. They were often as strictly formalized, and governed by hierarchy and conventions, as any festival element at the host court itself, providing potent propaganda opportunities for travelling guests. Both Platters considered them eminently noteworthy. Thomas Platter describes watching the 100-horse retinue of the Connétable of Tournon, Henri, duc de Montmorency and his wife Louise de Budos wending its way towards Tournon for his formal entry into the city in October 1595:

> At Fontagier we saw around 100 horses, they were those of the Connétable, riding to Tournon. [...] Then we saw the Connétable of Tournon make his entry into the town on horseback, and enter the castle. After we had eaten supper in

---

[15]   *Thomas Platter d.J*, 194–5 (16 February 1597, Marseille). As the second husband of Henriette-Catherine de Joyeuse, he added to his own lands those of her father, Henri, duc de Joyeuse, who in March 1599, as Père Ange, entered the Capuchin monastery of the rue Saint-Honoré in Paris, where he was seen begging and preaching by Thomas Platter (580: 28 July 1599, Paris).

[16]   Guarinonius, *Grewel*, 200, 204.

[17]   Innsbruck UL, Cod.110, IV, ff.421–2, 428–9, 515.

the town, a citizen of Tournon, M. Sarrazin, and I climbed up to the castle, where they had also already eaten supper. The Connétable and his wife were there, with the Colonel or Marshal Alphonse [d'Ornano], M. [Pomponne] de Bellièvre, chancellor of the Royal House of France, the king's secretary M. [Pierre Forget, Seigneur] de Fresnes and his wife, M. de Saint-Geniès, who was dancing with the Comte de Tournon's little daughter, the Comte de Tonnerre, who danced voltes, courantes, gaillardes, and other foreign dances, [Claude de Guise] Prince de Joinville, and many other noble lords and ladies. [...] The chamber in which the feasting and dancing took place was beautifully furnished with tapestries embroidered in gold and silver and lit with 40 lamps and torches. [...] And I was all the more impressed by all this because it was the first French court that I ever saw.[18]

He was surprised that only three musicians accompanied the dancers, on a soprano, tenor and bass violin, although he found them very good, and enjoyed watching the Connétable's four- or five-year-old son, wearing a showy plume of feathers, skilfully dance voltes and galliards with his six-year-old sister, while many of the adult nobility threw dice for high gold stakes. In March 1596, he viewed the formal mounted entry into Montpellier of the Connétable's son-in-law and daughter, Anne de Lévis, duc de Ventadour and Marguerite de Montmorency, accompanied by numerous high aristocrats. That evening, he also watched the games of chance and dancing at the reception held for them.[19] In August 1599, he witnessed Charles-Philippe de Croy, Marquis d'Havré, riding out of Edingen with numerous horses and coaches, for the entry into Brussels, a day later, of a notable visitor, the imperial cousin, Cardinal Archduke Andreas of Habsburg, 'with two troops of his soldiers, all well and impressively armed' (Diagram 2). That December, he saw Charles-Emmanuel, duc de Savoie, entering Paris 'with around 200 horses, and his people were all costumed and presented in the most impressive manner. They went to huge expense with clothes and presents, which pleased the French greatly, but they had no wish to reciprocate, instead only making fun of the Savoyans for this'.[20]

Felix Platter's accounts of journeys to festivals with his patron Georg Friedrich, Margrave of Baden reveal – more forcefully than any printed festival book – how tightly expectations governed court festival participants, not just within the host court, but from the moment they set foot outside their own territory. The margrave took 218 courtiers and over 200 horses to the 1598 Hohenzollern wedding. Eight pack wagons, 50 horses and 25 servants were sent on a day ahead of the main procession, whose hierarchical formation included a two-horse sedan for the

---

[18]   *Thomas Platter d.J*, 48, 52–4 (3 October 1595, Tournon). Claude de Guise (1578–1657) was the younger brother of Charles de Lorraine, fourth duc de Guise (1571–1640).

[19]   *Thomas Platter d.J*, 145 (15 March 1596, Montpellier).

[20]   *Thomas Platter d.J*, 655–6, 659 (20–21 August 1599, Edingen and Brussels), 897–8 (20 December 1599, Paris).

margravine.[21] The entourage for the margrave's six-day journey to the March 1596 Stuttgart court christening of Prince August of Württemberg was differently arranged but equally regimented. One hundred and fifty horses and 170 courtiers were led by a strict formation of around 50 noblemen, riding three to a row, preceded by a single mounted drummer, and followed by a row of three drummers. Directly behind rode the margrave, flanked by two footmen and followed by the margravine's steward on horseback, leading the coach of the margravine and her stewardess and noblewomen, driven by two coachmen and a footman. A further formation of some 60 courtiers, also riding in rows of three, separated this coach from that of the margrave, carrying Felix Platter and five senior courtiers and again driven by two coachmen and a footman. Following up the rear were the six-horse coach of the servants and the four-horse coach of the court musicians, four pack wagons flanked by footmen carrying the margravial silver and luggage, and two spare horses.[22] They were escorted from their last stopping place, Leonberg Castle, on the morning of 6 March 1596, and met shortly before they reached Stuttgart by a party of 150 horses led by the 14-year-old heir of their host, Friedrich, Duke of Württemberg. This was Prince Johann Friedrich, whose then three-year-old sister Barbara later married Friedrich of Baden, the son of Platter's court patron (Diagram 2).

Like many aspects of festivals, journeys were heavily dependent on weather conditions. The combined one kilometre long entry party continued in persistent rain to the Stuttgart court, where it was greeted with a mighty fanfare of military drums and pipes by 30 halberdiers, costumed in red damask trimmed with yellow silk and velvet caps with white feathers. By the time they finally reached their rooms, all the guests were soaking wet. The following morning, Sunday 7 March 1596, Prince August was carried to the court chapel on the arm of his oldest sister, on a cushion supported by two noblemen, for the christening service. Music was provided by 30 singers, cornet and trumpet players, and the organ. Then, they were escorted to the banquet by military drummers and 12 trumpeters, all with their instruments decorated with yellow damask banners sporting Duke Friedrich's arms. The banquet was served on some 120 tables in four separate rooms, strictly organized according to rank, to the music-making of singers, spinet players and harpists. The dances which followed, until late into the night, were accompanied by trumpets and shawms. To protect the gorgeous dresses of the noblewomen from the mud after the heavy downpours, the path to the chapel had to be specially covered with planks.[23]

Felix Platter reports that the running at the ring of 5 October at the 1598 Hohenzollern wedding was postponed for a day by rain.[24] Jakob Frischlin, the

---

[21] English translation: Chapter 16, this volume.

[22] *Felix Platter Tagebuch*, 467–9 (28 February 1596, Hochburg).

[23] *Felix Platter Tagebuch*, 470–2 (5–7 March 1596).

[24] English translation: Chapter 16, this volume. Unlike his brother Thomas, and Jakob Frischlin, Platter here dates according to the Swiss custom, then 10 days behind Swabia.

festival's official chronicler, notes that the tournament ground remained empty on Wednesday because it was such an overcast and rainy day, but unlike Felix does not reveal that yet more rain meant postponing Friday's hunt to Saturday 7 October.[25] Staged in Count Eitel Friedrich IV's enclosed wildlife park, supporting rabbits, foxes, oxen and 900 red deer, Felix describes an arrangement familiar from court hunts painted in the 1540s by the Lucas Cranach workshop,[26] in which gamekeepers and hunting dogs drive game into a bottleneck area of the park formed by several long shallow lakes. Here, strictly segregated in their own shelter, the noblewomen watched the noblemen slaughter the game, in a chivalric ritual whose gender-specific performativity is completely missed by Guarinonius's comment on a similar hunt, that 'the presence of women is as inappropriate here as in battle'.[27] Then Platter accompanied the Margrave of Baden back to his Hochburg court, arriving on 12 October completely soaked by the continuing heavy rain. Here, five further days of festivities included the usual banqueting, dancing and music-making and other courtly diversions of the type depicted in Plate 22, as well as tennis playing, a wild boar hunt, and a tournament whose waterlogged state seriously heightened its already hazardous health risks.

Official festival chronicles habitually make light of unfavourable weather. As revealed by Thomas Platter in unsparing detail, Boch's Latin festival book downplays its effect on the procession of guilds at the entry into Brussels of Archduke Albrecht of Habsburg and his wife Isabella:[28]

> As [the third] guild entered the square, such a bitter wind and rain whipped up that the Archduke and his consort, who were then by the great church of St Ergoul (Goedelen), had to dismount and take shelter in the dry refuge offered by the church. They waited there for at least a couple of hours until the rain had eased off. The companies on foot and on horseback divided themselves around, some took refuge in the King's court, others in the church, others here and there where they could, under roofs and in courtyards. So the entry was completely disrupted by the weather, and the pealing of the great bells was also interrupted until the rain eased off. When the rain stopped, the great bells began pealing again, and I returned again to my place on the square. [...] and this entry carried on into darkest night [...] After the evening meal we left our inn to return to the city [...] After midnight I returned to my lodgings.[29]

---

[25]   Frischlin, *Hohenzollerische Hochzeyt*, 215.

[26]   For example, *Hunting party in honour of Charles V at Torgau Castle* (variants: Madrid, Vienna, Stockholm, Copenhagen).

[27]   *Grewel*, 1220. Lötscher similarly comments on how nauseating it was that the spectators of such butchery included women (*Felix Platter Tagebuch*, 504n90).

[28]   Bochius, *Historica narratio*, 110–70. The couple became the rulers of the Spanish Netherlands through Isabella's dowry from her father, Philip II of Spain.

[29]   *Thomas Platter d.J*, 705–6, 709–10 (5 September 1599, Brussels).

Thomas Platter arrived in Brussels by canal boat on 30 August 1599 to see this entry, one of the most magnificent of an astounding number of court and civic festivals he was able to pack into the concluding Grand Tour of his half decade away from Basle. Often challenged by last-minute changes in timing or location, Platter had to rearrange his plans to accommodate the entry's postponement to 5 September 1599, by moving forward his visit to Louvain in order to allow time to return to Brussels after seeing the royal couple in nearby Hal.[30] Returning on 4 September to find Brussels full to bursting point with visitors, his group 'had to lodge with the innkeeper of a beer tavern, the Blue Ship, because we were unable to find reasonably priced accommodation in any other inn'.[31]

In late January 1599, Platter and a travel companion, Sebastian Schobinger of St Gallen, had joined numerous visitors attracted to Barcelona by news of the forthcoming double wedding of Isabella to Archduke Albrecht, and her half-brother King Philip III of Spain to his mother's (and Albrecht's) cousin, Margareta of Habsburg, with their associated royal entries and other public festivities (see Diagrams 2 and 5). He recorded with interest the citizens of Barcelona's preparations for the royal entry, noting that: 'In honour of the King, numerous very high wooden towers were constructed at great expense throughout the town, on which all manner of triumphs were to have been made, as we saw in the Fishmarket, not far from the warehouse.'[32] Official festival accounts rarely hint that festival architecture was anything other than ephemeral, specially designed and constructed for each occasion. Maybe, despite the event's relocation, the efforts of the Barcelona city fathers could be recycled, for later that year Thomas tells us that at the Palais des Seigneurs, in Antwerp in August 1599, he saw:

> next to St Michael's, also several arches and large constructed animals, which had been used for the entries of great noblemen into Antwerp. And it was explained to us there that these and many more would be put up for the entry of Archduke Albrecht, which people were preparing to get ready for because he was awaited shortly. As we then saw a large wooden (theatrum) spirally constructed construction already erected on the Meerbruck, on which many people could sit, and several skilful, diverting things were to be performed during the Archduke's entry. [...] In the city hall is an extremely large, gigantic and fearsome statue of an elephant.[33]

Possibly, this is the striking over-lifesize elephant statue depicted in Boch's account of the couple's 1599 Antwerp entry, of which Platter saw evidence on his return from London: 'we also saw several tall (theatra) stages and gateways, that

---

[30]   *Thomas Platter d.J*, 690, 703 (1 and 3 September 1599, Brussels and Hal).

[31]   *Thomas Platter d.J*, 704 (4 September 1599, Brussels).

[32]   *Thomas Platter d.J*, 343 (28 January 1599, Barcelona).

[33]   *Thomas Platter d.J*, 675–6 (24 August 1599, Antwerp).

had been put up for the enjoyment of Archduke Albrecht and his wife during their entry into Antwerp, which took place shortly before our arrival'.[34]

Thomas Platter also provides details on the entry tradition and its importance in Catalonia.[35] The protests raised by Philip's misgivings reveal both how anxious Barcelona's authorities were to host this prestigious event, and the degree of seriousness invested in the exact protocol of the performance of legally binding ceremonies:

> But when the King learned that they were not planning any modifications for his entry from their traditional way of receiving a Duke of Catalonia, he decided to welcome his bride in Valencia, where he is King, which is indeed what happened. But on several occasions we saw numerous of the queen's coaches, servants and coach horses arrive in Barcelona, and unload, all sent there in order to await the queen. But when the people of Barcelona realized that the King did not want to receive his queen there, they are said to have sent him news that they were willing to pay for everything, and to present him with 200,000 crowns on top of this, if he wished to receive his queen in their city. Their only stipulation was that he should make his entry into their city only after the wedding, and that he would have to knock three times on the city gates, before they could be unlocked and he could be presented with the keys. I was told this by a local resident, who saw for himself how stubbornly they clung to their traditional rights.[36]

Thomas Platter's account of Isabella's September 1599 entry into Brussels illuminates possible expectations of her brother King Philip III in Barcelona: 'At this gate, on the city boundary, the key to the city gates were presented to Archduke Albrecht in an elaborate ceremony, through which he was appointed absolute ruler over the city and its inhabitants.'[37] Boch's account of Isabella and Albrecht's Antwerp entry illustrates such a legally-binding key-presenting ceremony, staged on a specially erected ceremonial structure outside the city gate, raised to maximize spectator visibility.[38]

Thomas Platter notes Don Giovanni de'Medici's entry into the port of Barcelona, with a gift for Philip III from the ruling Duke of Florence, his half-brother Ferdinando de'Medici, in a galleon from Tuscany accompanied by 12 ceremonial trumpeters.[39] He was received with banquets and festivities by Barcelona's civic authorities, but when they demanded an excise tax, he sailed off to another port.

---

[34]   Bochius, *Historica narratio*, 272; *Thomas Platter d.J*, 874 (2–5 November 1599, Antwerp).

[35]   *Thomas Platter d.J*, 385–6 (24 February 1599, Barcelona).

[36]   *Thomas Platter d.J*, 343 (28 January 1599, Barcelona).

[37]   *Thomas Platter d.J*, 713 (6–7 September 1599, Brussels).

[38]   Bochius, *Historica narratio*, 171–316 (illustrated with 28 etchings).

[39]   Commoners too required them. A Savoyan trumpeter was engaged by the small party with whom Thomas Platter shared a boat up the Rhône, to deliver the formal

Unwilling to take part in a ceremony whose details he perceived as undermining his authority, Philip III too cut short his negotiations with the intransigent Barcelona authorities, who evidently rated the expression of political power more highly than broader economic factors, and relocated his festivities to Valencia.[40] At his next destination, the Benedictine Abbey of Santa Maria de Montserrat, Platter told the porter who asked him to identify himself and explain where he came from and what he wanted, that he and Sebastian Schobinger were Germans who had travelled to Barcelona for the King's entry and wedding, and the hermits that they intended to wait for the weddings.[41] In the end, the only wedding they saw in Barcelona was that of an unidentified wealthy local couple at the height of the carnival festivities.[42] Margareta's fleet sailed from Marseille into Collioure a fortnight after Thomas Platter left Spain, and the Spanish double wedding finally took place in Valencia on 18 April 1599, the day Platter made his final farewells in Montpellier, before leaving for England and the Spanish Netherlands.[43]

Thomas Platter's account of Albrecht and Isabella's Brussels 1599 entry emphasizes the economic potential of such events, which attracted great crowds to their host cities. He personally encountered all manner of visitors keen to pay for board, lodgings and souvenirs flocking to Brussels. High-born visitors he had seen earlier, and recognized again taking part in the entry itself, included Vincenzo di Gonzaga and his cousin Charles, duc de Nevers, who had left Antwerp together in warships whose cannons saluted Platter's boat as they passed it on the Schelde.[44] Unlike Boch, Platter provides visual evidence of the Brussels entry: five annotated pen-and-ink sketches of triumphal arches, and several smaller sketches.[45] He describes its music and plays, and its 'living pictures', featuring live actors among their figural decorations:

> Daily for many days, on a stage in front of the city hall, amusing comedies were performed in Flemish, on all sorts of things that were happening in the Netherlands. Additionally they staged other diverting performances elsewhere, and held dances and other social gatherings. Every square and corner of the city was full of celebration at the arrival of their prince of peace, as they hoped [...] Outside the church of St Nicholas sat a bishop (he was a small *live* boy, dressed in bishop's clothes) and he had three small carved children sitting next to him

---

announcements of their passports demanded by soldiers levying the numerous river tolls (*Thomas Platter d.J*, 30: 28 September 1595, Seyssel).

[40] *Thomas Platter d.J*, 341–3 (28 January 1599, Barcelona).

[41] *Thomas Platter d.J*, 356, 358 (5–6 February 1599, Montserrat).

[42] *Thomas Platter d.J*, 374–5 (21 February 1599, Barcelona).

[43] *Thomas Platter d.J*, 390, 397 (2 March, 18 April, Collioure and Montpellier).

[44] *Thomas Platter d.J*, 664–5, 707 (23 August and 5 September 1599, Antwerp and Brussels).

[45] Bochius, *Historica narratio*, 110–70. Most reproduced in: *Thomas Platter d.J*, 704–744 (5–7 September 1599, Brussels: 712, 714, 717, 732, 736, 740).

in a bath, very skilfully depicted. [...] Right in front of the city hall they had constructed the stage for the actors, on it stood a completely naked little live boy (Cupidinem) representing the god of love, and this same little boy shot an arrow at each of Albrecht and Isabella as they rode past. Also on it were St Ergoul and two young women, living people, one held a round mirror and a script, the other a bow, on either side stood a man with a burning torch or nightlight. There was also a statue standing with them, stamping on the head of the Devil. Another statue held a lantern in its hand, and the Devil was secretly lighting the light in this lantern, it was all depicted in the most skilful way [...] I bought some Latin verses expressing anticipation and longing for the lasting freedom heralded by the archduke's arrival, and hope that the Spaniards in the fortresses would be sent home and replaced with Netherlanders instead. But this hasn't yet happened, because the Spaniards have continued to stay since then, and the war has intensified the longer it has continued.[46]

Festival masquerade costume habitually drew on classical mythology. Often, as here, or as at the court christening and Hohenzollern wedding attended by Felix Platter in 1596 and 1598, they included a Cupid played by a young boy.[47] Representations of such mythological characters did not meet with universal approval. Guarinonius articulates his repugnance for artistic and stage representations of this 'naked, blind child of a whore', in diatribes attacking paintings of 'Cupid with a burning torch', 'devilish Venuses' and other heathen, 'godless and sinful' classical nudes, of a type he was shocked to see exhibited at the 1594 Regensburg Reichstag. Exposure to the sinfulness of such characters, he asserts, leads to 'the certain destruction of physical health', whether seen in pictures or on stage, because 'what has been said here of paintings applies equally to indecent plays and suchlike comedies, or other kinds of performances and diversions'.[48]

Thomas Platter watched Albrecht and Isabella round off the very long second day of their Brussels entry festivities incognito in the main square, in a coach unrecognized by the crowds because it was unaccompanied by the customary ceremonial torch-bearers. Here, seated hand in hand, they watched a firework display of the type depicted in Plate 25, staged on a house-height galley-ship specially constructed for this purpose opposite the City Hall.[49] Platter's festival accounts draw on second-hand information as well as eyewitness experience.

---

[46]   *Thomas Platter d.J*, 710, 728–9, 735, 744 (6–7 September 1599, Brussels).

[47]   *Felix Platter Tagebuch*, 474, 498 (9 March 1596, Stuttgart; 5 October 1598, Hechingen).

[48]   Guarinonius, *Grewel*, 191, 225, 232, 1303 (Cupid and Venus are illustrated in the bottom right-hand corner of *Grewel's* titlepage illustration: Plate 6); see also Bücking, *Kultur und Gesellschaft in Tirol*, 94–5; Brückle and Müller, 'Die unzimblichen *Gemåhl'*. On English stage Cupids, see Jones-Davies, Hoenselaars and Jowett, 'Masque of Cupids', 1030–2.

[49]   *Thomas Platter d.J*, 710 (6 September 1599, Brussels).

Unlike the official recorders, he could and did speculate on the shortcomings, informal actions or private thoughts of rulers. Enquiring about the circumstances of Henri IV's 1595 royal entry into Lyon, for which he saw evidence in Lyon during his initial journey to Montpellier that September, he uncovered a telling anecdote unrecorded in the official festival books to which he alludes:

> The whole town [of Lyon] was still full of visitors. They had come here in order to see the King make his entry, which had taken place shortly before. Consequently, in many streets, and especially in the Place du Change, I saw tall arches, pyramids, towers and walls, with tiles, cloths and large plaster statues, all decorated with beautiful colours and ingenious inscriptions, verses and inlays. Nothing had yet been cleared away. And I was told that, some eight days before his entry, the King himself was in this same place. He had watched the workmen construct and put up everything, and had also asked when the King would be making his entry, what they thought of him & etc. Everything incognito. When everything had been arranged, he is said to have secretly ridden away, and afterwards, to have made his entry on the Connétable's horse, with an extremely impressive company in white silver-gilt. And the facade of every house – from the gates to his lodgings – is said to have been completely covered with tapestries. [...] As I crossed the Saône, still up there on a slightly raised cliff not far from the Port de Paris, I saw the decoratively constructed wood, straw and grass pavilions from which the musicians were said to have played extremely impressive music during the King's entry. Just as this will doubtless all have been published.[50]

Thomas Platter attended court festivals as a tourist. Felix Platter's involvement with court festivals, dating back to his student lute-playing and dancing, intensified in 1563, when he helped organize Emperor Ferdinand I's entry into Basle. His journal provides an overview of civic preparations and arrangements for the entry, and one of his most detailed *Observations* records his treatment of Lazarus Sween, a member of the imperial retinue, for kidney stones.[51] In his capacity as court physician, Felix Platter's personal attendance at court festivals was part of his professional duties. Integral to the festival itself, it was vital for the protection of a patron exposed to risk of serious injury by participation in martial arts, at tournaments routinely bursting the predictable confines of choreographed spectacle (Plates 22–4, 27). Felix Platter considered Henri II's fatal tournament accident of 1559 noteworthy.[52] Nicodemus Frischlin concludes his official festival account of the wedding of Ludwig, Duke of Württemberg, to Dorothea Ursula von Baden by recording the death and burial of Albrecht, Count of Hohenlohe, mortally wounded

---

[50] *Thomas Platter d.J*, 37–8 (20/30 September 1595, Lyon).

[51] *Felix Platter Tagebuch*, 392–9 (8–9 January 1563, Basle); Platter, *Obseruationum*, 763–6.

[52] *Felix Platter Tagebuch*, 365 (1560, Basle).

by Joachim Ernst von Anhalt during one of the festival's tournaments. Attended by the court physicians Paul Phrygio and Johannes Kielman, Count Albrecht died on 15 November 1575, the day after these festivities ended.[53] Guarinonius recalls seeing a foot tournament as a Prague schoolboy, in which:

> One knight crushed the helmet of another onto his head so forcefully with a mighty sword blow that the knight who had been hit was so badly injured that he lost his reason. I myself many times handled the tournament sword with which this blow was delivered, and discovered that it weighed no less that fifteen pounds. It was used by an extremely strong knight whom I could name, built like a giant.[54]

These were not isolated incidents. In 1600, the riding teacher Alessandro Malatesta writes of festival tournaments: 'all sorts of jousts and combats lead to, and ultimately have to do with, real warfare',[55] and Felix Platter was well aware of the court physician's obligations and challenges.

Sometimes, the physician himself required medical attention. Travelling to the 1577 Hohenzollern wedding, Felix Platter had been playing his lute in the carriage of the noblewomen when the bad state of the road led their coachman to try his luck on the fields. The vehicle fell onto its side, crushing Felix's left foot, which swelled up to the knee and had to be cut out of his riding boot, wrapped in linen cloths and placed on a velvet cushion before the journey could continue. He spent most of it unconscious, receiving small doses of local red wine along the way as a painkiller. At their destination, his injuries needed constant treatment from a series of barber-surgeons, and, once no longer bedridden, still in great pain, he participated in the festivities on crutches. Although this injury kept him from the first performance of five excellent singing miners, a type of choir he had appreciated from childhood, he recovered sufficiently to enjoy their later performances.[56] The Schwaz miners' choir, which had performed at court since at least 1567, is highly praised by Hippolytus Guarinonius, who explains that its singers became popular performers at grand court festivities through singing so cheerfully at work, and describes songs and ritual ceremonies miners traditionally performed with outsiders, of whatever rank, who entered their mines.[57] As an invited guest, Felix Platter experienced performances by these miners and others who did not primarily earn their living as performers, as well as by full-time professional performers such as

---

[53]   Frischlin, *De nuptijs illvstrissimi principis*, 165–7. The theologian Paul Constantinus Phrygio (c.1483–1543), a friend of Platter the Elder, officiated at Felix Platter's baptism (Platter the Elder, 'Thomas Platters Lebensbeschreibung', 126, 133).

[54]   Guarinonius, *Grewel*, 1195.

[55]   Watanabe-O'Kelly, *Triumphall shews*, 24 (in translation).

[56]   *Felix Platter Tagebuch*, 73, 459–61, 465 (1544, Basle; August 1577, Sigmaringen).

[57]   Guarinonius, *Grewel*, 170–1, 1177–8; Senn, *Musik und Theater*, 177; Drexel, 'Quelle zur Musikgeschichte', 58–9.

the internationally-acclaimed instrumentalist and singer Pauli of Zell. This star among the comic entertainers of both the 1577 and 1598 Hohenzollern weddings variously recited his hugely popular improvised comic rhymes or sang them to his lute. In 1577, he had great success accompanying his own crying and laughing on the lute. In 1598 Pauli, whose act now involved spoken and sang verse drawing attention to the shortcomings of, even ridiculing, certain aristocratic guests, was rewarded with rapturous applause and an honorarium of over 100 crowns.[58]

Felix Platter took a professional interest in the genuine physical dangers facing tournament contestants. Official printed festival books were generally addressed to courtiers already familiar with the rules of combat and theatrical conventions of specific types of tournaments. Platter, by contrast, spells out their dangers and niceties. Unlike the main festivities, the concluding tournament of the 1598 Hohenzollern wedding was held not at Hechingen but at Hochburg, the court of Platter's patron, the Margrave of Baden. Continuing heavy rain forced its postponement for two days to 17 October, and relocation from the waterlogged tournament ground to a raised meadow. Virtually turned into an island by the flood waters, this had to be specially laid with planks and surrounded by protective cloths, to keep the horses out of deep water. Here, 15 noblemen engaged in one-to-one mounted sword combat resulting in at least four minor and two major injuries. The bride's father Rheingraf Friedrich, in the dangerous role of first challenger, sustained multiple injuries. In a spirited first encounter, the Margrave of Baden dented his helmet, and was himself injured under his arm. Weighed down by heavy protective armour, the Rheingraf was toppled from his horse by his next opponent, Eberhard von Rappoltstein. His fifth clash became his last, when a wound to his hand by his son Johann forced his withdrawal from the contest. The seventh encounter ended similarly, when Jacob von Rotburg was seriously wounded in his right hand. A combatant in a late encounter drove his opponent through the protective cloths with such force that he and his horse had to be pulled out of the flood waters.[59]

In March 1596, Felix Platter accompanied the Margrave of Baden to the Stuttgart court, to celebrate the christening of Prince August. A grand and expensive christening festival attracted powerful godparents and guests, contributing towards a solid foundation for dynastic success. Prince August's position as fourteenth child of the ruling duke, Friedrich von Württemberg, was no guarantee against his playing a major dynastic role in later life. High early modern infant mortality meant that every noble child had to be appropriately christened. However, August, born in January 1596, and christened with so much spectacle in March, died on 21 April 1596. Platter's detailed descriptions of the festival's four days of tournaments, respectively a costumed running at the ring, burlesque tournament, courtly combat

---

[58]   *Felix Platter Tagebuch*, 465, 496 (19 August 1577, Sigmaringen; 1 October 1598, Hechingen); Schmid, *Musik*, 44, 103, 597.

[59]   English translation: Chapter 16, this volume.

and professional combat (Plates 22–4, 27), highlight the importance of the court physician's role at tournaments.[60]

The most stylized, and consequently least dangerous, form of tournament was the running at the ring, of a type depicted in Plate 23. That of the 1596 christening was contested in the tournament square in the court gardens on Tuesday 9 March, by 10 impressively costumed companies of knights, with special safety precautions protecting their horses. Before the start of the contest, they paraded past the numerous spectators, including the noblewomen in the summer-house alongside the tournament square, and the judges on a special raised velvet-covered stage. The first masquerade company was that of the host, Duke Friedrich. It included five camels, each led by two lackeys in Turkish costume, the first carrying a globe which periodically opened to reveal two violin-playing court fools, the others masked mythological couples. While parading, the camels went down on their knees at the ladies' stand, afterwards they were tethered out of sight to avoid frightening the horses. Nine further companies were costumed as monks and nuns, or as classical and mythological characters,[61] musicians, planets, Moors and Turks. Each paraded in turn, escorted by the host's trumpeter and two mounted cuirassiers, before challenging the host's group at running at the ring. One trumpeter announced the start of each run, and 12 announced each ring scored. The tournament was injury free, the host winning 32 cups. A final parade of all 10 companies was followed by an evening banquet, dances, and the judges' presentation ceremony, during which the prize-winners, having made acceptance speeches, were crowned with wreaths by the noblewomen.[62]

The second tournament of the 1596 christening was a more accident-prone burlesque tournament, of the type depicted in Plates 24 and 27.[63] Alluding to their physical dangers three decades earlier, Massimo Troiano emphasizes the novelty and ridiculous satirical humour of these 'new tournaments'. He describes contestants at the 1568 Munich wedding festivities, with bodies and arms thickly padded with thick layers of straw, wearing not regular helmets but bulky garishly-painted protective wooden headgear, and wielding long thick sticks tipped with large round buttons instead of regular lances.[64] Held on Wednesday 10 March, the 1596 burlesque tournament involved two teams, each of 10 knights, all protected by grotesquely decorated armour padded on the outside with cushions and on the inside with straw.[65] As in Munich in 1568, they were mounted on rundown horses

---

[60]   *Felix Platter Tagebuch*, 467–83 (28 February to 2 April 1596, Hochburg-Stuttgart-Hochburg). This twentieth-century edition of Felix Platter's account is a modern reconstruction, compiled from partial eighteenth- and nineteenth-century transcriptions of this festival's only known record, Platter's lost manuscript.

[61]   Including Janus (see Chapter 11, this volume).

[62]   *Felix Platter Tagebuch*, 472–6 (9 March 1596, Stuttgart).

[63]   Known as the 'Kübelturnier'.

[64]   Troiano, *Dialoghi*, sigs.123ᵛ, 139ᵛ–143ᵛ.

[65]   *Felix Platter Tagebuch*, 476–7 (10 March 1596, Stuttgart).

with minimal tack, and armed with long blunted wooden spears. They confronted each other in opposing groups of five at a time, and every time a knight was knocked off his horse, the spectators roared with laughter. Felix draws attention to participants' not inconsiderable risk of injury, pointing out that despite their comic nature burlesque tournaments are 'not without danger'. Although there were no serious accidents in 1596, many combatants complained for several days after the event of the extensive bruising routinely suffered after participating in such tournaments.

Thursday 11 and Friday 12 March contrasted aristocratic chivalric skills with brute mercenary force. The noblemen's foot tournament was on Thursday; the combat of the professional gladiators – contractually obliged to fight until blood was drawn – on the concluding day. The courtly combat was preceded by costumed parades of the four competing companies, accompanied by military musicians, on the tournament square.[66] One-on-one combat preceded a concluding half-hour battle, in which two sets of two companies fought each other at full strength, with the sole aim of breaking as many lances or swords as possible on their opponents' helmets. According to the rules, blows were delivered with maximum force. Each contestant was shadowed by a second, who handed out replacement weapons as needed, and by two referees, who enforced the rules and restrained unacceptable aggression, such as attempts to exceed the permitted maximum of five sword blows in one-to-one combat. This tournament concluded with the customary closing procession, banquet, dance and presentation of prizes. Held in the palace courtyard, Friday's tournament, officially styled a fencing school, dispensed with the niceties of musicians, costumes and processions.[67] On behalf of Duke Friedrich, who 'let it be known that there had to be red blood, otherwise it did not count', 24 mercenaries had been recruited from Strasbourg and elsewhere. Ten were blooded during this event, their wounds ranging from minor cuts to the loss of a goldsmith's apprentice's eye.

Such fencing schools, of which one is depicted on the right-hand side of Plate 22, attracted considerable condemnation. In *Grewel*, Guarinonius surveys classical manifestations of 'fencing', including wrestling and other hand-to-hand combat. He follows Galen in rejecting such sports as largely worthless in terms of discernible health benefits, relating, as a warning to parents, two unfortunate early encounters of his own ending in near loss of his opponents' eyes. One involved a fight with another boy's miniature weapons during his Viennese childhood, the other his fight with staves against Hannibal, a tall young Bohemian mercenary fencer challenging allcomers in St Procopius' Caves.[68] Having learned the German style of using rapier and dagger in Prague from the highly rated fencing master

---

[66] *Felix Platter Tagebuch*, 477–9 (11 March 1596, Stuttgart).

[67] *Felix Platter Tagebuch*, 479–80 (12 March 1596, Stuttgart).

[68] Guarinonius, *Grewel*, 1192. My thanks to Richard Šipék for identifying St Procopius' Caves as Prokopské údolí, a wooded valley in the south-west suburbs of Prague, formerly inhabited by hermits.

'the little Schlosserle', the Italian fencing Guarinonius saw in Padua compelled him to reject his theatrical German approach and start anew.[69] Praising Italian fencing schools for their genuine attempt to teach pupils using safe techniques and weapons, he regards German fencing schools as 'more heathen than Christian', mercenary displays whose valuable prizes tempt apprentices to sinfully neglect their work and recklessly risk injury to their proper means of livelihood, their 'fists, hands and arms'.[70] He highlights these contests' physical and moral dangers, to combatants often pitted against each other on unequal terms. Unlike the contestants of healthy sports, who are motivated by concerns for 'diversion and mutual trust', German fencing school participants, Guarinonius claims, are recruited through the twin sins of avarice and gluttony. Their unhealthy desire for money and alcohol is used to goad them into dangerous encounters in which bloodshed is expected and rewarded, and serious injury or death are genuine dangers. Felix Platter confirms that those contestants of the 1596 fencing school who drew blood were richly rewarded in coin by the judges, and that their opponents' sometimes serious injuries in no way dampened the spirits of the guests. The day's celebrations closed with a banquet and a two-hour firework display in a burning galley-ship constructed on the tournament square, of the type witnessed by Thomas Platter at Isabella's 1599 entry into Brussels, or depicted in Plate 25.[71]

One of the four competing companies at the tournament of 11 March 1596 was led by Friedrich von Württemberg's heir, 14-year-old Johann Friedrich. He succeeded in 1608, the year in which Felix Platter's patron the Margrave of Baden joined the German Protestant Union. In November 1609, the Margrave of Baden was in Stuttgart for Johann Friedrich's marriage to Barbara Sophia of Brandenburg. One of the Union's founding court festivals, it has been identified as articulating 'a specifically German Protestant political programme', through iconography that was 'a statement of the hopes and aspirations of the German Protestants'.[72] To what extent is this agenda reflected in the costumes of its attendant festivities? Balthasar Küchler's official festival book of 1611, one of several commemorating this wedding, features over 200 plates depicting costumed tournament entries, including those contributed by the Margrave of Baden to a running at the ring and a foot tournament.[73] Overwhelmingly, Küchler depicts tournament participants wearing either contemporary or historical military costume, or the non-military nationally or classically-inspired costumes that, influenced by Italian festivals, had become increasingly fashionable at German tournaments since the Munich court wedding of 1568. 'Ancient German costume' is much in evidence.[74] But, at a time when the theatrical use of religious costume was widely discouraged on European

[69]   Guarinonius, *Grewel*, 1255.
[70]   Guarinonius, *Grewel*, 373, 1192, 1254–5. See also Innsbruck UL, Cod.110, I, f.540ᵛ.
[71]   *Thomas Platter d.J*, 709 (5 September 1599, Brussels).
[72]   Watanabe-O'Kelly, 'The iconography of German Protestant tournaments', 47.
[73]   Küchler, *Repræsentatio*.
[74]   Watanabe-O'Kelly, 'The iconography of German Protestant tournaments', 51, 54.

stages,[75] and Wilhelm V, devout father of Maximilian of Bavaria, the Catholic ruler whose actions precipitated the formation of the Protestant Union, was living out his lengthy abdication in Jesuit robes, Küchler illustrates a remarkably negative use of Catholic vestments (Plate 26). It occurs in the first entry, sponsored by the host and groom himself, Johann Friedrich, of the festival's opening tournament, a running at the ring. While Felix Platter has left no account of the 1609 Stuttgart wedding, a second-hand report by Hippolytus Guarinonius not previously cited in this connection, offers swift, solid evidence that this rare exception to the festival's hundreds of traditional tournament costumes, far from going unnoticed, made an extraordinarily immediate, sensationally shocking negative impact on devout German-speaking Catholics. In an eight-page chapter of *Grewel*, apparently written up even before the final guests had left Stuttgart, Guarinonius records, in dialogue form, a discussion with a local Tirolean merchant who, while returning to Hall, 'eight days ago, in this month of November, in the present year 1609', had witnessed a publicly-staged tournament held in celebration of 'a German court wedding [...] a performance not staged at any Catholic place'.[76] Guarinonius's concern is neither to offer a factual account of the 1609 tournament, nor even, given that it occurs in a section of his treatise concerned with health issues relating to physical exercise, to discuss the hazards of festival tournaments. Concentrating on an item of information considered specially diverting and newsworthy by the merchant, namely that one tournament participant was costumed as a Jesuit priest,[77] he returns to his favoured subject of spiritual health.

Guarinonius informs the merchant that Jesuit religious robes should not be thought incongruous in tournaments, given the Jesuits' tireless defence of the Catholic Church in spiritual tournaments. The merchant retorts that this particular Jesuit's visual emblems were defamatory. In one hand, he carried a foxtail, which the common people took to mean that he was a sycophant, the merchant takes as a sign of Jesuit ability to flatter the nobility, and Guarinonius interprets as a triumphant symbol of Jesuit renunciation of bestial vices and follies in favour of Christian virtue, signifying their virtuous loyalty to their only leader, God. In his other hand, he held poisonous snakes, as a sign of the Jesuits' cunning and poisonous nature. Taking this opportunity to teach the merchant that the flesh of poisonous snakes was a key ingredient of the opiate-based poison antidote and universal medicine theriac, Guarinonius, by contrast, proclaims that those closest to Jesuits are physically and spiritually the healthiest and strongest, and compares this Jesuit with the heroic young Hercules, also depicted holding snakes. The

---

[75] Religious costume and objects had been banned from the plays of Hall's Jesuit college since 1586 (Senn, *Aus dem Kulturleben*, 372).

[76] Guarinonius, *Grewel*, 1195–1203 (6, XIII: 'On the foot tournament, and an exquisite, beautiful, brand new parade'), 1196, 1198. Bücking notes the passage without comment (*Kultur und Gesellschaft in Tirol*, 161).

[77] In 1632, the Elector Frederick V of the Palatinate wore Jesuit robes in a court masque organized by the King of Sweden (Norbrook, 'The masque of truth', 100).

merchant's revelation that 'painted around the lower seam of his long coat, this tournament Jesuit had all sorts of poisonous and cunning animals' is glossed by Guarinonius as yet further mythologically-inspired imagery symbolizing Jesuit superiority, and he enthusiastically applauds the merchant's suggestions regarding carnival costumes lampooning Protestant preachers and their wives.[78]

A later dialogue, in which Guarinonius refers back to this event as 'the foot tournament of the recent court wedding', reveals both his professional interest in the health dangers of tournaments, and his own acute sensitivity to the mockery of physicians by tournament masqueraders:

> Only seldom does such a public tournament take place without several accidents or injuries. And additionally, sometimes there are other contributing factors inappropriate to honest knights, as for example making fun of the learned, as when, as I have often seen, several costumed like medical doctors raised their urine flasks in front of the womenfolk and looked into them.
>
> *Reader*: And what could they tell from their own urine?
>
> *Doctor*: That they are fools.[79]

His earlier dialogue continues by warning the merchant – and his readers – to renounce foolish gluttony, excess drinking, and lust, and recommends that they lead sober, sensible and moderate lives, by following the Jesuits in rejecting all heresy and sinful dissidence, and fully embracing the virtuous teachings of the Roman Catholic Church. The merchant concludes that 'most of the world is mad and foolish [...] and that's why it praises what is in its own mad likeness, namely folly'.[80]

In Küchler's depiction of the 1609 Stuttgart entry discussed by Guarinonius, Adulatio, wearing Jesuit robes, walks in front of two mounted women, Germana Fides and Sinceritas (Plate 26). Adulatio's robes are plain and undecorated, and he holds not a snake and a foxtail, but an open book and a rosary, while a snake writhes at his feet. However, many of the attributes noted in Guarinonius's dialogue are distributed between three further characters. Directly in front of Adulatio stands Simulatio, brandishing a foxtail, and wearing a costume richly festooned with foxtails. Securitas, standing at the front of the group, holds a second writhing snake. Between these two men walks a female warrior, Diffidentia. Discrepancies between Guarinonius's account and Küchler's picture raise questions regarding interpretation of the latter, and of court festival iconography more generally. Is Guarinonius's account misreporting both costume and context, or is it an indication that Küchler's published depiction of this entry is not literal? Does Küchler's

---

78   Guarinonius, *Grewel*, 1198, 1200.

79   Guarinonius, *Grewel*, 1223.

80   Guarinonius, *Grewel*, 1199–1203.

illustration unpack complex metaphorical references – originally incorporated into the Jesuit's own costume – into three further characters not originally present: Securitas, Diffidentia and Simulatio?[81] Did Johann Friedrich's entry really involve 'no less than' 118 people?[82] Or is Küchler here iconographically unpacking into four separate unmounted figures what was performed in the festival itself by a single pedestrian preceding the two mounted figures? In short, were some of the characters depicted by Küchler iconographic representations rather than actually enacted by separate participants at the festival itself? Guarinonius's account provides a valuable reminder of some wider issues regarding the interpretation of pre-photographic festival illustrations, and correlations between their iconographic conventions and the events they depict.

Only grand courts could afford to employ full-time physicians. Physicians represent an exceptional category of educated commoner, with routine privileged access to many spheres of the ceremony, spectacle and routines of court festivals. Their festival descriptions provide rare alternative perspectives to official court-sponsored festival books. Guarinonius's identity as a physician is relevant to his account of the 1609 tournament Jesuit, which raises challenging questions for the interpretation of festival texts and pictures. The Platter brothers' medical education and professional practice inform the insights into court festivals offered by deviations from, and additions to, official accounts reviewed in this chapter, and in the following chapter, in Felix Platter's description of the 1598 Hohenzollern wedding.

---

[81] Watanabe-O'Kelly reproduces this plate without commenting on the four unmounted figures (*Triumphall shews*, 52).

[82] Watanabe-O'Kelly, *Triumphall shews*, 52.

Chapter 7

Commedia dell'Arte Costumes at a German Court Wedding of 1598[1]

This chapter examines Felix Platter's account of one particular tournament entry at the 1598 Hohenzollern wedding, at which Johann Georg, Count of Hohenzollern, married Franziska von Salm. Through the quartermaster sergeant's records, he had access to the exact details of the 984 guests and 865 horses brought to Hechingen for this festival (Diagrams 1 and 2).[2] The festival's official chronicler, Jakob Frischlin, was a writer, dramatist and teacher at the school in nearby Reutlingen. He translated into the vernacular Latin plays and festival books by his more gifted older brother Nicodemus Frischlin, who had died in 1590 as a murder suspect fleeing from custody, and staged at least one carnival play with Hechingen's court musicians, in 1599.[3] Thousands of doggerel couplets separate the conclusion of his printed account of the 1598 Hohenzollern wedding, explaining it as a pious bid to immortalize his rulers, from his description of the bride's arrival.[4] In her party, Frischlin notes a man who has left a crisper and more sophisticated version of this festival, neither mentioning Frischlin, nor written as an enduring public monument to his patron's family. This was Felix Platter, characterized by Frischlin as a fellow writer and historian, and court physician to the bride's brother-in-law.[5] In the year of Johann Georg's birth, 1577, Felix Platter had attended the court wedding, in Sigmaringen, of his uncle, Christof von Hohenzollern, to Katharina von Welsperg. Still dressed in mourning, she and her two sons were among the wedding guests in Hechingen in 1598. The devout Catholicism of the groom's grandfather, Karl I, Count of Hohenzollern, and his willingness to be of service, strengthened his dynasty's links to the Habsburg and Bavarian courts (Diagram 2). Born in Brussels and named after his godfather Emperor Charles V, at whose Madrid court he was partly brought up, Karl I was King Philip II of Spain's official envoy to one of the most culturally influential of all early modern German court festivals, the 1568 Munich wedding. Here his prominent ceremonial role included receiving Duke Albrecht V of Bavaria's prospective daughter-in-law Renée of Lorraine with

---

[1]   *Felix Platter Tagebuch*, 484–513 (28 September to 18 October 1598, Hochburg-Hechingen-Hochburg); English translation: Chapter 16, this volume. See also Katritzky, 'The autobiographical writings'.

[2]   *Felix Platter Tagebuch*, 488–92 (1 October 1598, Hechingen).

[3]   Bumiller, 'Die Brüder Frischlin', 9, 23, 27.

[4]   Frischlin, *Hohenzollerische Hochzeyt*, 251.

[5]   Frischlin, *Hohenzollerische Hochzeyt*, 136.

an elaborate French speech greeting her on behalf of her future husband Prince Wilhelm, and presenting her with a diamond necklace from the Spanish king.[6] In 1560 and 1570, on behalf of Emperors Ferdinand I and Maximilian II, Karl I led entourages escorting their daughters Eleonore and Elisabeth of Habsburg to their respective weddings in Mantua and Paris.[7]

The sole tournament held for the 1598 wedding in Hechingen itself took place on Thursday 5 October. As noted in the previous chapter, Felix Platter's account emphasizes its waterlogged conditions. Both Platter and Frischlin describe its seven costumed entries. Of special interest to scholars of transregional theatre are their descriptions of the second company, organized by the groom's paternal uncle, Karl II von Hohenzollern. Platter's account names the company's 10 knights, two defenders and two seconds. This and further information provided by Platter and Frischlin reveal the extent to which Karl II's choice of his 14-strong company was guided by matriarchal dynastic ties. Both his seconds, the counts Friedrich von Fürstenberg and Georg or Frobenius von Helfenstein, and his fifth and sixth knights, Heinrich von Limpurg-Sontheim and Frobenius Truchseß, were sons of sisters of the groom's mother, Sybille von Zimmern.[8] Karl II took the part of first knight himself. His second knight, the Count of Holach, may have participated in the costumed unmounted combat at the 1596 christening attended by Felix Platter, and led a masquerade of monks and nuns in the running at the ring. The day before Karl II's 1598 masquerade tournament, he displayed impressive horsemanship skills on a dappled mount he had trained in dressage, acrobatic tricks and jumping; and he also participated in the hunt.[9] Karl II's third and fourth knights were the bride's brother, Wild- und Rheingraf Otto zu Kyrburg, and the Count of Zeiningen. The seventh knight, Carl von Schornstetten, represented Ernst Friedrich, Margrave of Baden-Durlach, occasional patient of Felix Platter and oldest brother of his patron Georg Friedrich, Margrave of Baden. Husband of Juliane Ursula von Salm, the bride's oldest sister, Georg Friedrich was, with Eberhard von Rappoltstein, defender to Karl II's company.[10] The eighth and ninth knights, Wolf and Christoph Fuchs, had left their native Tirol after finding that, following their conversion to Protestantism, their services as courtiers were no longer required in Innsbruck.[11] Karl II's tenth and final knight is an otherwise unidentified court accountant.

Frischlin associates the costumes of Karl II's company of 'challengers' with those of Turks, Hungarians, Tartars and Croatians:

---

[6]   Troiano, *Dialoghi*, sigs.22ᵛ–26ᵛ, 93ᵛ; Wagner, *Beschreibung*, sig.31.

[7]   Frischlin, *Hohenzollerische Hochzeyt*, 94–5; Schmid, *Musik*, 15.

[8]   Sybille and five of her sisters attended the 1598 Hohenzollern wedding (Frischlin, *Hohenzollerische Hochzeyt*, 270n245; *Felix Platter Tagebuch*, 489–92, 501).

[9]   *Felix Platter Tagebuch*, 473, 478, 498–9, 504.

[10]   Frischlin, *Hohenzollerische Hochzeyt*, 150–1; *Felix Platter Tagebuch*, 482, 489. See also Diagram 2.

[11]   Hirn, *Erzherzog Ferdinand II von Tirol*, I, 136.

There followed a very strangely behaved bunch. They arrived wearing hoods, they were little red hats, bonnets or caps, all very tight-fitting. They rode in on their horses wearing baggy white breeches. These men looked pretty horrible in their little hats of red, blue, yellow cloth. Such people can be found in Hungary. They rode up in the Turkish fashion, several with twisted moustaches. [...] Some wore masks as if they were in Turkey. They had horrible expressions like Tartars or Croatians. And two in particular looked really horrible when they got closer. They ran up on the green meadow, gnashing their teeth and had such large noses that everyone who saw them running had to laugh at them. [...] They arrived looking like Hungarians and ran around frighteningly on the grass with the big round noses that they had on their masks, making gruesome gestures. There were two with long noses, who also gnashed their teeth while they played their tricks, so that everyone laughed at them.[12]

Frischlin's mistake reflects the popularity of Turkish, Hungarian and Tartar masquerade costumes at previous court festivities, including the Stuttgart wedding of 1577, where, as recorded by his brother, they featured in the third, fourth and ninth entries of the tournament on the fifth day.[13] Turkish masquerade costumes featured at the 9 March 1596 running at the ring of a Stuttgart christening described by Felix Platter, and were equally popular at other courts.[14] Thomas Platter records the use of Turkish costume on 9 June 1597, at Emmanuel de Crussol, duc d'Uzès's[15] coming of age entry into Uzès. This festival featured the ubiquitous classical costume: 'three nymphs or goddesses' played on a raised stage, by 'three young, beautiful boys, without masks, beautifully and extremely daintily costumed as young girls, each differently from the other', who delivered lengthy speeches to the Duke in French, Latin and Occitan; but also Eastern costume:

item, one company all dressed in the Turkish manner and armed with Turkish bows and sabres, they also had several kettle drums and other improvised instruments which they played, so that it sounded like a Turkish battle. The second company was costumed after the Arabic and Moorish fashion, they also shot with bows, and all wore face masks.[16]

In naming all 10 'challengers' of 1598, and providing their stage names for this masquerade, Felix Platter, who has the inside information on their real identities, reveals a surprising correction to Frischlin's reading of their masquerade disguises. They are not based on ethnic national and regional costumes, but on that of Zanni, a stock theatrical role:

[12] Frischlin, *Hohenzollerische Hochzeyt*, 222–3, 240.
[13] Frischlin, *De nuptijs illustrissimi principis*, 143, 146.
[14] See Chapter 6, this volume.
[15] 1570–1657
[16] *Thomas Platter d.J*, 221, 223 (9 June 1597, Uzès).

Ten knights, riding in pairs, costumed like Zannis, especially the two last, who wore ugly masks or makeup. [...] They wore blue or in several cases brown nightcaps, with white caps underneath, with attached cowls and aprons down to their boots, short cloaks like collars, blue, brown or yellow in colour. The first called himself Joan Badello, and placed a ten gulden wager with the judges in order to take part in the tournament. The second, Joan Frimocollo, [...] the third Scherisepho [...] the fourth Peterlino [...] the fifth Jhan Fourmage [...] the sixth Joan Fritada [...] the seventh Francotrippo [...] the eighth Pergomasco [...] the ninth Zani [...] the tenth Zani.[17]

Lötscher footnotes Zanni as a generic theatrical stage clown, without specifying the connection with the commedia dell'arte.[18] Schmid identifies Zannis as 'Harlequin figures', but explicitly describes the group as 'Hungarian-Turkish'.[19] In fact, as the masked comic servant figure of the commedia dell'arte, Zanni is its most important stock role. The 1598 masquerade's grotesquely masked big-nosed tooth-gnashing final pair were generic Zanni, and at least seven of the other eight are Zanni variants. During the half-century from around 1570, Zanni costume became an essential element of public and private Mediterranean carnival practice, dominating the theatrical masquerade costumes then a popular subject for depiction in friendship albums.[20] Alliterative lists of stage names varying the Zanni role are the defining feature of one genre of early modern popular printed ephemera. Unlike the Zanni names in late examples, many of which are purely literary, with seemingly little or no connection to genuine stage roles,[21] sixteenth-century examples of the genre often name genuine performers. I believe that the Zanni variants of the 1598 wedding tournament are not fantasy names, randomly created for this masquerade, but all or mostly inspired by genuine actors of the time.[22] Most obviously, Peterlino and Francotrippo are the stage names of two internationally known and widely documented commedia dell'arte stars, Giovanni Pellesini da Reggio[23] and Gabriele Panzanini da Bologna,[24] creators of the stage servants Pedrolino and Francatrippa.

---

[17]   *Felix Platter Tagebuch*, 499–501. For the full translation and a note on currencies, see p.291, this volume.

[18]   *Felix Platter Tagebuch*, 499n77.

[19]   Schmid, *Musik*, 604.

[20]   See, for example, frontispiece, Plates 7, 11–19. On the friendship album as a source of early modern depictions of stock characters engaged in comic routines, see Katritzky, *Women, medicine and theatre*, 67–9, 'I costumi della commedia dell'arte', 'Franco Bertelli' and 'Was *commedia dell'arte* performed by mountebanks?'.

[21]   Raparini, *L'Arlichino, poema carnevalesco* and *L'Arlichino poema*.

[22]   Katritzky, *The art of commedia*, 98–102.

[23]   c.1526–1612.

[24]   Active 1571–1609.

Jhan Fourmage is possibly inspired by Jean Potage, an English stage version of the Zanni variant John Posset or Jan Bouset, created and introduced to Germany by Thomas Sackville, an internationally renowned English actor based at the court of Wolfenbüttel during the 1590s, when he also played several seasons at the Frankfurt Fair.[25] Joan Frimocollo, Joan Fritada and Joan Badello are genuine stage names not yet firmly linked to specific actors. Joan Frimocollo, also variously recorded as Zan Frogniocola or Frignochola, is Zan Fargnocolo, the stage name of an actor in Pisa in July 1581 with the Desiosi troupe of commedia dell'arte actors, where Montaigne saw them act and won some of the impoverished Fargnocolo's belongings in a raffle.[26] Joan Fritada is the street entertainer recorded by Ben Jonson, Tomaso Garzoni and others in the decades around 1600 as Fritata or Zan Fritada.[27] Joan Badello is identifiable with Zan Padella, Gradella or Badil, recorded in *Contrasti* of 1613 and 1617 and by Garzoni, and depicted as Padelle on the French mountebank stage of Gille le Niais, with Harlequin and others (Plate 33).[28] Pergomasco may be the 'Gianni bergamasco' noted in Nicola Rossi's *Discorsi sulla commedia*, of 1589, or a generic bergamasque Zanni.[29] Scherisepho's context also indicates a Zanni variant. Possibly there is some connection with Zan Panza di Pegora, the stage persona of Simon, the Zanni of the Gelosi Company, thought by some to have inspired Sancho Panzo. *Lachrimoso Lamento [...] di Zan Panza di Pegora, alias Simon Comico Geloso*, published on his death in 1585, and the previously referred to *Contrasto* of 1617 both name Panza di Pegora himself, as well as Zan Padella, Pedrolin, Zan Frignacola and Zan Fritada. Giulio Cesare Croce's poem of 1621, 'La Gran vittoria di Pedrolino', adds Francatrip to these latter four.[30] Several of the names used in 1598 by Karl II's masqueraders appear together in publications of 1597. The cast list of Oratio Vecchi's *L'Amfiparnaso* includes Pedrolin, Zane Bergamasco and a Francatrippa who recites a list of Zanni variants including Fritada, Pedrolin, Padella, Gradella and Frignocola, while a *sonneto* in Adriano Banchieri's *Il donativo di qvatro asinissimi personaggi* lists Pedrulì, Fregnocola and Francatripp.[31] A late sixteenth century *Genologia di Zan*

---

[25]   On Jean Potage, see Hansen, *Formen der commedia dell'arte*, 42–7; Katritzky, 'Zan Bragetta a Jan Potage'.

[26]   Giovanni Gabrielli, *Il novo Maridazzo alla bergamasca de M. Zan Frogniocola con Madonna Gnignocola*, Verona 1611; *Stanze alla venitiana d'vn bravo*, Venice 1582 (both in Pandolfi, *La commedia dell'arte*, I, 339 and IV, 37); Montaigne, *Complete works*, 1231, 1236.

[27]   Jonson, 'Volpone', II.ii (*Workes*, 469); Garzoni, *La piazza universale*: Discorso CIV, 910. Further references in Henke, *Performance and literature*, 118–19; Katritzky, *The art of commedia*, 100.

[28]   Garzoni, *La piazza universale*: Discorso CIV, 911. See also Pandolfi, *La commedia dell'arte*, I, 286, 349; V, 416; Katritzky, *The art of commedia*, 100.

[29]   Magni, 'Il tipo dello zanni', 113.

[30]   Pandolfi, *La commedia dell'arte*, I, 223–4, 286; II, 24–9.

[31]   Pandolfi, *La commedia dell'arte*, II, 266, 275, 302.

Capella unites Frittada, Zan Padella and Pedroli, and Camillo Conti's *Partenza di Carnevale* of 1615 adds Francatripp to these three.[32] Felix Platter's identification of Karl II's group as professional Italian stage names is of theatre-historical value in itself, and for confirming them as the subjects of Frischlin's account of this group. It also reveals as courtiers rather than noblemen the group's final pair, whose outsize noses and ugly masks struck spectators as so grotesquely comical when they ran across the meadow gnashing their teeth at them.

In March, May and July 1598, the groom's father, Count Eitel Friedrich IV, sent a succession of courtiers, including his tailors Jakob Maurer and Jakob Flies, and his director of music Narcissus Zängel, to Milan.[33] On his instructions, they ordered, purchased and transported back to Hechingen bales of cloth of gold, velvet and silk, tapestries 'for the running at the ring', masquerade costumes, 24 theatrical face masks, musical instruments and other luxury items for the wedding festivities, to the value of over 3,000 florins. The Sigmaringen archives preserve a small sample of cloth of gold tucked into some correspondence relating to this journey, its richly patterned sophisticated weave of red and gold thread still glowing vividly after over four centuries.[34] Many German masquerade costumes were inspired by iconographic sources in ephemeral publications, or by engravings in emblem (Plate 29) or costume books (Plate 1), and in turn impacted on the iconographic record through costume and festival book illustrations. But more directly than to iconographic sources, or even than to Eitel Friedrich IV's Milanese and other Italian contacts and suppliers, the search for the source of this unprecedented array of Zanni variants north of the Alps before 1600 points directly to the February 1568 Munich wedding festivities of Wilhelm of Bavaria. Johann Georg von Hohenzollern's grandfather, father and uncle substantially contributed to these, and the Stuttgart and Munich courts maintained close cultural links, lending and passing on musicians and other performers to each other. One such was a dwarf in the service of Archduke Ferdinand of the Tirol, whose signature act, evidently as well-received at court in Stuttgart as in Munich, later entertained Felix Platter:

> *A third Dwarfe.* At the wedding of the Duke of *Bavaria* about forty years since, there was a Dwarfe whom after I saw in the Court of *Wittemberg* when I was at *Stutgard.* He was armed all over with a short spear and a sword, and put into a Pie or pastry, and brought to the table. He brake the Pie-crust, and with his sword drawn, fenced up and down upon the table, and made all laugh and admire.[35]

---

[32]   Pandolfi, *La commedia dell'arte*, I, 253–7; IV, 32, 37.

[33]   Schmid, *Musik*, 256–60.

[34]   Sigmaringen StAS FAS HH1-50 T1-5 A696 (unfoliated).

[35]   Platter, *Obseruationum*, 546 (this translation: Plat[t]er, Culpeper and Cole, *Platerus histories*, 359). This then six-year-old 65cm tall dwarf's virtually identical act at the 1568 Munich wedding is described by Wirre (*Ordenliche Beschreybung*, f.54ᵛ) and Troiano (*Dialoghi*, sig.81ᵛ; see also Katritzky, *The art of commedia*, 49).

Images and festival books relating to the 1568 Munich wedding are among the most significant records suggesting that, less than a decade after the first definite records of professional commedia dell'arte performances in Italy itself, it was established and popular at the Bavarian court.[36] Two fresco cycles of the 1570s at the Bavarian court's country seat, Castle Trausnitz at Landshut, represent some of the most important early iconographic records of the commedia dell'arte. At Wilhelm's 1568 Munich wedding, commedia dell'arte contributed to the festivities in three contexts. Some of its costumes were used in masquerades; the commedia's stock comic pair, the old Venetian master and his young manservant Zanni, entertained together on several occasions as masked clowns; and on 8 March 1568 there was a full-length play, of which Massimo Troiano's account is the earliest substantial description of a commedia dell'arte performance.[37]

As Spanish envoy, Karl I von Hohenzollern was an honoured guest at the 1568 Munich wedding, invited to take part in the dances and masquerades, seated near to the head of high table at banquets and feasts, and permitted the exceptional distinction of eating with his head covered.[38] His sons Eitel Friedrich IV and Karl II, then recent graduates of the University of Bourges, were among the young noblemen chosen to wait at high table. Eitel Friedrich IV was one of four carvers, while Karl II had probably already been Duke Albrecht V of Bavaria's trusted personal cupbearer since at least November 1565, when a Hohenzollern count accompanied Prince Ferdinand of Bavaria to Italy.[39] On 24 February 1568, one masquerade group of a costumed running at the ring featured six mounted knights, including Eitel Friedrich IV and Karl II, who respectively lost and won their rounds of the contest. With the groom Wilhelm, and his brother Ferdinand, the Hohenzollern brothers paraded on richly covered horses, in a party of six, all costumed in Moorish fashion, in cloth of gold and silver, with feather plumes on their show helmets, accompanied by seconds, pages and trumpeters in matching costumes.[40] Karl II officiated with Ferdinand of Bavaria, as two of four *Mantenadores*, or defenders, at the unmounted lance and sword tournament of 25 February, and as *Padrino*, or second, at the tournament of 1 March.[41] An emblem designed by the court musician Massimo Troiano for Karl II, who also served for a while at the court of Archduke Ferdinand, identifies him as 'Duke Albrecht's faithful cupbearer', and he was presented with a trophy after this tournament by Euphrosyne, Countess of Öttingen-Wallerstein, the bride he brought home on his return from Munich in 1569.[42]

---

[36] Wagner, *Beschreibung*; Wirre, *Ordenliche Beschreybung*; Troiano, *Dialoghi*.

[37] Troiano, *Dialoghi*, sigs.146ᵛ–152ᵛ; Heck, *Commedia dell'Arte: a guide*, 37.

[38] Troiano, *Dialoghi*, sigs.52ᵛ, 57ᵛ–8ᵛ, 74ᵛ, 89ᵛ.

[39] Troiano, *Dialoghi*, sigs.59ᵛ, 137ᵛ; Munich BHStA.GHA, Korr.Akt 924, f.1ʳ.

[40] Troiano, *Dialoghi*, sig.88ᵛ; Wagner, *Beschreibung*, sig.40ᵛ, f.41ᵛ, f.43ʳ.

[41] Troiano, *Dialoghi*, sigs.106ᵛ, 143ᵛ; Wagner, *Beschreibung*, sig.45ʳ.

[42] Troiano, *Dialoghi*, sigs.134ᵛ–5ᵛ, 137ᵛ; Schmid, *Musik*, 15–17, 32.

On Monday 8 March 1568, the renowned composer Orlando di Lasso, who counted several commedia dell'arte roles among his performing skills, acted the part of the elderly Venetian merchant Pantalone in the first extensively documented commedia dell'arte performance either side of the Alps.[43] Regardless of whether Karl I saw this, or stayed long enough at the Munich court to routinely experience its commedia dell'arte performances, it is clear that waiting at high table and participating in tournaments gave the Hohenzollern brothers excellent opportunities to see the commedia dell'arte entertainments that played such an integral part in the 1568 Munich wedding festivities. Its banquets featured, to great acclaim, *intermezzi*, brief one-act entertainments performed by the central duo of the commedia dell'arte, the masked servant–master pair Zanni and Magnifico, recorded by Troiano on 22 and 27 February.[44] All three official festival chroniclers, Massimo Troiano, Hainrich Wirre and Hans Wagner, record the Italian comedians who followed the Hohenzollern brothers' group at the costumed running at the ring of 24 February. According to Troiano, the antics of these six Zannis in Bergamasque clothes, accompanied by a Venetian Magnifico, stole the show.[45] Wirre notes that: 'they were lewd [...] Magnifici, each wearing a big, wide blue beret on his head'.[46] Wagner notes of them: 'sixteenth came several in long red robes, in the manner of Magnifici, they wore big blue caps, beside them ran four Zannis in Bergamask costume'.[47] According to Wagner, this group included the tournament's *Mantenadores*, the groom's uncle, Archduke Ferdinand of the Tirol, and his chamberlain, Giulio de Rivo. They had also led the masked procession, entering on a triumphal wagon, in long red damask robes, red caps and full-face masks complete with long grey wigs and false beards, surrounded by five music-playing goddesses or muses. The concluding group was perhaps drawn from those surrounding this first wagon, who included four footmen 'in red satin jackets and caps, and Moorish masks', and 'four on white Spanish horses in long red scarlet cloaks, with long hair and grey beards, with red Venetian caps, like the Magnifici'.[48] Archduke Ferdinand's group probably also provided the Zannis and Magnifici who entertained at table. They performed in Italian, and may have been members of a professional Italian troupe engaged by Archduke Ferdinand for the Munich wedding, rather than amateur performers chosen from amongst his Innsbruck courtiers.

Both Frischlin and Felix Platter praise the music at the 1598 Stuttgart wedding, and comment on the specially-composed music of Orlando di Lasso's son Ferdinand di Lasso, who returned from Munich to play at the wedding in Stuttgart,

---

43   Katritzky, *The art of commedia*, 55–8.

44   Troiano, *Dialoghi*, sigs.68ᵛ, 121ᵛ –2ᵛ.

45   Troiano, *Dialoghi*, sig.88ᵛ.

46   Wirre, *Ordenliche Beschreybung*, sig.40ᵛ.

47   Wagner, *Beschreibung*, sig.41ᵛ.

48   Troiano, *Dialoghi*, sig.85ᵛ; Wagner, *Beschreibung*, sig.40ᵛ.

where he had been court musician to Eitel Friedrich IV during the 1580s.[49] Three decades after taking part in the Munich wedding tournament masquerade, letters of September and October 1598 from Karl II, organizer and leader of the 10-strong Zanni group at the 1598 wedding, to Eitel Friedrich IV, assure his brother that he is having his own masquerade and tournament costumes designed and made for him in Munich.[50] It seems probable that Karl II himself provided the impetus for his tournament masquerade group's commedia dell'arte costumes, drawing on Munich experiences such as his 1565 journey to Italy with Prince Ferdinand of Bavaria, and his experience of masked Italian comedy at the 1568 Munich wedding. Similar characters at the wedding festival of Eitel Friedrich IV and Karl II's kinswoman, Jakobe von Baden, also have a Munich link (Diagram 2). A cousin of Wilhelm V of Bavaria, Jakobe grew up at the Munich court before leaving for Düsseldorf in 1585 to marry Johann Wilhelm von Jülich. Diederich Graminaeus's official festival account of her wedding records a tournament masquerade featuring two buffoons in the guise of a Venetian Magnifico and his servant. Although the servant is not identified by name, his peasant clothes, wide sailor trousers and 'strangely large hat' amply confirm him as a Zanni. The servant–master pair at Jakobe's wedding – evidently Italian professionals – performed various diverting tricks during the otherwise tedious entry of six similarly costumed noblemen.[51]

Comparative analysis of Jakob Frischlin and Felix Platter's contrasting interpretations of Karl II's tournament group emphasizes yet again that, for any number of reasons, not least lack of specialist knowledge, authors of official festival accounts are far from infallible. Even when describing festivals also known from officially-sanctioned publications, private reports such as those of the Platters offer valuable independent perspectives. While the commedia dell'arte master–servant duo of Magnifico (or Pantalone) and Zanni had become a commonplace stock fixture of the Italian stage well before 1600, the roles remained, at this time, an exotic rarity in much of German-speaking Europe. The eight specific Zanni variants named in Platter's 1598 festival account represent the most substantial evidence for Zanni types familiar in the German-speaking regions before 1600, and significant further evidence for the crucial role played by the Munich and Habsburg courts in diffusing commedia dell'arte stock roles. Karl II's group made a considerable impact in 1598, even though many of its spectators were unaware of the source of its costumes. These German descriptions of Zanni, by Felix Platter, who recognized them as such, and by Frischlin, who did not, chart transregional influences that helped promote and diffuse the commedia dell'arte beyond Italy. They are excluded from Alberto Martino's comprehensive overview of the commedia dell'arte's early German sources, and previously disregarded in connection with the commedia dell'arte. Felix Platter's accurate

---

[49]   *Felix Platter Tagebuch*, 494–5; Frischlin, *Hohenzollerische Hochzeyt*, 184–5; Schmid, *Musik*, 226–7, 238–9.

[50]   Schmid, *Musik*, 58.

[51]   Martino, 'Fonti tedesche degli anni 1565–1615', 17.

identification of their theatrical costumes reveals that they augment the known pre-1600 documentations of Zanni north of the Alps, and offer vivid insights into early modern German reception – and expectations – of the early modern Italian professional stage's most influential stock role, its comic stage servant.

PART III
Healers and Performers

Chapter 8
Queen Elizabeth, Shakespeare, and English Actors in Europe

The focus of Part II was politically motivated ceremony and spectacle promoted by religious and educational groups, civic communities and courts concerned with controlling its content and impact. The writings of Guarinonius and the Platter brothers also indicate key economic intersections and interdependencies between medicine and theatre. They contain passages relevant to health-related themes on the professional itinerant stage, and Guarinonius's stylistic choices offer insights into some literary uses of theatrical themes. Parts III and IV focus on some aspects of these issues.

Professional performers were primarily motivated by the need to earn a year-round living. They drew on a range of economic activities, including the sale of entrance tickets, and medical or non-medical trading and practice. Early modern Europe's most successful professional actors were the mixed-gender Italian commedia dell'arte troupes. While some were financed by court and civic engagements, many relied on quack medical activity. The focus of Part IV is Hippolytus Guarinonius and Thomas Platter's substantial descriptions of the medical and theatrical activities of such commedia dell'arte quack performers. Part III contextualizes these accounts within a consideration of the three physicians' writings on a wide range of professional performers and itinerants, in London and on mainland Europe. Chapter 9 overviews their accounts of the deployment of medicine and theatre by marketplace healers and performers. Chapter 10 surveys mutual influences between supernatural, medical and theatrical practices, taking as a case study the impact of magical impotence on Jacobean drama, in the light of Thomas Platter's account of its practice in Languedoc. Chapter 11 examines the three physicians' references to a group then regarded as highly significant supernatural omens, monstrous humans: as curiosity cabinet specimens, medical patients and live performers, and as performed roles.

The present chapter takes as its point of departure the brief references to English actors through which Thomas Platter and Hippolytus Guarinonius first became known to theatre historians. In contrast to their Italian rivals, itinerant English troupes relied on non-medical commercial strategies to fund mainland tours.[1] Because year-round outdoor performances are impossible in northern

---

[1] Itinerant English actors with medical training included the qualified apothecary John Buggs, who served in the troupe of the former Queen of Bohemia (Princess Elizabeth Stuart) in 1631 (Pelling, *Medical conflicts*, 161–2; Pelling and White, 'BUGGS, John').

Europe, court patronage was even more crucial to English travelling troupes than it was to the Italians. Their rise in Europe received a tremendous boost with Anna of Denmark's marriage to King James VI/I in 1589, which confirmed the courts of Anna's brother and sisters, at Kronburg Castle in Helsingør (near Copenhagen), Dresden, Wolfenbüttel, and Schloss Gottorf in Schleswig, as financially viable destinations for English actors.[2] Guarinonius, who never visited England, has achieved a minor place in mainstream theatre history through a single reference to the all-male English acting troupes touring German-speaking Europe for over a century from the 1580s, while the attention of English-speaking theatre historians was drawn to Thomas Platter through his brief eyewitness reports of two performances at unidentified London theatres in 1598. The present chapter revisits these references to English actors: Guarinonius's within an examination of the paragraph on Italian professional actors within which it occurs; Platter's within his account of his tour of England, and notably his journal entry for 21 September 1599, recording his impressions of London culture, including a performance of *Julius Caesar*.

From 18 to 26 September and 1 to 20 October 1599, Thomas Platter and several travel companions lodged in Mark Lane EC3, at Monsieur Briard's Fleur de Lys inn, near the Tower of London and Aldgate.[3] Platter spoke no English. His group was with an unidentified interpreter at Hampton Court on 27 September, and it is unclear whether Mr Button, their interpreter at the Lord Mayor's residence and Richmond Palace in mid-October, had already been engaged by 21 September.[4] That day's journal entry begins by describing two theatre performances. Platter saw *Julius Caesar* at a South Bank theatre that afternoon. The other performance, seen on an unspecified date, perhaps in Bishopsgate, is presented in the context of his detailed immediately following summary of London's taverns, theatres and other commercial leisure attractions.

Thomas Platter knew Jacob Rathgeb's account of Duke Friedrich of Württemberg's 1592 England tour, published in 1602, and perhaps also manuscripts or reports of the visits to England of Lupold von Wedel, Samuel Kiechel, Philip Duke of Stettin, and Paul Hentzner's account of chaperoning the young Silesian nobleman Christoph von Rehdiger around England in 1598, published in 1612.

---

[2]   Anna's oldest brother succeeded as King Christian IV of Denmark; her sisters Hedwig, Elisabeth and Augusta respectively married Christian II (Elector of Saxony), Duke Heinrich Julius of Braunschweig-Wolfenbüttel, and the Duke of Schleswig-Holstein-Gottorp.

[3]   *Thomas Platter d.J*, 778, 862 (18 September and 1 October 1599, London); Platter, *Englandfahrt*, XXVII; Williams, *Thomas Platter's travels in England*, 224.

[4]   *Thomas Platter d.J*, 784, 834, 865 (27 September, 13 and 17 October 1599, London). Platter's language skills (German, Latin, French and Spanish) suggest the still marginal role of English in Shakespearean Europe. According to Guarinonius, 'nothing good can be said of the recently deceased godless Queen Elizabeth of England apart from her learning and skill in all languages, notably Latin and Greek' (*Grewel*, 266).

His journal drew on personal impressions, those of previous London visitors and, above all, on the standard reference works quoted at length by such travellers.[5] He closely observes the immediate effects and *post-mortem* symptoms of heavy tobacco use by English smokers:

> which they take as a special medicine for catarrh and for pleasure. It is such a common habit with them that they always carry their instruments with them, and strike flame, light up and drink it everywhere, at the plays, the inns and elsewhere. They have it brought to each other, as we do wine, and it also makes them foolish and merry, so that they become dizzy, as if they had drunk too much wine. But it soon wears off, and because it is so enjoyable they indulge so heavily that their preachers shout about how they are ruining themselves with it. I was told that, after his death, one such was found to have the inner surfaces of all his blood vessels coated with soot, like a chimney. The leaves are brought from the Indies in large quantities, and some are much stronger than others, as one can immediately taste on the tongue. They make strange gestures while they drink it. And they first learned this medicine from the Indians, as Mr Cope, a citizen of London who spent a long time in the Indies, explained to me, whose cabinet I visited with the London doctor Matthias de Lobel.[6]

Next, Platter describes a visit to Walter Cope's curiosity cabinet, and summarizes many London tourist sights and public attractions. These include 'a large live camel in a house on the Thames Bridge' (evidently Mr Holden's famous dancing camel on old London Bridge), and several of the 37 types of male and female street trader depicted in *Parte of the criers of London*.[7] This large coloured engraving, interleaved into his journal, suggests that such prints found a ready market as popular tourist souvenirs. His account of Paris twice refers by title to an example of this genre he acquired there, the printed booklet *Cris de Paris*, detailing 136 Parisian street traders.[8] This genre originated in Italy, where examples often featured street healers, such as the toothdrawer in the lower middle of Plate 40.

Extracts from Thomas Platter's journal entry for 21 September 1599 were first published by Gustav Binz in 1899.[9] No Shakespeare specialist is unaware of its

---

[5]   Platter, *Englandfahrt*, 171–3; *Thomas Platter d.J*, XXII–XXIV; Williams, *Thomas Platter's travels in England*, 102, 136–40; Deutschländer, 'Allein auß begirdt', 57–8.

[6]   *Thomas Platter d.J*, 795–6 (21 September 1599, London). Like Felix Platter, the distinguished botanist de Lobel (1538–1616) had been a pupil of Rondelet in Montpellier (see also Dulieu, *La médecine a Montpellier: La Renaissance*, 396).

[7]   *Thomas Platter d.J*, 798–800 (21 September 1599, London).

[8]   *Thomas Platter d.J*, 555 (28 July 1599, Paris). The London print supports Sean Shesgreen's hypothesis that the earliest *Cries of London* prints predate 1600 (*Images of the outcast*, 19–21).

[9]   Binz, 'Londoner Theater', 458–62; see also Platter, *Englandfahrt*; and for further

first sentence (albeit often in second- or even third-hand translation), recording Platter's visit to a performance of *Julius Caesar*:

> On 21 September, after lunch, at around two o'clock, I travelled across the water with my companions. In the house with the straw-thatched roof, we watched the tragedy of the first emperor Julius Caesar very skilfully acted with around fifteen parts. At the end of the play they danced wonderfully with each other, extremely gracefully after their fashion, always two dressed in men's with two in women's clothes.[10]

Literary scholars share an understandable sense of dismay at this casual treatment of what is almost certainly Shakespeare's play. Platter's passport confirms that the internationally renowned English celebrity who drew Platter across the perilous Channel was not the 35-year-old playwright, still largely unknown in 1599, but Queen Elizabeth I. Bearing Elizabeth's own red wax seal, it identifies its bearers as: 'Jean Joachim Stuber, Petrus Julius, Andreas Pucher, Paulus Holtzbecher,[11] Martinus Pissetius, Thomas Platerus, high Almaynes gentilemen and schollers came latelie over, moved with à desier to see her Mayeste an the conntrey'.[12] Platter obtained this passport from the Blackfriars residence of Henry Brooke, Lord Cobham, on 20 October for himself and the five German travel companions with whom he left for Dover that same afternoon. Platter and Ludwig Jaske of Danzig had been joined in Paris by two Silesians, Andreas Bucher of Breslau[13] and his Polish tutor, the recently qualified physician Martin Pisecius. In London they were joined by Peter Julius of Denmark and Hans Joachim Stüber von Battenheim of Eisch in Franconia, two fellow lodgers at the Fleur de Lys inn. Known to Platter from Languedoc, Julius and Stüber continued with him from Calais.

Family connections and medical expertise helped Thomas Platter achieve his main aim in England, an audience with Queen Elizabeth. His future wife Crischona Jeckelmann's older brother Heinrich was born in 1565, the year in which their barber-surgeon uncle Franz Jeckelmann[14] died of the plague, deeply regretting ever entering the family practice, and having 'been extremely melancholy for a long time, saying that although he was an operator, he had no wish to be a murderer'.[15] Rejecting surgery, Heinrich Jeckelmann studied theology and languages and travelled widely, spending nine years with the governor of Dover, and staying in

---

English translations of the passage, Williams, *Thomas Platter's travels in England*; Schanzer, 'Thomas Platter's observations', 466.

[10]   *Thomas Platter d.J*, 791 (21 September 1599, London).

[11]   Perhaps an otherwise unidentified servant; or possibly Jaske, who signed Platter's friendship album as 'Ludwich Kuene Jaschky genandt', travelling under yet another alias.

[12]   *Thomas Platter d.J*, 868 (20 October 1599, Dover).

[13]   Now Wrocław, Poland.

[14]   Older brother of Felix Platter's wife Madlen.

[15]   *Felix Platter Tagebuch*, 438 (9 January 1565, Basle).

London with Lord Cobham's brother, George Brooke.[16] Within 24 hours of Platter's arrival in England, Edward Kempe, the elderly mayor of Dover, was brought to his inn with aches and stomach cramps. Uzès, the small town where Platter started his medical practice, supported a spice merchant, three barber-surgeons and no less than eight apothecaries.[17] Dover had none, and Platter's prescriptions had to be made up and delivered by the Canterbury apothecary Joseph Calf. They swiftly alleviated the suffering of Kempe, totally cured when Platter returned to Dover five weeks later. Kempe's appreciation earned Platter a letter of introduction to Lord Cobham, who issued his passport to France and a document authorizing his group's access to private inner chambers of royal palaces.[18] This facilitated two personal encounters with Elizabeth.

At the now destroyed Nonsuch Palace, the Lord Admiral[19] authorized access to the 66-year-old queen's audience chamber:

> Soon we were led up to the reception chamber, and placed well to the front, so that we would be able to see the queen all the better [...] After we had waited there a short while, perhaps between twelve and one o'clock, several men with white maces came out of an inner chamber, and behind them many high ranking great lords, and they were closely followed by the queen. Alone, unescorted, she still walked quite steadily and upright, sat down in the reception chamber on a chair padded with many gold embroidered red damask cushions. The cushions lay almost on the floor, the chair was so low, under a canopy that was most magnificently attached to the top of the stage. She was decoratively dressed in the most expensive manner.[20]

Platter's account, an exceptionally comprehensive record of Nonsuch Palace and its gardens,[21] offers observations on Elizabeth's apparel, her courtiers, servants and guards, and how she read, listened to a sermon, commanded the preacher to hurry up and finish it, left with her maid of honour, and returned shortly to take her midday meal and listen to some music played by her trumpeters and shawm players before withdrawing to her inner chambers with her courtiers. Two days

---

[16]   Executed for treason in 1603. *Thomas Platter d.J*, 811–12 (25 September 1599, London).

[17]   *Thomas Platter d.J*, 218 (21 April 1597, Uzès). In the 1660s, John Ray marvels that 'the number of apothecaries in this little city [Montpellier] is scarce credible there being thirty shops, and yet all find something to do' (Mortoft, *His book*, 25n3).

[18]   *Thomas Platter d.J*, 775, 869 (17 September and 23 October 1599, Dover).

[19]   Charles, Lord Howard of Effingham, patron of the distinguished professional English acting company, The Lord Howard's Men, later known as The Admiral's Men.

[20]   *Thomas Platter d.J*, 827 (26 September 1599, Nonsuch).

[21]   Chambrier, 'La relation', 174.

later, she received and imprisoned Robert Devereux, second Earl of Essex on his return from Ireland.[22] Platter, meanwhile, returned to Lord Howard, who:

> commanded his (*secretario*) scribe to write me a letter addressed to all those living in royal residences, that they must show me and my group not just the gardens, large halls, chapels and chambers, but also the small royal cabinets and the precious things kept in them. Which we afterwards used now and again. Because shortly before, an attempt had been made to poison the queen by sprinkling powder on the chair that she sat on and touched with her hands, she never again wanted to allow anyone into her rooms without the Lord Admiral's authorization.[23]

During the following weeks, Platter visited Hampton Court, enjoyed music in Windsor Castle's chapel, inspected Eton College, stayed at The Bear (then as now in Bear Lane, Oxford) while viewing 10 of Oxford's 16 colleges, and toured further royal residences, including Woodstock Manor and Greenwich.[24] At Richmond Palace, he was advising a Montpellier student friend, Kaspar Thomann, on the niceties of applying for an Oxford scholarship when:

> the queen came out of her reception chamber alone, unescorted, with all her lords, councillors, bodyguards and court servants. She walked closely past us, and most of the onlookers fell to their knees. When, through a window in the corridor, she looked at her people outside in the courtyard, they all fell to the ground on their knees together in the courtyard, and she spoke in English to them: God bles mi piple! [...] And all together they cried in reply: God save the Queen! [...] and remained motionless on their knees until she gave a sign with her hand that they should stand up, which they did with the greatest reverence they possibly could. Because this much is certain: the English don't simple regard her as their queen, but also as their god.[25]

Platter's astonishment at the reverence the English showed for their queen does not mask his own enthusiasm for watching her. His audiences with Elizabeth fulfilled a planned aspiration; his attendance at the 21 September 1599 performance of *Julius Caesar* was a random act of chance. His description of its concluding jig, like the accounts of other London visitors such as Paul Hentzner, contributes to our understanding of theatrical jigs, excluded from published playtexts, as the integral conclusion to Elizabethan theatre performances, with the clown as their master of

---

[22]   Platter, *Englandfahrt*, XXXII.
[23]   *Thomas Platter d.J*, 831–2 (26 September 1599, Nonsuch).
[24]   *Thomas Platter d.J*, 843–65 (27 September – 17 October 1599, England).
[25]   *Thomas Platter d.J*, 866–7 (17 October 1599, Richmond).

ceremonies.[26] One specialist imaginatively conjures from this 'jarring and bizarre' report of a 'naive theatre critic' the image of 'the elegant jig of Caesar and the boy dressed as Caesar's wife'.[27] A more straightforward interpretation suggests that Platter is describing a jig danced by several groups, each of four male actors costumed as two couples in contemporary dress. Interrogation of Platter's reference to *Julius Caesar* has largely focused on the single issue of whether or not it refers to the Globe production of Shakespeare's famous play. Even the exact placing of one particular hyphen in E. K. Chambers' translation has generated conflicting opinions on the extent to which 'a shocking mistranslation' of 'the reflections of a late sixteenth-century German tourist' may or may not be regarded as 'dangerous'.[28] Binz identified the theatre as 'almost certainly' the Globe, whose construction on London's South Bank was initiated on behalf of The Chamberlain's Men on 20 January 1599. He inclined towards identifying the play as Shakespeare's *Julius Caesar*, rather than a *Julius Caesar* play by another playwright, such as one he notes in the 1594 repertoire of Shakespeare's own company.[29] The majority verdict, that Platter is describing 'what was obviously Shakespeare's play at a theatre obviously the Globe',[30] in an account providing the most important *post quem* for the Globe's completion, seems a victory for common sense.[31] Some scholars cite Platter's passage without articulating a clear verdict on this issue.[32] Inconsistencies in Platter's account, not least that Shakespeare's *Julius Caesar* has more than 15 parts, lead others to alternative theories. Schanzer notes that the two variables are not unrelated: if the theatre was the Globe, then by definition the actors were The Chamberlain's Men, staging Shakespeare's *Julius Caesar*. His suggestion that an unidentified *Julius Caesar*, performed by The Lord Admiral's Men at the Rose, could equally plausibly fit Platter's description is rejected by Taylor but accepted by Egan.[33] Noting that the 1599 autumn equinox fell on 13 September, eight days before its official date of 21 September, according to the Julian calendar then used in England, Sohmer suggests that Shakespeare wrote *Julius Caesar* specifically to

---

[26]   Hentzner, *Travels*, 29 ('Without the city are some Theatres, where English actors represent almost every day tragedies and comedies to very numerous audiences; these are concluded with excellent music, variety of dancers, and the excessive applause of those that are present'); Wiles, *Shakespeare's clown*, 53–6; Holmes, 'Time for the plebs', para.14.

[27]   Wilson, 'Is this a holiday?', 31, 35

[28]   Chambers, *The Elizabethan stage*, II, 364–6; Schanzer, 'Thomas Platter's observations', 465; Tiffany, 'Review', 42; Spong, 'Bad quartos', 66–9.

[29]   Binz, 'Londoner Theater', 462–3.

[30]   Kermode, 'Julius Caesar', 1147 (see also 1964–5).

[31]   Platter, *Englandfahrt*, XXX, 151; *Thomas Platter d.J*, 791n2; Deutschländer, 'Allein auß begirdt', 61; Wilson, 'Is this a holiday?', 31; Aaron, 'The Globe', 281; Holmes, 'Time for the plebs', para.32.

[32]   Sohmer, '12 June 1599', paras.5 and 6.

[33]   Schanzer, 'Thomas Platter's observations', 466–7; Wells and Taylor, *William Shakespeare*, 121; Egan, 'The Lords Howard's Men', 234.

comment on the Elizabethan calendar controversy, for performance at the opening of the Globe, on the summer solstice 1599.[34]

Platter immediately follows his account of *Julius Caesar* with his fuller description of an undated visit to an unidentified London play: 'On another occasion, also after the [midday] meal, I saw a play not far from our inn, in the suburbs, I seem to remember at Bishopsgate'. Given his limited English language skills and preference for group sightseeing in London, he is unlikely to have attended it unaccompanied.[35] Platter, who habitually identifies himself as German, and is described in his passport to England as a 'high Almaynes gentilemen and scholler',[36] continues:

> In this, members of diverse nations presented themselves, each of whom an Englishman had to fight for a girl. And he conquered all of them except for the German. He won the girl by fighting, sat himself down next to her, and because of this drank himself into extreme drunkenness with his servant, until they were both drunk. Then the servant threw a shoe at his master's head, and they both fell asleep. Meanwhile, the Englishman climbed into the camp and abducted the German's prize. In this way he even outwitted the German. At the end, they also danced most gracefully, in English and Irish fashion.[37]

Binz, unable to identify this comedy, is convinced that it was staged at the Curtain.[38] With reference to its concluding jigs, and to the clownish Carlo Buffone's threat in *Every man out of his humour*, first staged in 1599: 'I warrant you: would I had one of *Kemps* shooes to throw after you', some specialists accept Creizenach's suggestion that the shoe-thrower Platter saw in September or October 1599 was played by Shakespeare's celebrated clown, William Kemp.[39] Kemp was still with The Chamberlain's Men when they finalized plans to move from the Curtain. He signed the lease for a one-tenth share in the Globe on 21 February 1599 with Shakespeare, Thomas Pope, Augustine Philips and John Heminges, but sold his share back to them shortly afterwards and is thought to have stayed at the Curtain when they moved to the Globe.[40] Renowned for his comic jigs, in February 1600 he famously danced the morris all the way from London to Norwich. Hecht agrees that the theatre was the Curtain, while noting that the EC2 location of The

---

[34]   Sohmer, '12 June 1599', para.14.

[35]   *Pace* Egan, 'Thomas Platter's account', 55.

[36]   *Thomas Platter d.J*, 356–8 (5–6 February 1599, Montserrat), 813 (25 September 1599, London), 868 (20 October 1599, Dover); Deutschländer, 'Allein auß begirdt', 64–5.

[37]   *Thomas Platter d.J*, 791–2 (21 September 1599, London).

[38]   Binz, 'Londoner Theater', 463.

[39]   Jonson, *Workes*, 154 (IV.viii); Creizenach, *Das englische Drama*, 344, and 'Verloren gegangene englische Dramen', 42; Chambers, *The Elizabethan stage*, II, 365; Wiles, *Shakespeare's clown*, 36.

[40]   Wiles, *Shakespeare's clown*, 34–6, 117; Aaron, 'The Globe', 279–81.

Mermaid, in Bread Street near St Paul's, was close to Platter's inn.[41] Noting that shoe-throwing is not unique to Platter's comedy, Egan suggests yet another theatre not excluded by Platter's vague geographic indications, the Boar's Head, known to have used stage booths of a kind possibly indicated by Platter's phrase 'die zelten'.[42]

Platter's journal entry for 21 September provides valuable contextualization for London's theatre culture:

> Thus, at two in the afternoon, two, sometimes even three plays are performed daily in various places in the city of London, each ridiculing the others, because those who perform best get the most spectators. The places are constructed in such a way that they act on a raised stage, and everyone can see everything well. However there are separate galleries and seats where it is more entertaining and comfortable to sit, for this reason one also pays more. For he who remains standing below pays only one English penny, but if he wants to sit, he is then allowed to enter a door on payment of another penny; but if he desires to sit on cushions in the most entertaining place, where he not only sees everything well but can also be seen, then he pays a further English penny at a second door. And during the play, food and drink is carried around among the spectators, so that in this way anyone can also refresh themselves at their own expense. The actors are most expensively and elegantly costumed, because it is the custom in England that when eminent aristocrats or knights die, they bequeath and donate almost their best clothes to their servants. Because it is not proper for them to do so, they do not wear such clothes, but rather offer them for sale cheaply to the actors. Anyone who has ever seen them perform or act is well aware of how long they could merrily spend every day at the plays. [...] The English pass their time with such and many other diversions. At the plays they find out what is going on in other countries, and neither men nor women hesitate to go to the aforementioned places, because most English are not much given to travelling, but are content to learn of foreign matters and enjoy their diversions at home. There are very many inns, public houses and beer taverns distributed around the city, in which one can also be greatly diverted by eating, drinking, music and the like; in this way, performers came to our inn nearly every day [...] There are also strict municipal regulations regarding prostitutes [...] But despite stringent attempts to control them, large crowds of such women swarm up and down the city, and in the beer taverns and playhouses.[43]

---

[41]   Platter, *Englandfahrt*, XXX, 36–7, 151–2.

[42]   Generally translated as 'the tents', 'a tent' or even 'the tent', but in this context here translated as 'the camp'. Schanzer, 'Thomas Platter's observations', 465; Egan, 'Thomas Platter's account', 54–6; Egan, 'NTQ book reviews', 290.

[43]   *Thomas Platter d.J*, 792, 794–5, 799 (21 September 1599, London).

Because the regulation of theatrical performances was especially stringent within the City of London, many London theatres were located just outside the legal limits of its city walls. The performers who came almost daily to Platter's inn are almost certainly musicians, not 'fugitive inn-playing' actors staging performances of the type officially banned within the City of London.[44] His explicit inclusion of women as well as men at these diversions is rare and significant evidence for regular female play-going in pre-1600 London.[45] Strikingly, Platter's account of London refers to theatrical venues as places ('örteren', 'örter'), or playhouses ('comoedien plätz'), using 'theatrum' only for commercial blood sports arenas:

> There is also in the city of London, not far from the horsemarket,[46] which is a great square, a house, in which [...] cockfights are held, and I saw this place, which is constructed like a (theatrum) theatre. In the middle of the same, on the floor, is a circular table covered with straw and surrounded by high ledges, on which the cocks are set against each other and incited, and those who are betting against each other on which cock will kill the other, sit the very closest around the round platform, however, the spectators who have paid to enter are seated round above.[47]

Comments such as 'the inhabitants [of Barcelona] often told us about such things at the plays and elsewhere' or 'Castilians and Catalans do not much like each other, as I saw from their plays'[48] suggest that Platter visited the theatre frequently while in Spain. His account of Catalan theatrical culture proves his familiarity with the use of the term 'theatre' as a playhouse, and illuminates yet another major economic intersection between medicine and commercial theatre:

> In Barcelona much entertainment is also to be had at the plays, for which special places (*theatra*) have been built, in which many can watch what and how they are (*agieret*) performed, because the actors present them on raised stages. When many people are present, the young boys who have been raised in the [foundling] hospital bring many comfortable armchairs for which there is room on the floor, as there is no seating. The gentry sit down in these, each paying at least half a real for one armchair, this is a little more than one batzen, many pay more. This money, which amounts to a very large sum each year, is used to the best effect by the hospital, which does not just provide the armchairs, but also these (*theatra*) theatres, from which they also receive a rental income. At all such plays and performances of this type, alms are levied, in order to demonstrate that people who don't mind paying to see such diversions should not forget the poor. And

---

44   *Pace* Menzer, 'Tragedians', 176.
45   See also Mann, 'Female play-going', 62; Lough, *Paris theatre audiences*, 19.
46   Keiser identifies this as West Smithfield (*Thomas Platter d.J*, 792n2).
47   *Thomas Platter d.J*, 792–3 (21 September 1599, London).
48   *Thomas Platter d.J*, 346, 381 (28 January and 24 February 1599, Barcelona).

even though Barcelona has an exceptionally large, well-built hospital, which I saw, and by whose quality I was greatly impressed, I was still informed that this same hospital, like the others in Spain, has little or no regular income. Rather, they receive a great deal from the aforementioned places, and the nobility and rich people send daily contributions of enough meat, bread, wine, money and the like, that the hospitals always have more than enough, and even a lot left over. In the aforementioned places I saw many good comedies excellently played by the Spanish, with all sorts of unusual plots. And once, when a valuable diamond was mislaid at a gathering of this type, in order to get it back again, after stern threats about how everyone would be searched, each person was forced to plunge their closed hand into *one* tub of bran, and pull out their open hand. When everyone had done this, the ring lay in the bran.[49]

Platter's account of London's cultural diversions is all the more valuable for being contextualized within the broader perspective of his journal. It informs current understanding of early modern theatre practice, and continues to inspire innovative Shakespeare scholarship.

Both Thomas Platter and Guarinonius refer to itinerant troupes of English players in northern Europe. English actors drew heavily on commedia dell'arte stage practice but rejected quackery as a basis for their commercial activities. Instead, they charged spectators a fee to see their shows, and supported the high cost of touring the European mainland with various non-medical commercial activities. Their travels between English and northern Europe courts often facilitated the exchange of people, goods and politically sensitive information. Robert Browne's troupe dealt in arms, livestock, and boy and adult performers. As early as 1595, Queen Elizabeth I made Browne responsible for transporting from England to her 'Cousin the Lantgrave of Hessen [...] one hundred longe Bowes of Ewe and two thousand Arrowes', and a second, even larger shipment of similar arms.[50] In 1604, Browne carried an embassy pass facilitating exports confirmed by English diplomatic correspondence from Paris: 'the king hath at this present signed a warrant under his hande, to one Browne an English Comedian, for ye transporting of doggs Beares and Apes etc. for his specyal pleasures, a sure argument of his martial intentions'.[51] Several broadsheets of around 1621 depict an English stage fool, or Pickelhering, as an arms merchant claiming: 'Unlike other fools, I don't deal in expensive Italian silk goods' (Plate 31). This alludes to the commercial activities of English actors such as Robert Browne, George Vincent, and especially Thomas Sackville. Sackville retired from his successful acting career to become a full-time cloth merchant in Wolfenbüttel, where the

---

[49]   *Thomas Platter d.J*, 347–8 (28 January 1599, Barcelona). On the directly preceding description of performances by the French acrobat Buratin, see Chapter 9, this volume.

[50]   Brand, 'Robert Browne', 41, 108. Maurice, Landgrave of Hessen-Kassel (1572–1632) was an accomplished musician and composer, and a great patron of English actors.

[51]   Yates, 'English actors in Paris', 402.

imposing half-timbered house in which he lived with his family from 1602 to his death in 1628 stills stands at Kanzleistrasse 1, just off the town's main market square.[52] George Vincent imported goods and performers to the Polish court from at least 1617, when London Privy Council passes permitted him to bring eight musicians, including Richard Jones and the 10-year-old boy-player John Wayde, to Warsaw. In 1618, Vincent brought assorted luxury goods, five musicians, his own wife and children, and Richard Jones's wife Harris Jones, to Warsaw.[53]

Thomas Platter's only reference to English travelling troupes occurs in his description of Parisian theatre life, where he notes them among foreign troupes sometimes sharing the stage of the Hôtel de Bourgogne with Valleran-le-Conte's French troupe.[54] Guarinonius's sole reference to English actors of any type is a digression on such English travelling troupes, within an account of itinerant Italian actors, in his most sustained theoretical consideration of the stage.[55] Guarinonius's aside on the English players, and the chapter of *Grewel* in which it occurs, won wide recognition by being quoted almost in full in the opening pages of an influential early monograph on English actors in German-speaking Europe, which, however, makes no reference to his far more significant commedia dell'arte descriptions.[56] The relevant passage contrasts the performances of Italian comedians with those of itinerant English players:

> Similar plays and spectacles can now be seen in Germany, and their actors, as I myself have seen, are from Netherlandish and English cities. They travel around, from one town to another, performing their amusing farces and acrobatics (but without unseemliness) to a considerable extent, as far as they can, in German and with the use of mime, in exchange for payment by those who wish to watch and hear them.[57]

At which point Guarinonius returns to describing Italian commedia dell'arte troupes staging their performances in the context of quack activities, as free shows attracting potential customers for medical products and services. Guarinonius's

---

[52]   The 'water poet' John Taylor and his actor brother William Taylor (an accomplished lutenist based at the Saxony court of Count Ernst III zu Holstein-Schaumburg in Bückeburg c.1607–30) stayed with Sackville in this house for two days in September 1620, en route to a court christening in Prague (Taylor, *Trauels*, sig.B4ᵛ).

[53]   Riewald, 'English actors', 89–90; Schrickx, 'Pickleherring', 140; Limon, *Gentlemen of a company*, 100–102.

[54]   See Chapter 12, this volume.

[55]   Guarinonius, *Grewel*, 213–15 (Book 2, Chapter 17).

[56]   'Guarinonius über die Schauspielkunst in 1609'. (Meissner, *Die englischen Comoedianten*, 1–12. The monograph quotes Guarinonius's reference to English players three times: 6, 10, 51).

[57]   Guarinonius, *Grewel*, 214. See also Innsbruck UL, Cod.110, I, f.308ᵛ; Chapter 13, this volume.

substantial index lists this passage under the terms 'Engellåndische Comedianten' and 'Teutsche Comœdianten' but has no entry for Netherlandish troupes.[58] By 1610, Netherlandish professional troupes were not yet touring Germany, although some prominent English actors were permanently settled in German courts or Netherlandish cities, often with local wives. Guarinonius was more probably acknowledging the Netherlands as a popular European base for English troupes at this time, than anachronistically referring to Netherlandish as well as English troupes.

According to Bücking, Guarinonius saw English players after 1600 in 'an unidentified south German city', which Dörrer thought to be Munich.[59] Specialists have generally followed Meissner's lead in seeking the source for Guarinonius's familiarity with English actors in the performances of John Green's renowned itinerant troupe at the court at Graz in November 1607 and February 1608.[60] Correspondence between its ruler, Archduke Ferdinand (II), and his kinsman Duke Wilhelm of Bavaria, kept Graz courtiers well-informed of the Bavarian court's anti-theatrical tendencies (Diagram 2). In 1597, religious melancholy led Wilhelm to abdicate in favour of his heir Maximilian and spend the last two decades of his life in reclusive contemplation. In a letter of January 1595, he had exhorted Ferdinand (II) to observe the Lenten prohibition of carnival pursuits and theatrical entertainments, and to punish and renounce 'unseemly households and other bestial sins, all manner of wanton people, such as buffoons, jesters, actors, and suchlike wretches, and not to tolerate them at court'.[61] While representing Graz at the Diet of Regensburg in February 1608, Ferdinand (II) received a very different type of letter, describing the visit of John Green's troupe to his court. From his 18-year-old sister Archduchess Maria Magdalena, it particularly emphasizes the English actors' propriety and lack of lewdness.[62] The longstanding tradition of linking Guarinonius's reference to the English players to performances by John Green's troupe at Graz in the winter of 1607 to 1608 persists in this context.[63] Hippolytus Guarinonius, whose brother Johann Andreas Guarinonius was a courtier at Graz, served Archduke Ferdinand (II) in Hall, but was never, as is sometimes suggested, the court physician at Graz. Regardless of whether Guarinonius saw Green's troupe perform, or was even kept informed about his Graz visit, my examination of the manuscript version of *Grewel* definitively excludes all but three words of it from referring to John Green's 1607–8 Graz season. The manuscript's format and internal dating confirm that he wrote it sequentially from start to finish,

---

[58]   Guarinonius, *Grewel*, 'Register: E' and 'Register: T'.

[59]   Bücking, *Kultur und Gesellschaft in Tirol*, 97; Dörrer, 'Guarinoni als Volks-schriftsteller', 141.

[60]   Meissner, *Die englischen Comoedianten*, 10.

[61]   Valentin, *Theatrum Catholicum*, 28–9.

[62]   Meissner, *Die englischen Comoedianten*, 76–82; Morris, 'A Hapsburg letter', 14; Murad, *The English comedians*, 4–11.

[63]   Morris, 'A Hapsburg letter', 17; Limon, *Gentlemen of a company*, 120.

one chapter after another, from first to last, from 1604 to 1609, with revisions likewise sequential, and relatively few changes from the revised manuscript to the published version.[64] Both sentences referring to the English actors appear in the main body of the text of a manuscript section written in 1606, over a year before Green's arrival in Graz.

The phrase 'doch ohne Ungebuehr', found neither in the main text nor *addenda* of the manuscript, may have been added by Guarinonius when the section was revised in 1608, or possibly even just before publication in 1610. Discrepancies between the manuscript and the published version (including omission of a manuscript *addendum* criticizing masquerades and mumming at the court of Prague, and addition of a further comment concerning seemliness on the stage not to be found in the manuscript, both later in this same paragraph), indicate the possibility of minor but conscious authorial or editorial toning-down of polemic, perhaps attempting to exclude Habsburg courts from the negative implications of Guarinonius's criticism of travelling players. A suggestion that it indicates that the English players were not required to pay taxes on their entrance money is unconvincing.[65] More likely, Guarinonius was favourably contrasting non-Italian performances with the bawdier commedia dell'arte, perhaps adding this phrase to guard against his remarks concerning the English comedians from being read as criticism of Habsburg cultural politics. Whether or not this three-word parenthetic note commenting on the non-Italian players' lack of unseemliness refers directly to Green's Graz performances, the rest of the passage predates them. It is unlikely that Guarinonius was even kept well-informed on Green's troupe. *Grewel*'s section on fencing, written in November 1609, the year after their visit, notes a fencing accident between two young noblemen at Graz, but not the rapier and dagger fight described in Maria Magdalena's letter to Ferdinand II, in which the English player 'with the long red hair' (probably John Green himself), stabbed a Frenchman to death and was himself seriously wounded.[66] Thomas Platter and Hippolytus Guarinonius's brief allusions to the English players achieved integration into mainstream theatre history a century before their substantial commedia dell'arte descriptions attracted specialist interest. Before turning to these latter in Part IV, the remaining chapters of this section examine the wider context within which the Italian professionals, and other marketplace itinerants, healed and performed.

---

[64]   *Grewel*'s references to dates include: 'last year, 1604' (49); 1605 (53, 74); 'last year, 1605' (159, 293, 310, 318, 376); 1606 (100, 125, 136, 148, 200, 347); 'last year, 1606' (469); 1607 (409, 444, 446, 545, 615, 705, 775); that the page in question was being revised in 1608 (54, 238); 1608 (440, 900, 934); that serious illness had forced a break of several weeks from 7.2.1608 (791); 1609 (969, 1011, 1071, 1173, 1074, 1196, 1224, 1296); author aged 37 (1156); 'next year, 1610' (1208); 31.12.1609 (1330).

[65]   *Pace* Limon, *Gentlemen of a company*, 120; Balme, 'Cultural anthropology', 50n44.

[66]   Guarinonius, *Grewel*, 1192; Murad, *The English comedians*, 8–11, 24.

Chapter 9
Marketplace Healers and Performers

In the decades around 1600, healers and performers, and their striving towards increasing economic prosperity and professionalism, were richly intertwined. On mainland Europe, itinerant theatrical and medical economies did not merely overlap, but were so interdependent that one cannot usefully be considered without the other. The most visible and public economic interface between healing and performance is offered by early modern charlatan or quack troupes, many of whom aimed to seamlessly integrate their medical practice or trading with their performances.[1] For the English actors considered in the previous chapter, trading activities were supplementary to their performances, carried out in different times and places from them, and non-medical. The most common type of commercial activity associated with itinerant French and Italian acting troupes was quackery. On their stages, healing was performance. Especially when they harnessed the healing power of music and laughter, performance often also became their most effective medicine. Quacks were the least respectable and respected early modern healers. Situated on a broad continuum seamlessly bridging the gaping chasm between the solidly respectable municipal merchant or medical practitioner and reviled, rootless mountebanks and beggars, quacks combined, in widely varying proportions, three elements: the medical, the itinerant and the theatrical. Quack activity involved the broad health areas of healing, hygiene and cosmetics. Some quacks sold herbs, drugs, pharmaceuticals, patent medicines and other portable products. Others also provided services, prescribing and administering medications and treatment to patients, either for a variety of ailments or as specialists. Some travelled the length and breadth of Europe, from one annual fair or public spa to another, many stayed within their own country or region, or travelled only intermittently.

---

[1]   For a nuanced consideration of the early modern licensed London physician as being separated from the quack by an 'excluded middle' of 'so-called irregular practitioners' qualified in an extensive range of recognized medical occupations, including barber-surgeons and apothecaries, see Pelling, *Medical conflicts*, 12–13, 148–65, 332–43. On specifically Italian quacks, see Gentilcore, *Medical charlatanism*. See also Katritzky, *Women, medicine and theatre*, 5n7: 'The area of overlap between mountebanks, charlatans and quacksalvers is great and disputed. Broadly speaking, mountebanks are itinerant performers who may or may not sell medical products or services, charlatans are itinerant performers who sell medical products and services, and quacksalvers are sellers of medical products and services who may or may not be itinerant or perform in public'.

Thomas Platter's account of Zan Bragetta's Avignon performances of 1598 and Guarinonius's descriptions of professional comic stage routines are two of the relatively rare detailed eyewitness accounts explicitly linking healing and spectacle within the same early modern Italian itinerant troupe. These texts, which contain some of the most substantial and significant evidence for the degree to which commedia dell'arte and quack troupes were not discrete performing and healing groups, but could profoundly synthesize the two spheres of economic activity even at the level of celebrated acting troupes, are the subject of Part IV. Early modern quacks were not a tightly defined group. In many municipalities, itinerant traders, healers and performers were covered by the same regulations. The present chapter provides an overview of how and where quack troupes performed, practiced and traded. It considers some descriptions of market traders and performers by the three physicians which do not clarify whether or how they combined performing and healing. It concludes with Guarinonius's account of how he, as a qualified physician, drew on overtly quack methods to treat a patient whose health had been gravely compromised by an ignorant itinerant healer.

Professional theatre and fairground spectacle were staged by independent travelling troupes. Only the most successful received long- or short-term acting engagements from prestigious public or private sponsors enabling them to earn their living independently of non-performing commercial activity. Most were financially dependent on alternating between making arrangements to rent suitable venues privately and cover their costs with entrance tickets to their performances, and setting up their stages in public places and paying their way by trading. Each community had its own definition of itinerant traders, and its own municipal bye-laws for regulating their healing and performing activities. Early modern itinerants could no more perform or sell how, where, what or when they wanted to than modern street traders. Quacks, non-medical traders and performers generally underwent the same standard procedure for gaining the right to perform in public, administered by the same officials. North or south of the Alps, they were required to compete and pay for short-term licences, authorizing them to perform for a set period in a specified public place. Troupes had to supplicate in advance, in writing, for licences from the civic authorities who controlled the territories in which they wished to perform. If successful, the troupe was required to pay a licence fee, and to adhere to strict regulations covering their activities, which varied from one city to another. In some regions it was obligatory to display the appropriate licence. Troupe leaders, especially those ambitious to be regarded as contenders in the fierce competition for regular concessions at the larger trade fairs, generally played by the rules. They were well aware that respect for local regulations and payment of the licence fee were the main reasons most civic authorities tolerated their activities at all.

Civic authorities kept accurate records of supplications. The granting of trading and performing licences was primarily economically motivated. Both authorities and performers were concerned to maximize their profits. The fee obtained from the troupes for their licences, and any payment they received from the authorities, was entered in the city accounts and all the paperwork, including these accounts and the annotated supplications, was filed for reference in the city archives. Licences were valid for a set period in a specified public place. Troupes often exported their shows across regional and national boundaries, arranging tours to minimize travel expenses and maximize earnings, touring from one trade fair, marketplace or spa resort to another. Locations with the greatest potential for attracting profitable crowds, such as market squares at the time of lucrative annual trade fairs, were hotly contested by performers capable of earning enough to cover their expensive licence fees.

Consummate self-publicists, quacks were essentially itinerant commercial showmen who drew on a combination of medical and theatrical strategies to attract customers, and to promote and advertise their pharmaceuticals and healthcare services. Some were also promoters of theatrical spectacle, and they have earned wide recognition as a significant influence on the rise of professional acting and popular entertainment, through their employment of performers to attract customers for their wares. Only the poorest, most uneducated or most unworldly itinerant medical traders did not support their commercial activities with at least minimal theatricality. Herb-sellers, charlatans, toothdrawers and pedlars habitually deployed animals or props such as a chain of drawn teeth (Plate 40), monkeys, exotic parasols, showy costume, or prominently displayed licences, handbills, posters and other promotional material (Plate 37), speeches and other spectacle. Many travelling salespeople integrated their trading with shows sometimes or always performed in public and for free, to attract potential purchasers for the products or services whose sale provided their actual income. Travelling quack troupes sweetened their 'commercial breaks' with free shows involving anything from brief comic, musical or animal routines to full-length plays. They recognized spectacle encouraging laughter as an excellent and cost-effective way of attracting potential customers for medical goods and services, and often closely integrated their performing and non-performing activities into the same session. Some operated alone, others travelled in large troupes with their own sophisticated managerial and manufacturing infrastructures. Numerous depictions of quack troupes can be identified, not least through the most characteristic visual indicator of their activity, the medicine chest from which they typically marketed their wares on their public benches or stages (frontispiece, Plates 5, 33–8).

As a major economic threat, performing quacks suffered a relentless and increasingly coordinated three-pronged establishment attack from medical, performing and religious rivals. Sedentary musicians and actors did their utmost to discourage competition from itinerant performers. Considering its authority undermined by both their theatrical and medical activities, the Church deployed increasingly sophisticated rhetoric to differentiate quack performances from approved dramatic options. Itinerants staging all-male performances were savagely criticized for featuring actors cross-dressed in female roles, while troupes including actresses were accused of employing prostitutes. Substantial areas of quack healing were condemned as heretical witchcraft. If Lutherans were on occasion theatre-friendly, some other Protestant sects, including Calvinists, condemned all theatre. The Catholic Church discouraged attendance at the free performances of itinerant performers, which it recognized as dangerous competition for Church-sponsored all-male Jesuit and other religious school plays, sermons, music, ceremony and ritual. A third source of opposition was from the medical establishment. Qualified sedentary physicians routinely criticized unlicensed healers for their inability to understand Latin, denigrating them as 'mad and rash' rabble, lousy vermin, even as murderers.[2] That they also viewed them as a serious economic threat is tellingly highlighted by Guarinonius's anecdote of an eminent local merchant. Worth 'a hundred thousand florins and more' but too avaricious to invest a fair fee in a qualified doctor or apothecary: 'when he fell ill, he did not call for a qualified, educated physician, but eventually put his trust in a runaway stableboy who had taken up healing. Who, perhaps not without his heirs' extreme satisfaction, dispatched him to the cemetery within two days'.[3]

Concerned to curb unlicensed activities, physicians denigrated the activities of itinerants and promoted aggressive anti-quack measures. Those of Montpellier, a stronghold of the medical profession, were known for their strictness. Felix Platter's journal paraphrases his father's comments, in a letter of August 1556, on the harsh treatment of quacks breaching Montpellier's regulations:

> He also warned me not to let the Germans I was medically treating take advantage of me, so that I would not run the risk of being punished in the way that is traditionally meted out in Montpellier to those who practice medicine without a qualification. Namely, they are mounted backwards on an ass and made to hold its tail in their hand as reins, and in this way, they are mockingly led around and out of the city, with boys throwing mud at them.[4]

Thomas Platter encountered the custom, similar to the punishment of quacks in fourteenth-century London,[5] during his first semester at Montpellier. He was one of several medical students unsuccessfully attempting to banish a quack:

> No itinerant (*empiric*) or quacksalver or theriac seller is permitted to sell or practice in the city, and neither is any foreign doctor who has not previously obtained the university's authorization. Item, no apothecary is permitted to dispense anything to the sick without the advice of a doctor, on pain of considerable punishment, with the exception of a few insignificant things, such as suppositories, standard

---

[2]   Guarinonius, *Grewel*, 93, 109, 132, 206, 319, 823. Referring to the most characteristic theatrical prop of commedia dell'arte playing quacks as a symbol of deceit, Guarinonius also lables them 'ignorant, stupid, clumsy, uncouth, mad empirics and mask-doctors' (*Grewel*, 965).

[3]   Guarinonius, *Grewel*, 341.

[4]   *Felix Platter Tagebuch*, 251 (25 August 1556, Montpellier). The original letter is lost.

[5]   Mellinkoff, 'Riding backwards', 160.

clysters or worm tablets, etc, as specified in Joubert's Montpellier *Pharmacopee* [of 1581]. And once someone has served as an apothecary's assistant, he can no longer qualify as a medical doctor in Montpellier. If, however, an itinerant or quacksalver or suchlike is found practicing medicine there, then the doctors and their students have the immediate right, without any further formalities, to place him backwards on a donkey. He is made to hold the ass's tail like reins, and is led around the whole city in this manner, while being loudly ridiculed. All the common folk run to see him, and pelt him with dirt until he becomes as filthy as if he had rolled in mud. Once, on 19/29 December 1595, we caught someone like this and wanted to put him on a donkey and treat him like this. When his wife found out that we were holding him in the anatomy theatre, she broke out into howling and weeping, loudly crying that the students wanted to dissect her husband alive. This moved the whole neighbourhood to such compassion that he was forcibly taken from us and freed. After that he was never seen again.[6]

Meanwhile, under Felix Platter's deanship, the University of Basle's medical faculty was actively lobbying for the strengthening of local municipal regulations against quacks and empirics, including Jewish and female practitioners, as indicated in a supplication of the mid-1590s:

In the year 1460 the authorities drew up a mandate explicitly forbidding any doctor, whether male or female, who had not been examined by the faculty of medicine to practice any kind of medicine in the city of Basle, whether uroscopy, purging and prescription or the like, or any surgeon, apothecary, barber-surgeon, herbalist or empiric to practice medicine, unless they are similarly certificated by the aforesaid faculty. [...] Most recently, on 11 March of the year 1594, the council ratified a public mandate against such false doctors, barber-surgeons, itinerants, theriac merchants and other vagrants, and posted and publicized it throughout the city and region.[7]

Felix Platter's *Observations* records the hard line he took with patients who went to quacks. He dropped one altogether after she consulted 'a Chirurgion and [...] a Mountebank', when her husband reinfected her with the pox of which Platter had already once cured her.[8] Even so, he only identifies by name one of the surgeons, midwives, Jews, meddling mountebanks, quacks, empirics, Paracelsians and other 'ignorant imposters' against whose medical incompetence the book's readers are repeatedly warned.[9] This is Dr Adam Bodenstein, a former pupil of Paracelsus

---

[6]   *Thomas Platter d.J*, 70–1 (October 1595, Montpellier).

[7]   *Supplicatio ad magistrans contra empiricos*, post-1594 (Huber, *Felix Platters 'Observationes'*, 226).

[8]   Platter, *Obseruationum*, 685 (this translation: Plat[t]er, Culpeper and Cole, *Platerus histories*, 450).

[9]   For example, Platter, *Obseruationum*, 15, 309, 411, 622, 684–5, 718, 822.

featured in the list of local medical practitioners Platter compiled when he started practicing in Basle in 1558.[10]

The forthright language Platter uses to describe Bodenstein's practice indicates both the strength of his feeling regarding misguided medical rivals, and the fluidity of quacks as a category. Having 'tormented' a patient who complained of 'Suffocation from Copulation' whenever attempting conjugal relations with his wife with sweat cures and 'fruitless' Paracelsian medicines for several weeks, Platter reports that the Paracelsian celebrity Bodenstein charged the unfortunate man 200 crowns and sent him home, where he shortly choked to death while engaged in testing the efficacity of his alleged cure.[11] A later case-study reports Platter's palpable sense of satisfaction regarding two quacks whose own plague remedies could not save them from dying in Basle plague epidemics. An unidentified 'Impostor or Mountebank with a Ball of Stibium' with which he 'bragged that he cured all of the Plague' succumbed in the epidemic of 1593–4. Bodenstein, who fled to Frankfurt during the great Basle plague of 1563–4, during which Felix Platter served his city with great distinction, and it lost a third of its population of 4000, died in 1578, shortly after publishing a book recommending his 'treacle which he made of Chymical Medicines', for the prevention and cure of victims of the great Basle plague epidemic of 1576–7.[12]

Despite such professional misgivings, Felix and Thomas Platter are more open-minded about quack activities than Guarinonius. Their journals give some indication of the wide range of itinerants open to profiting from the hawking of medicines and medical services. An example of one with a strong medical background was Samuel Hertenstein. Son of a Lucerne physician, he had abandoned his medical studies to practice around Toulouse, where he was well known as an empiric. In 1557, loudly singing in German while returning on foot from a short spell as a mercenary in Piedmont, he encountered and recognized Felix Platter, with whose father he had boarded in the 1540s, and invited him to sign his friendship album, and to a meal in Toulouse.[13] Only rarely is there explicit documentation concerning the medical activities of those, such as pilgrims, whose itinerant commercial activities, primarily intended to encourage donations to support specific journeys, might have little or nothing to do with their trade or training. On 25 May 1598,

---

[10]   *Felix Platter Tagebuch*, 335–7 (1558, Basle: quoted in Chapter 2, this volume). Bodenstein (1528–77) matriculated at Basle University in 1537, and studied medicine there and elsewhere from 1548, qualifying as a physician in Ferrara in 1550. His father, the theologian Andreas 'Carolostadius' von Bodenstein, moved his family from Karlstadt, a small town just north-west of Würzburg in Franconia to Basle, where he died in the plague epidemic of 1539–41.

[11]   Platter, *Obseruationum*, 171–2; Plat[t]er, Culpeper and Cole, *Platerus histories*, 104–5; Huber, *Felix Platters 'Observationes'*, 199–200.

[12]   Platter, *Obseruationum*, 308–9 (this translation: Plat[t]er, Culpeper and Cole, *Platerus histories*, 199–200).

[13]   *Felix Platter Tagebuch*, 267 (3 March 1557, Toulouse).

Thomas Platter delayed leaving Avignon in order to view 'all sorts of rare items' laden on the mule of Herr Freytag of Laer, a German pilgrim returning from Jerusalem who was sharing his lodgings.[14] Without specifically noting medicinal applications, Platter records that Freytag presented him with several small lumps of 'some earth from the field on which Adam was created'. Felix Platter notes his embarrassment at the old and ugly German women among the Companions of St James passing through Montpellier, begging and singing for their supper on their way to and from Santiago de Compostela.[15] In May 1555, he learned that one such 'Jacob's brother' he heard singing at dinner, Heinrich Müller, was from near Basle. Entrusting him with letters (which reached their intended recipient, Platter the Elder), he bought Müller a meal, and gave him a small sum of money and a tin of theriac to sell while he was travelling.[16] It was manufactured and sold in the Catelan's apothecary, where the famously sweet-toothed Felix, perhaps motivated as much by its high sugar content as by any actively addictive ingredients, often secretly helped himself, by his own account without suffering any ill effects.[17]

Itinerant performers unable to compete for municipal licences enabling them to travel from one previously arranged engagement to another, often earned a precarious living targeting public diners. They were not always conventionally recompensed. In September 1553, Felix Platter was paid a surprise visit in Montpellier by Heinrich Pantaleon, recently qualified as a physician in Valence, but known to him as a Basle cleric and teacher, amateur singer and director of school plays. After entertaining Pantaleon to supper, several medical students, including Platter, played games of chance with an itinerant singer staking his songs. Having lost, the singer was made to perch precariously on a window ledge while singing: 'according to the custom, by which they sing abundant songs *alla chambre* etc. Dr Pantaleon was amazed at this, telling us he had never seen anything like it.'[18] Later that year, Platter busked on the streets of Montpellier with two other German medical students, his bed and board fellow Johann Friedrich Ryhiner, and Johann Jacob Huggelin.[19] They 'played three lutes together. The householders were on the point of chasing us away, but eventually they allowed us to take to the streets after all'.[20]

---

[14]   *Thomas Platter d.J*, 239–40 (25 May 1598, Avignon).

[15]   *Felix Platter Tagebuch*, 246 (1 June 1556, Montpellier).

[16]   *Felix Platter Tagebuch*, 219 (29 May 1555, Montpellier).

[17]   *Felix Platter Tagebuch*, 75; Platter, *Obseruationum*, 223. Catelan's grandson, Laurent III Catelan, published the family recipe in a treatise of 1614, *Discovrs svr la theriaqve et ingrediens d'icelle*.

[18]   *Felix Platter Tagebuch*, 184 (27 September 1553, Montpellier).

[19]   Both Ryhiner (future father-in-law of Felix's half-sister Magdalena) and his older brother Johann Heinrich Ryhiner studied medicine in Montpellier; Huggelin died in the great Basle plague epidemic of 1563–4.

[20]   *Felix Platter Tagebuch*, 189 (11 December 1553, Montpellier). This term for night-time street busking ('gaßathum gehen') recurs in Felix's summary of a letter in which his

Disagreement over one such busker aggravated a bitter argument that spoiled a seven-week family holiday of 1563.[21] It was undertaken so that Thomas Platter the Elder could introduce Felix to relatives he had left behind when he moved from the Valais, while the childless Madlen visited Leuk, whose medicinal spa waters were renowned for curing infertility, with her father, Franz Jeckelmann. This wealthy barber-surgeon and sometime city councillor was a neighbour and close family friend, on whose family business Felix had relied for haircuts and minor surgery since childhood.[22] In Solothurn on the return journey, Jeckelmann harshly criticized Felix during dinner for socializing with some Catholics he knew from Montpellier. Hurling the crayfish he was eating back into the communal dish, Felix stormed out. The following evening, a fiddler came to their dining table and asked Felix for permission to play: 'I said yes, he should go ahead and play. But that angered my father-in-law so much that he rose from the table again, mounted his horse, and rode off towards Liechstall on his own.'[23] Lötscher blames Felix's loss of temper squarely on Jeckelmann's domineering bullying. Dictated nearly half a century later to Thomas Platter, and perhaps, as Hochlenert suggests, drawing on earlier records, this account still betrays raw resentment at what Felix perceived as Jeckelmann's uninvited intrusion into this Platter family holiday.[24] Repeatedly referred to, but never by name, in *Observations* as 'my Father in Law a famous Chirurgion',[25] Jeckelmann, who had assisted at Andreas Vesalius's public dissection in Basle in 1543,[26] and whose family business instrumentally supported the young physician in establishing his flourishing medical practice, may well have been sensitive to elements of professional rank-pulling in Felix's unsubtle manoeuvrings to take control of his group's dinner table, by imposing Catholics and itinerant entertainers on them. A day later, the physician and surgeon entered Basle separately. Their quarrel rumbled on for over a year, until Jeckelmann, during the epidemic that claimed his son Franz, helped Felix cure his parents of the plague.[27]

---

father identifies lute busking, dancing, performing in carnival plays and womanizing as elements of the scandalous behaviour that had Felix's former school friend, the student Hans Beat Häl, jailed, then banished from Basle (199, 22 May 1554, Montpellier). On occasion, Felix also busked by day (*Felix Platter Tagebuch*, 272 (11 March 1557, Bordeaux). Guarinonius too remembers spending half the night going 'cassatum' in his youth (*Grewel*, 1286). There was an attempt to ban night busking in Hall in 1612 (Senn, *Aus dem Kulturleben*, 466, 473).

[21]   *Felix Platter Tagebuch*, 401–26 (2 June – 19 July 1563, Valais).

[22]   *Felix Platter Tagebuch*, 70, 80–1 (1544–6, Basle).

[23]   *Felix Platter Tagebuch*, 425 (17–18 July 1563, Solothurn and Balsthal).

[24]   Lötscher, *Felix Platter und seine Familie*, 115; Hochlenert, 'Das "Tagebuch" des Felix Platter', 96–7, 118, 199.

[25]   Platter, *Obseruationum*, 489, 726 (this translation: Plat[t]er, Culpeper and Cole, *Platerus histories*, 325, 475).

[26]   Trinkler, *Pathologie*, 25–6.

[27]   *Felix Platter Tagebuch*, 436, 438 (August 1564 and 9 January 1565, Basle).

Another itinerant fiddler gave Thomas Platter grief of a different kind in July 1599, when he and two travelling companions stopped for the night at a French inn:

> As we were at our evening meal, a lone fiddler entered, dressed in a masked harlequin costume, and played for us, as well as executing unusual acrobatic leaps and performing amazing tricks. After dinner we made arrangements with our drover, we wanted to get up right after midnight and so we asked the chamber-boy to wake us at midnight, we should leave our door unlocked for him, which we did. On 28 July, right after midnight, the chamber-boy woke us. When I was dressed I checked both my purses to see whether all the money was still in them, which I could easily detect by feeling them. In a small black velvet purse, I was missing several small silver coins and a Turkish gold coin that I had collected for my honourable brother [Felix] because of its unusual design. But in the other purse, which I used for my daily keep, I was unable to find anything missing, except that the thief had taken two large pennies from the daily keep purse and packed them into the velvet purse in place of those he had stolen. In similar fashion, he had stolen two gold Spanish double crowns (worth exactly the same as my loss) from the purse of my countryman Hieronymus Curio, and placed two smaller coins wrapped in paper in their place. He too could find nothing else changed. From another, he had thieved a whole franc. We were all as surprised as we could possibly be that he had managed to reach our purses, because all three of us had hidden them in the pockets of our clothes, under our pillows, on which we slept. And nothing at all was taken from Ludwig Jaske, who had left his clothes, in which he had a gold chain and many gold crowns, lying openly on the table. We complained amongst ourselves and immediately suspected the performer, but because it was not a high sum and we were in haste to get to Paris, and also because the innkeeper told us that we would find it very hard to prove anything, we left things as they were and went on our way.[28]

Regardless of whether Thomas Platter made the connection with Harlequin in 1599, or only in 1604 when writing up his journal, his exceptionally early German record of this key commedia dell'arte role indicates the remarkable extent to which it achieved international recognition within two decades of being created by the actor Tristano Martinelli.

The Platter brothers shared a fascination for two attention-grabbing staples of itinerant quack repertoire, human acrobatics and exotic performing or show animals. Like many iconographic records, such as Plate 39, their accounts do not always clarify possible connections between such spectacle and quack activities. The day after being robbed by the Harlequin, Thomas Platter records acrobatics performed by a Spanish strongman at the University of Paris. He carried:

---

[28]   *Thomas Platter d.J*, 544–7 (27 July 1599, Montlhéry).

a mighty stave, of the type we put across haywains at our hospital, around the courtyard with his teeth, on his forehead and on his chest, one after the other, without the help of his hands, and in the same way also a heavy oak gallows and extremely high fire ladders on the specified three places, of which no piece would not have strained the strongest man even to have carried on his shoulders, or however he found most convenient. And I observed that it caused the veins on his neck to bulge as thick as a little finger, and become so full of blood, that one might have thought they would burst. He also carried around a dozen drawn swords all wedged together by their hilts, by a single blade tip on his bare tongue. Then he balanced the same drawn sword, into which all the others were wedged, on his bare hand, carried it around in this fashion, and spun it around on his hand like a spindle, without injuring himself in any way. He also performed more rare tricks, not all of which I saw. He was a blackish-brown, strong young male, born in Spain, as he said.[29]

The following month he visited the Halles de la Boucherie: 'a fine large butchers' market with broad spaces and rooms in which I have seen plays performed, high stilt-walking, and strange dances, as people of this type often come to Antwerp'.[30]

Earlier that year, in the large ground floor hall of the 'Barau' house in Angers, Thomas Platter had been diverted by a matachin, a type of acrobatic armed *moresco* dance much performed by itinerant troupes:

I saw the most amusing dancing apes I ever saw in my life. An itinerant showman, who was travelling round with them, played the fiddle while five fully costumed apes, all five with their front paws raised up towards each other, danced the branle together in excellent time to the music played by the man. Then two rested while three danced a matachin or dance of death, in such good time to the music, and with such human gestures, that many were highly amazed by them. They also performed a lot of unusual monkey business and acrobatics with each other, all at the command of their master.[31]

In 1597, he had seen various exotic creatures in Marseille, including 'an animal that looked like a very large ape, but whose build was somewhat different, and it performed very strange, diverting tricks, they called him Bertram', and a live ostrich 'capable of pushing over a boy with its feet' that effortlessly swallowed horseshoe nails.[32] Far from being exceptional, this dietary eccentricity had become an expected element of the repertoire of a species of whom John Lyly wrote 'remember that the Estrich disgesteth harde yron to preserue his healthe'; routine

---

[29]   *Thomas Platter d.J*, 587 (28 July 1599, Paris).
[30]   *Thomas Platter d.J*, 675 (24 August 1599, Antwerp).
[31]   *Thomas Platter d.J*, 484 (22 May 1599, Angers). The left foreground of Plate 20 features six *moresco* dancers.
[32]   *Thomas Platter d.J*, 186–7 (14 February 1597, Marseille).

behaviour aggressively invoked in the murderous threat of Shakespeare's rebel draper Jack Cade to Alexander Iden: 'I'll make thee eat iron like an ostridge, and swallow my sword like a great pin'.[33]

Acrobats documented by Felix Platter in France in the 1550s include a Moor who raised mighty stone blocks before letting them fall onto his head and shoulders, 'a pregnant woman walking on a rope suspended up high, in the manner of tight-rope walkers',[34] and a troupe combining show animals with acrobatic routines:

> On 6 January, itinerant showmen were in Montpellier, who performed amazing acrobatics, they also had a lion, who was meant to fight a bull. They bought a not very robust bull, sawed off the tips of both his horns, and first brought the lion to the arena and tied him with a thick rope to a post that had been sunk into the earth in the middle of the arena. Then they also tied the bull to the post with a rope, and pricked the lion to goad him into attacking the bull. The lion sprang at the bull, but he repeatedly gored him with his horns so aggressively that if his horns had been sharp, he could easily have killed him. In the end, when the lion kept repulsing him, and the bull started tiring, the lion sprang as fast as a cat over his horns and onto his back, biting and pushing him to the ground so that he could not move, although even this was not enough to kill him, and he had to be slaughtered.[35]

Although this account of 1556 does not indicate quack activity, the iconographic record suggests that by the 1570s, carnival bullfights were routinely staged by professional commedia dell'arte acting troupes of the type associated with quack activity (Plate 11).

Guarinonius's opposition to superstition and quackery, unusually vigorous even for an early modern physician, drew inspiration from Carlo Borromeo, who accused quacks of spreading heresy by printed publications, fortune-telling, magic and witchcraft.[36] In his vernacular plague treatise of 1612, Guarinonius rhetorically asks 'whether it is possible to produce a plague medicine that can protect people for specific days, weeks, months or years?'. His answer refers to a quack whose activities seriously impinged on the business of the local doctors of Hall, even though he dressed and behaved like a pig-castrator:

> Among those who came here to Hall during the current epidemic was a quacksalver with a strange black powder, who claimed that anyone who dosed themselves with it would not just be protected from the plague for that particular day, but for many days, weeks, months and years to come. Item, because the

---

[33] Lyly, *Euphves*, 40–1; Shakespeare, *2 Henry IV*, IV.x.28–9.

[34] *Felix Platter Tagebuch*, 228, 262 (21 September 1555, Marseille; 18 January 1557, Montpellier).

[35] *Felix Platter Tagebuch*, 239 (6 January 1556, Montpellier).

[36] Guarinonius, *In memoria æterna*, 609–10.

powder was a sure cure for the plague. This his deceptive novelty gained far more attention than the medicines that the physicians had invented, produced, classified, and, by the grace of God, thoroughly tested and proven in the treatment of numerous patients. He even harangued the authorities themselves into buying it off him in huge quantities at a high price, namely for a ducat per dose or *presa*.[37] Soon after, when his deception came to light, they sold it off cheaply within a few days, silencing the mighty outcry that nobody had ever desired or wanted it. Thereafter, of all those who were infected who used it, all but two died, having neglected to follow the proper remedies, such as blood-letting and the rest. And it was also just as useless for all those who took it as a preventative measure against the plague. As indeed I could list the names of several here. Among them are several who held the powder in such high regard as a remedy that they were convinced it would protect them from the plague for a full year. Two of them have already died. One survives, and is even now preparing to meet his God. So to believe this is not just madness but also a major sin against God, and impossible in the natural world.[38]

In conclusion, Guarinonius comments harshly on city officials who fail to regulate unlicensed health practitioners, and undermine his profession by trusting 'the unknown quacksalvers bearing sealed licences who travel here from every corner'.[39] The first volume of *Grewel*, on health, discusses the destructive impact of medically incompetent quacks, and records plans for more detailed criticism in the second volume.[40] Two chapters specifically target quacks. One, 'On the abomination of the frightful, fanatical, antimonian, sulphurous, mercurial and other similar risible medicines for spirits and inhuman horses and cattle', warns readers off quack medicines. Pointing out that every well-governed German city has strict laws preventing the entry of quacks or their life-threatening remedies, it refers to their medications as:

> wild, untamed, poisonous, devilish, not medicines, but spirits that monstrously strangle and destroy human nature. [...] whether taken in a small or large dose, in sweet, sour or other form, because in every form, they certainly, truly and unfailingly represent bitter death or a life shortened by many years.[41]

The other, 'Outline of the extremely destructive, unhygienic and also unchristian teachings and methods of several unhygienic horse and cow doctors', alludes to quacks' theatricality and itinerancy. Dismissing them as 'blustering empirics, or

---

[37]   Guarinonius, *Pestilentz Guardien*, 124*. An early modern reader was sufficiently impressed by this high price to underline the phrase in ink (HAB, 128.3 Med).

[38]   Guarinonius, *Pestilentz Guardien*, 123*–251 [*sic* 125*].

[39]   Guarinonius, *Pestilentz Guardien*, 126*.

[40]   Guarinonius, *Grewel*, 639, 909, 962.

[41]   Guarinonius, *Grewel*, 962 (V, Chapter 29, 961–2).

masked- and horse-doctors, who wreak their damage on many poor people, of whom many hold their fluent sayings in high regard in the same way that the Jews do those of their Rabbis and Pharisees, because they sing their people a satisfying little song', it notes that they travel from patient to patient 'with many horses, carriages, women, and practically all their servants, just like vagrants, staying for quite a few weeks'.[42] Chapter 19 of *Grewel*'s unpublished second volume, on pathology, targets 'itinerant marketplace quacks who trick simple folk out of their money by means of all sorts of plays and entertainments'.[43]

Physicians routinely unmasked panaceas as an excuse for the alcoholic excesses of quacks' clients. Guarinonius, whose physician father was a prominent landowner with productive vineyards in the Etschtal region, sharply criticizes itinerant quacks' deceitful pharmaceutical marketing of bad wine and spirits as good medicine, denouncing their vermouth and malmsey based panaceas as dangerous poisons for the healthy, prescribed by empirics and 'mask-doctors'.[44] Convinced of the medicinal and spiritual dimensions of wine, he condemns this as a gross perversion of the healing professions. His readers are warned to distinguish between the true physician, who 'cures according to the venerable, praiseworthy and proven methods of Hippocrates, Galen, Avicenna, Celsus, and Mesuæ', and the unqualified 'empiric, alchemist, laboratory experimentalist, itinerant, deceiver of patients', peddling immortality but spreading disease, insanity, even death, with his pinch of '*Flores* (yes) *dolores antimonii*' in wine and 'suchlike deceitful nonsense [...] Paracelsian murderous poison, cow and horse medicine' to the uneducated fools crowding round him.[45] Declaring quacks 'alchemists and magicians who should be burnt at the stake', public murderers masquerading as doctors, whose 'monstrous' chemical and alcohol-based medicines are poisonous works of the Devil that dispatch the old and the weak to their fate and kill unborn children and mothers, fit only to treat animals and unbelievers, he warns that 'water is the first and noblest path to health [...] Christ the Lord himself decreed wine not as a regular drink, but as a medicine for happiness [...] But medicines must be taken with extreme care'.[46] Guarinonius compares quack medical practice to that of 'old wives', attacking them as drunken, heathen sinners without professional or personal regard for social laws or Christian commandments, who promote serious alcohol abuse amongst their patients.[47]

---

[42]   Guarinonius, *Grewel*, 97–8 (Vortrab, Chapter 27, 97–101).

[43]   Innsbruck UL, Cod.110, IV, ff.471ᵛ–473ᵛ.

[44]   Guarinonius, *Grewel*, 617–18, 676, 850; Mayr, 'Volksnahrung', 136.

[45]   Guarinonius, *Grewel*, 58. Unlike the prolific Greek physicians Hippocrates and Galen or the Arab philosopher and physician Avicenna, Ioannis Filii Mesuæ (*In antidotarium*, 1550) and the Roman physician Aulius Cornelius Celsus (*De medicina*, c.50 AD) are best known for one work.

[46]   Guarinonius, *Grewel*, 109, 609, 909, 912–13, 1327.

[47]   Guarinonius, *Grewel*, 98–101.

Guarinonius follows *Grewel*'s first description of the deceptions of the false healers with a general warning: 'Not only such practices and trickery themselves, but simply having unquestioning trust in deceitful fabrications of this type, can suffice to enable their predictions to depress and frighten the spirit and sap bodily strength, following which people must rapidly deteriorate.'[48] The respected physician illustrates this point with a remarkable autobiographical digression from early in his professional career. It reveals that he was not above deploying supernatural quackery himself, having successfully treated a patient in an unprecedentedly theatrical demonstration of the placebo effect, disguised as an itinerant astrologer. Before examining this, it is relevant to briefly consider early modern attitudes to astrology, with particular reference to those of Guarinonius himself. Astrologically-based foretelling of the future represented a significant confluence of medicine, magic and performance. Felix Platter had come into personal contact with the most notorious astrologer of his age, as one of 13 German students who set off from Montpellier on 15 September 1555 to gather medicinal herbs in Provence. A week later, returning via Salon de Craux, the small Provençal town between Arles and Marseille that was home to Michel de Nostradamus, several of the group spoke with the 52-year-old 'famous calendar and horoscope maker'. Within a month Felix, who was not one of them, was sent a horoscope by one of his father's boarders, Johann Heinrich Kneblin.[49]

Prophetic astrology was condemned as heresy by the Church, a harshly punishable crime in Elizabethan England, and denounced by sceptics such as Montaigne and Reginald Scot, and by scientists, physicians and clergy, some of whom viewed astrologers as their professional rivals.[50] In 'Discorso VIII' of his compendium of the professions, the churchman Tomaso Garzoni exposes astrologers and their ilk, from Nostradamus downwards, as madmen, ruffians and charlatans.[51] Guarinonius's *Grewel* repeatedly attacks astrologers and astrology-based medicine. He abhors the common man's 'superstition and folly' in being taken in by the over-inquisitive follies of almanac writers, whom he accuses of drawing on white, even black magic in the production of their 'almanackish, deceitful, superstitious falsehoods', which lead to 'innumerable superstitions and their associated magic practices and godless vices [...] that go against the laws of God and drill the whole German nation in superstition and idolatry'.[52] He warns against reliance on the astrologically determined dates for carrying out medical practices or health procedures, such as bloodletting or bathing, and shocks

---

48   Guarinonius, *Grewel*, 33.

49   *Felix Platter Tagebuch*, 229, 232 (23 September and 6 October 1555, Avignon and Montpellier).

50   Smith, 'Judicial astrology', 161–2; Thomas, *Religion and the decline of magic*, 283–321.

51   Garzoni, *La piazza universale*, 157–66 ('De' formatori de' pronostichi, tacuini, lunarii, et almanachi').

52   Guarinonius, *Grewel*, 301, 375, 992, 997, 1006, 1021.

his gullible readers by unmasking the almanac writers identifying these dates as superstitious, heathen confusers and deceivers of fools, whose predictions have the accuracy of a blind man shooting at a target:[53]

> *Reader*: Are you not aware of the single and double red crosses in our regular German almanacs?
>
> *Doctor*: Of course. And what of them?
>
> *Reader*: They are the signs for when bloodletting is necessary, and indicate when it is good or best to let blood.
>
> *Doctor*: Yes, when its good or best to strangle and murder people. It is customary to designate bloodletting with single and double red crosses because compared with that authorized by regular German almanacs, which are deceivers of fools, no other type of bloodletting leads to more red, bloody and murderish crosses, swiftly followed by the black crosses in the cemetery.
>
> *Reader*: That can't be God's will.
>
> *Doctor*: Of course it is neither the will of God nor reason, but of common ignorance, common madness and folly […]
>
> *Reader*: Truly you have not called almanacs deceivers of fools without reason […] I am the mayor of the city […]
>
> *Doctor*: I praise your humane reason […] Now, as a good start, arrange that in your city none of your citizens, whether healthy or ill, are permitted to undergo bloodletting except by prior authorization of a qualified physician.[54]

This is reiterated in his denunciation of the incompetence of barber-surgeons who follow the 'superstitious, calendrical follies' of almanacs:

> the municipal authorities should not authorize anyone to let blood unless they are expressly certified by a qualified doctor […] I speak the truth when I say that I have often laughed no less heartily at the deceiving antics […] of the bathmasters and barber-surgeons with their bloodletting, than at the diverting tricks of the Zannis of the Italian comedy.[55]

---

53 Guarinonius, *Grewel*, 908, 988–1026.
54 Guarinonius, *Grewel*, 989, 992.
55 Guarinonius, *Grewel*, 1004, 1040.

Two chapters on astrology in the published volume of *Grewel* pair each of its seven planets and 12 signs with a particular sin, and suggest replacing the 'heathen' zodiacal signs with virtuous Christian symbols, and the second volume revisits the subject.[56] Guarinonius professes intense incredulity regarding astrology's degree of influence.[57] He expresses a deeply negative attitude towards this pre-Christian belief system, identifying it as a dangerous challenge to Catholicism, an idolatrous folly rooted in heathen traditions that posed a particular threat to women, whose sinful inquisitiveness (which he brackets with that of apes) and 'frivolous character makes them especially susceptible to magic, superstition and similar godless manifestations'.[58]

Guarinonius's own impersonation of an astrologer arose when a patient from a neighbouring town persuaded him to pass himself off as an astrological quack. This sorrowful husband begged him to travel from Hall to the nearby town of Schwaz, in order to cure his sick wife, plunged into great misery by the negative diagnosis of an 'alchemical, greedy itinerant quack' who had predicted that she would die within nine months. Distraught at the physical deterioration suffered by his previously healthy wife during the following four months, he requested Guarinonius's intervention in the persona of an itinerant fortune-teller.[59] Guarinonius, an intent student of acting methods well aware of the close relationship between theatre and healing, elsewhere rhetorically asks his readers: 'Have you never observed the behaviour of actors and comedians in plays, maintaining such control over their eyes, face, mouth, forehead, fists, feet, voice, shouting and whole body that they seem to be behaving quite genuinely, although it means nothing to them?'[60]

Using his knowledge of astrologers' 'superstitions [...] strange customs, clothes and habits' to disguise himself as an 'excellent horoscope reader, astrologer and fortune-teller', Guarinonius took up his customary lodgings in Schwaz, at the inn of Hans Thernhauser.[61] Here he arranged for the woman to be brought to him:

> together with another woman. I read her palm, and then told her that she had a
> great sorrow of the heart, and was mired in sad thoughts day and night, unable
> to enjoy any happiness, and feared an early death, etc. Finally, that a deceitful

---

[56]   Guarinonius, *Grewel*, 1026–38 (Book 5, Chapters 42–3); Innsbruck UL, Cod.110, IV, ff.446^v–452^v.

[57]   According to Millar, Richard Dawkins is 'horrified that 25% of the British public has some belief in astrology – more than in any one established religion – and that more newspaper column inches are devoted to horoscopes than to science' ('The gullible age', 1). As a former president of The Medical Society of London drily put it in 1957: 'Even today I am sometimes asked to operate on days when the stars are favourable and I readily accede, it helps to spread the responsibility' (Wright, 'Quacks', 164).

[58]   Guarinonius, *Grewel*, 71, 1033.

[59]   Guarinonius, *Grewel*, 33.

[60]   Guarinonius, *Grewel*, 366.

[61]   Guarinonius, *Grewel*, 30, 921.

quack had plunged her into great misery. Whereupon the good woman heaved a deep sigh. Moreover, I informed her that she would recover from this deceit, and regain her health and strength, live in happiness, and reach her seventieth year. Whereupon the woman suddenly threw both her arms up towards the heavens, and with tears in her eyes cried with a ringing voice "O may God bless you, my dear Sir, for telling my fortune so truthfully". Thus I let her keep her good opinion and belief, and joyfully go home. On my return, after fourteen days, I called her to me again, and prescribed good food and drink, and allowed her to drink a little malmsey wine every morning, and a good traminer wine in moderation with meals, which she did. But when I returned again fourteen days later, the woman was already such a changed person, that I hardly recognized her any more. When the nine months were up and she had recovered really well, and fully regained her strength, I called her. I revealed the trickery of my fortune-telling to her, and that her health had previously deteriorated due to her irresponsible superstition, and had been restored to her through her present positive, fickle superstition. She could not be convinced of this, believing (to this very day) that I am a fortune-teller. Following this, many other women were sent by her up to me in Hall, and even some men, all wanting me to predict their fortunes.[62]

While warning his readers and patients against the spiritual dangers of enjoying the rhetorical and theatrical marketing techniques of itinerant performing quacks, Guarinonius drew on them to his own advantage and profit. As this autobiographical passage reveals, he deployed them effectively in his own medical practice, and was himself prepared to impersonate the costume and methods of precisely the type of quack that he himself most reviled, the astrological fortune-teller who, like some of those examined in the following chapter, based his medical practice not on scientific knowledge, but on magic and superstition.

---

[62]   Guarinonius, *Grewel*, 33; see also Rapp, *Guarinoni, Stiftsarzt*, 26–7.

Chapter 10
Medicine, Magic and Superstition

Early modern occult practices attracted various overlapping explanations, notably the legal (criminal fraud), the theatrical (generally benign human deception), the medical (psychological and pathological causes) and the religious – their actual agent was demonic rather than human. They were so closely associated with performance that, as the renowned professional commedia dell'arte actor Nicolò Barbieri complained in 1628, 'simple folk only have to hear you mention actors to think you are discussing witches and sorcerers; and in certain regions of Italy they think that actors make rain and tempests, and are more or less masters of the order of nature'.[1] Practitioners of magic commonly drew on medical or theatrical practices, or both, as with magical impotence, the occult practice here chosen as a case-study.

The previous chapter concluded by considering some supernatural medical practices. This chapter examines magic and superstition with particular reference to the relevance of the three physicians' writings to stage practice. An overview of some occult practices and stage magic they describe introduces an enquiry into the significance of magical impotence for the early modern London stage, in the light of Thomas Platter's account of its ritual practice in Languedoc. Medieval mystery plays established a sophisticated tradition of staging flaming hellmouths, devils, fireworks and other supernatural manifestations and magic on the religious stage. All magic was tainted with demonic associations. This included secular conjuring and stage magic, for which the early modern term was juggling. In his influential demonological treatise of 1580, *De la Demonomanie des sorciers*, the French lawyer Jean Bodin condemns jugglers who 'enchant peoples' eyes [...] by means of evil spirits'; noting that 'jugglers easily become sorcerers', and that sorcerers present juggling routines in between genuine magic to lull people into believing that they are merely performing idle stage tricks.[2] The Book of Deuteronomy was widely cited in condemnation of stage magic. The authoritative King James Bible translates the key passage as:

> There shall not be found among you *any one* that maketh his son or his daughter to pass through the fire, *or* that useth divination, *or* an observer of times, or an enchanter, or a witch. Or a charmer, or a consulter with familiar spirits, or a wizard, or a necromancer. For all that do these things *are* an abomination unto the Lord.[3]

---

[1] Barbieri, *La supplica*, 1628, 45.
[2] Bodin (1530–96), *Demonomanie*, sigs.47^r, 242^v.
[3] *King James Bible*: 'Deuteronomy' 18, vv.10–12.

The physician Johannes Wier (or Weyer), the English lawyer Reginald Scot and other sceptical demonological writers embraced anti-theatrical interpretations of such biblical passages.[4] They adapted them to their own ends, by vigorously pursuing a rational, science-based approach that routinely exposes allegedly supernatural phenomena as the cheap effects of stage jugglers.

The stage magic with the most venerable tradition is that enduring staple of magic shows, the decapitation routine. Integral to some medieval religious mystery plays, its earliest records go back to a papyrus account of around 2600 BC, describing a stage decapitation performed for King Cheops of Egypt.[5] A demonological treatise of 1608 relates that the Jewish physician Zedechias entertained royalty with a variety of magic routines in the year 876 AD, including one in which 'he used to cut off men's heads and hands and feet, and exhibit them in a bowl dripping with blood, and then suddenly he would restore the men unharmed each to his own place'.[6] Thomas Platter's account of the repertoire of the Italian commedia dell'arte quack troupe he repeatedly observed in Avignon in 1598 includes a description of a stage decapitation, in which the troupe leader, Zan Bragetta:

> hacked one young woman's head off behind the curtain, which he then drew aside, and there stood the head on its own in a bowl on the bench, and she stretched both arms down across the bench, so that one could see the stump at the neck very realistically. Anyone who didn't know this trick would not have suspected any irregularity, because of course it does not involve magic.[7]

Scot's demonological treatise of 1584 reveals the mechanics underlying professional stage decapitation routines of precisely this type, noting in a marginalia that 'this was done by one Kingsfield of London, at a Bartholomewtide, An. 1582 in the sight of diwerse that came to view this spectacle' (Plate 30).[8] His account may have directly influenced Philoclea's graphic description to Pyrocles of the mechanics of a fictional staged mock beheading for which her tormenters brought her:

> downe vnder the scaffolde, and (making me thrust my head vp through a hole they had made therin) they did put about my poore necke a dishe of gold, whereout they had beaten the bottome, so as hauing set bloud in it, you sawe how I played the parte of death [...] so as scarcely I could breathe.[9]

---

4   Wier, *De praestigiis daemonum*; Scot, *Discouerie of Witchcraft*, 111, 114–15.
5   Butterworth, *Magic on the early English stage*, xv.
6   Guazzo, *Compendium maleficarum*, 5.
7   *Thomas Platter d.J*, 305: see Chapter 17, this volume.
8   Scot, *Discouerie of Witchcraft*, 349–50, and the plate directly preceding 353.
9   Sidney, *Arcadia*, sig.339. Watson suggests that like Scot, Sidney may have witnessed Kingsfield's routine at the St Bartholomew fair of 1582 ('Sidney at Bartholomew Fair').

Factual accounts of stage decapitation based on Scot's include those in a treatise of 1634 on 'the art of jugling' by the actor and stage magician William Vincent (who toured England under the stage name Hocus Pocus), and the demonological treatise of 1655 with which Thomas Ady carried forward Scot's sceptical perspective. Ady does not illustrate his account of a 'Jugler's' mock decapitation of his 'Boy' involving a false head 'so lively in shew that the very bone and marrow of the neck appeareth, insomuch that some Spectators have fainted at the sight hereof'.[10] Vincent provides a new picture, from which the woodcut featured in a 1668 German edition of his treatise is derived.[11]

Scot's treatise also illustrates the specially adapted bodkins and knives some jugglers used to promote the illusion of cutting or stabbing themselves on stage, and alludes to those who make a public show of snake-charming, or profess to 'carrie burning coles in their bare hands, and dip their said hands in hot skalding liquor, and also go into hot ouens'.[12] The significant overlap between stage magic and the marketing of medicine is particularly apparent in such spectacular self-harming routines. They were pioneered by quacks, including some attached to commedia dell'arte troupes, who professed to publicly cut, burn or poison themselves before curing themselves with patent medicines thereafter sold to the astounded crowd.[13] Similar associations inform occult stage scenes such as that in which the Dame of Ben Jonson's *Masque of queenes* melodramatically proclaims to the witches of her coven, some of whom have ointment pots at their girdles: 'Reach me [...] a rustie knife, to wound mine arme; And, as it drops, I'le speake a *charme*'.[14]

While magic effects of the type popularized by the hellmouth scenes of medieval mystery plays became increasingly uncommon in seventeenth-century drama,[15] they continued to flourish on marketplace stages. Persisting supernatural associations in the 'Age of Reason' are indicated by observations such as one concluding a description of fire-eating marketplace quacks, in a German-Latin school textbook of 1719: 'We do not wish to discuss whether this is natural and enabled by the use of herbal extracts, or results from a demonic pact.'[16] The sinister reputation of stage magic is also illuminated by accounts of its offstage deployment. In July 1555, Felix Platter accompanied his Montpellier professor, Honoré Castellan, to the public execution of a peasant who, like three young Périgord hoaxers described by Montaigne, terrorized his neighbours. Montaigne's hoaxers, however, remained hidden, while imitating supernatural spirits only with their voices. Montaigne, writing in the 1570s, inclined towards ascribing such

[10]   [Vincent], *Hocvs Pocvs Ivnior*, f.E2ᵛ–3ʳ; Ady, *A candle in the dark*, 38–9; Bawcutt, 'William Vincent'; Butterworth, 'Brandon, Feats and Hocus Pocus'.

[11]   Piluland, *Vielvermehrter Hocus Pocus*, 136.

[12]   Scot, *Discouerie of Witchcraft*, 255 and plates between 352 and 353.

[13]   Katritzky, *Women, medicine and theatre*, 96–9.

[14]   Jonson, *Workes*, 946, 955.

[15]   Butterworth, *Magic on the early English stage*, xvi.

[16]   Comenius, *Orbis sensualium picti*, 46–7 ('XVII. Pyrophagus. Der Feuer-Fresser').

cases to the mental disturbance of their perpetrators rather than to evil intent or supernatural causes. Only briefly alluding to their jail sentence, he repeatedly situates their 'harmelesse devise or jugling tricke' in the theatrical sphere of stage magic.[17]

According to Guarinonius, who vigorously denounces 'superstitions and heresies', physicians get few opportunities to examine 'lying fortune-tellers, cheating astrologers, palm-readers and wound-blessers, harbourers of devils and spirits, destroyers of people, cattle and land, witches and similar monstrous patients', because most are of sound body when dispatched by the hangman.[18] His discussion of habitual abusers of distilled alcohol asks: 'How many become so drunk that, like monstrous spirits or like a living Lucifer, they spew fire and flames from their jaws?'[19] In publicly disguising himself as the Devil, the Montpellier peasant whose execution Platter witnessed in 1555 broke a taboo whose transgression during the carnival period was stringently regulated across Europe. Demonic carnival Devil masks were banned in Basle in 1432 and in Strasbourg in 1463 and 1483, while in the Tirol a regulation of 1618 accused masked carnival masqueraders of terrifying children and pregnant women.[20] Of the Montpellier peasant, Felix Platter notes that, having paraded in public in Devil costume, his nose, ears and mouth spewing fire, claiming that he was the Devil and would drag the local priesthood and population off at night if they did not give him money: 'He was hanged from the gallows in front of the city hall, then immediately taken down, and his head, arms and legs hacked off. Dr Honoratus [Castellanus], with whom I had eaten lunch, took me to a house in which there were many ladies and gentlemen, from which I watched it'.[21]

Felix Platter's *Praxis medica* classifies 'the cure of those possest with the Divel' as the business not of the physician, but of the Church: '*the preternatural cause* proceeding from *the Divel* as it doth no waies belong to the Physitian, so neither the Cure; for *the Divel* is forcibly expel'd by the Prayers of Divines and godly people'.[22] In the context of religious witchhunts, certain illnesses such as epilepsy, hysteria and melancholy acquired sinister non-medical connotations. Some early modern physicians, citing classical authorities, believed that melancholy afflicted body and soul, rendering both susceptible to the entry of evil spirits.[23] Those diagnosed with possession by evil spirits could be brought to trial and punished

---

[17]   Montaigne, 'Of the lame or cripple', *Essayes*, 580; Butterworth, 'The work of the devil?', 711, 720–2.

[18]   Guarinonius, *Grewel*, 425; Innsbruck UL, Cod.110, IV, ff.446ᵛ, 452ᵛ.

[19]   Guarinonius, *Grewel*, 663.

[20]   Aker, *Narrenschiff*, 276; Graß, 'Der Kampf gegen Fasnachtsveranstaltungen', 227. See also Lederer, *Madness, religion and the state*, 163.

[21]   *Felix Platter Tagebuch*, 220 (6 July 1555, Montpellier).

[22]   Plat[t]er, Cole and Culpeper, *A golden practice*, 35.

[23]   Gowland, 'Melancholy', 91–6; Klinnert, 'Johann Weyers "De Praestigiis Daemonum"', 104.

as criminals, or treated for insanity, generally by Church-organized exorcism. In 1560, Franz Venetz, an exorcist attached to Lucerne Cathedral, convalesced at the house of Platter the Elder,[24] during a lengthy unsuccessful treatment by Felix Platter of lameness caused by a painful injured hip. Eventually, Venetz told Felix Platter:

> "I want to go home again. You won't be able to cure me, because the ailment is supernatural. Through exorcism, I drove the evil spirit out of someone in Lucerne who, as he rushed out, confided in me. Saying: 'Priest, you have often cast me out, I want to reward you', he hurled me down onto the hearth, against which I knocked myself, and that's how I got to be lame". So he went.[25]

In *Observations*, Platter revisits the Venetz case, noting that 'After I had tried many things in vain, he confessed that the Devil had done it, when he laboured to drive him out of a man, by thrusting him violently against the chimney', exclaiming the following words in German as he did so: 'Priest! Now I'm paying you back for casting me out like this'.[26] According to his journal, Felix Platter was at Venetz's Lucerne home in 1561 to exact the Basle lodging fee still owing to his father, when two men threw in a possessed man afflicted with *stupor daemonicus*. Brought for treatment after going several days without food or drink, he was rigid and speechless, his head twisted backwards. Far from offering his professional assistance with Venetz's patient, the nauseated Platter tried to leave. As he did so, Venetz begged him not to tell his father that he was still casting out devils, as although Platter the Elder had often warned him against it, Venetz relied on the special payments he earned from it.[27]

In July 1599, Thomas Platter visited the Church of St Ursini, Bourges, where:

> the evil spirits are exorcised, and many are driven out, from those who are possessed, of whom rather a lot are to be found in this region. While I was staying in Sologne, gossip broke out that a young woman of Romorantin was possessed, but in the end it turned out that she was only dealing in deception,

---

[24] Who had travelled and studied with Anthonius Venetz in 1519 (Platter the Elder, 'Thomas Platters Lebensbeschreibung', 54–6, 126).

[25] *Felix Platter Tagebuch*, 362 (1560, Basle).

[26] Platter, 'Stupor dæmoniacus, in quo corpus immobile & insensile rigebat, & collum inuersum erat', *Obseruationum*, 18–19. The source of the first quote, the English translation of 1664 (Plat[t]er, Culpeper and Cole, *Platerus histories*, 12), omits all reference to the Devil's exclamation, exceptionally printed in German and in gothic script in Platter's original 1614 Latin edition: 'Exorcista quidam sacerdos An. 1560 [...] vti ante sæpe his verbis Germanicè minatum fuisse, 𝕻faff ich will dir noch den lohn geben / daß du mich also vertreibst / simulque ad focum adeò violenter se detrusisie'.

[27] *Felix Platter Tagebuch*, 362–3, 376 (1560, Basle and 1561, Lucerne); Midelfort, *A history of madness* 175, 180 1.

fooling many by behaving as though the evil spirit was working through her, for which she eventually received due punishment.[28]

Romorantin was a Loire village near Château Corborande, where Thomas Platter had recently been a guest, and the woman was 26-year-old 'Marthe la démoniaque'. Shown for money as a woman possessed by demons, by her father, the weaver turned mountebank Jacques Brossier, she became an international sensation.[29] Father and daughter fled to Rome when French bishops and court physicians exposed them as frauds, in effect elaborate stage magicians.[30]

During the early modern period, even very modest stage magic of the type of card tricks was widely viewed in a negative light.[31] Guarinonius deeply disapproved of 'the new political world, in which no-one believes in hell or the Devil any more'. Although himself unquestioningly accepting the physical existence of demons, devils, and 'God's ape, the Devil', like the sceptics, he went to great lengths to demystify the stage routines of professional magicians through rational explanation.[32] He unmasks one such trick in a section of *Grewel* defining three types of professional performer, namely acrobats, actors and juggling magicians, in the context of a consideration of physical exercise:

> Concerning itinerant entertainers, some can juggle so quickly simply with their hands that they can dupe the eyesight of the simpleminded, so that simpletons regard their juggling as miracles or even as magic. As when I was told, as if it were a great miracle, how one of them dealt playing cards onto the middle of a table, and found the King of Bells by tapping the arranged cards with a little stick. This card moved out of the pack by itself, and followed the little stick up and down the whole table in whichever direction the entertainer turned the stick. I said to him he could make himself a similar stick by fixing an iron nail at the front, and hammering it into the centre of its tip so that it is hidden and can't be seen. Then when the entertainer lays the card on the table again, he should confront him, pull his stick out from under his coat, and command the King of Bells to come out.[33]

The following day the spectator did just that; totally amazing everyone by getting two cards to follow his stick round the table, before the terrified performer gathered up his cards and fled, without divulging his secret. Guarinonius, however, eagerly does so:

---

[28]   *Thomas Platter d.J*, 525 (14 July 1599, Bourges).

[29]   Marescot, *A trve discovrse*.

[30]   Walker and Dickerman, 'A woman under the influence', 553.

[31]   Bodin, *Demonomanie*, sig.138ʳ.

[32]   Guarinonius, *Grewel*, 382, 1023.

[33]   Guarinonius, *Grewel*, 1255–6. In Alpine regions, the four suits are traditionally oak leaves, hearts, acorns and fools' bells.

The two cards had a layer of magnetic lodestone between their paper layers, which followed the iron in the stick. Such entertainment cannot be counted as exercise, but only as a foolish diversion for the eyes of the inquisitive. The second type of entertainers perform curious bodily contortions, such as strange leaps through hoops, above unsheathed weapons, and suchlike, and the more dangerous, the less diverting they are. The third type is the actors. Of all the many sorts of different types, those which are not to be tolerated at all are the ones who give sordid and voluptuous performances to the young, and stage shameless plays concerned with courting and etc.[34]

This last sentence refers to mixed-gender commedia dell'arte troupes, whose magic routines combined influences from classical, religious and secular drama. Whether represented as independent roles, or as temporary disguises for male or female stock characters, their typical occult characters were male necromancers, demons, spirits or astrologers.

Commedia dell'arte plots are preserved not in full-length playtexts, but as highly compressed indicative 'dramaturgical machines'[35] or scenari. Several of Flaminio Scala's 50 scenari, the only collection published during the early modern period, include real or supposed supernatural or magical plot elements. *Lo Specchio* features two ghosts, *Il finto negromante* a Harlequin disguised as a necromancer who inscribes circles on the stage and conjures up two fake spirits, *Flavio finto negromante* a necromancer, *Isabella astrologa* the heroine disguised as a male astrologer, *Rosalba incantatrice* four spirits and a silver vase containing the 'fire of truth', in which Arlecchino burns his hands, *Dell'Orseida* II a comic servant and maid who mistake each other for ghosts, and *L'Arbore incantato* two spirits and spectacular fire effects involving a whole range of props.[36] The concise, cryptic nature of scenari limits insights into the role of magic and superstition on commedia dell'arte stages. Designed to support professional actors and protect the trade secrets of their craft from censorship and rival performers, scenari often summarized their lazzi, or set-piece pre-rehearsed comic stage routines, in two or three sentences, or even words. The undefined relationship of most commedia dell'arte-related images to stage practice complicates interpretation of the iconographic record. Magic and supernatural themes are reflected in many of the titles of the only early modern scenari collection with illustrated titlepages, the 101 early seventeenth-century manuscript Corsini scenari.[37] *Il gran mago*, *Il mago*, *La maga*, *Il serpe incantato* and *Il fonte incantato* are pastoral dramas, and *Le teste*

---

[34]   Guarinonius, *Grewel*, 1256.

[35]   Robert Henke's expression (*Performance and literature*, 189).

[36]   Scala, *Il Teatro*, Days 16, 21, 28, 36, 44, 47, 49.

[37]   Corsini Manuscript, Biblioteca Corsiniana, Rome (all 100 title pages reproduced in: Pandolfi, *La commedia dell'arte*, V (unpaginated supplement between pp. 256–7); Katritzky, *The art of commedia*, plates 243–7).

incantate is a tragicomedy.[38] *Li spiriti, L'amorosi incanti, Il falso indovino, Li finti amici* and *La magica di Pantalone* (whose titlepage depiction shows a pastoral setting) are all styled as comedies.[39] The titlepage illustration to *La maga* depicts the hapless old master, Pantalone, being roasted in a fire attended by two comic servants, or Zanni, and presided over by a magician, an incident unexplained in the scenario text, and the Corsini illustrations' documentary value as records of the scenari to which they provide title-pages has persuasively been called into question.[40]

Scenari and other commedia dell'arte-related texts and images provide ample confirmation of the popularity of magic on early modern professional stages, but few facts on how this functioned in practice. Thomas Platter's description of a commedia dell'arte decapitation routine, quoted above, is exceptional for its detail. Another eyewitness account relevant in this respect is Hippolytus Guarinonius's description of a lazzo he saw in Padua in the 1590s. In this, the comic stage servant Zanni, wishing to take a closer look at a ghost above him, climbs a ladder to a window, from which flames and a young Devil shoot out at him, and one firework after another explodes onto his beard. Frightened and screaming 'murder', he tries jumping back down off the ladder, only to find himself trapped between another ghost chasing him up again and the ghost at the top trying to force him down.[41] This resembles a much later lazzo, performed in Paris in the 1660s by the comic star of the Comédie Italienne, Domenico Biancolelli:

> I climb a tree on which grows some beautiful fruit, when I go to pick it, a Devil comes out of the trunk and frightens me, I want to get down, but another Devil at the foot of the tree begins to climb. I climb up again and descend again several times [with the same lazzo], then the magician appears who touches me and leaves me in a ridiculous pose, then he gives me his wand and tells me marvels, etc.[42]

Ladders were popular professional stage props, featuring in numerous scenari recorded by Scala, Biancolelli and others. French courtiers at Fontainebleau in 1608 were impressed by a lazzo in which, as one recorded in his journal, the commedia dell'arte actor Cola 'climbed straight up a ladder that was not leaning against anything, and he fell its full length doing somersaults without getting a

---

[38]   Corsini MS I.5, I.13, II.57, II.73, II.77, II.97.

[39]   Corsini MS I.6, I.12, II.62, II.80, II.93.

[40]   Lea, 'Bibliography', 8–9; Mengarelli, 'Corsini Manuscript'.

[41]   Guarinonius, *Grewel*, 375 (lazzo no.8: for complete translation see Chapter 18, this volume).

[42]   *Arlechino creduto Principe* (Gambelli, *Arlecchino a Parigi*, II, 330; Scott, *The commedia dell'arte in Paris*, 143–4, in translation, bracketed phrase added from the original French by present author).

scratch'.[43] Ladder lazzi occur in the Parisian *Suite du festin de pierre* (1673) and *Colombine avocat* (1685), in more than one Scala scenario, and in several Corsini titlepage illustrations, including that for *Il Mago*, which also features devils.[44] The extravagant special effects of the Italian comedy in Paris routinely featured devils, ghosts or fire. For example, in *Le collier de perle* (1672), three devils with torches dance with five sorcerers; in *A fourbe, fourbe et demy* (1674), Arlequin's experiments with fire include setting alight the moustaches of the constabulary; and hell scenes feature in *Le voyage de Scaramouche et d'Arlequin aux Indes* (1676) and *La magie naturelle* (1678).[45] Guarinonius's description provides the detail to confirm that specific routines of a type standard to the repertory of the Italian comedians in late seventeenth-century Paris already had a well-developed presence on the travelling quack stages of sixteenth-century Italy.

The previous chapter surveyed some descriptions of itinerant acrobatics not specifically linked to medicine or magic. Thomas Platter's account of a handsome, strong young Frenchman called Buratin, whom he saw performing in January 1599 on a new stage, still under construction in a Barcelona suburb, indicates the care with which he observed and interviewed superlative acrobats, and the degree to which audiences viewed them less as talented, hardworking performers than as masters of the occult.[46] For several days, Buratin displayed astonishing tricks on a high horizontal tightrope, throwing himself around like an ape; hanging on, unfastened, just by an arm or a leg. Then, holding a long stave, he performed the *canario, gagliarda, branle* and other difficult, unfamiliar dances on the rope, executed numerous high leaps, then sat with the rope between his legs, and jumped up again, always keeping time with his instrumentalists on the stage below. Guarinonius, who contrasts skilful but safety-conscious Italian tightrope displays with the foolhardy, dangerous exploits of their German counterparts, explains the importance of the stave: 'As we know, and have repeatedly observed with tightrope walkers, they are able to perform their acrobatics much more easily and surely by carrying a weighted object in their hands, than without the weight.'[47]

Thomas Platter notes that Buratin then put aside his stave to dance a Spanish dance, gracefully and skilfully clicking the castanets with both hands. Then he walked up and down the rope and danced unusual dances such as the *passo e mezzo*, first with high slippers, then with round indoor tennis balls, fastened to the

---

[43]   Wiley, *The early public theatre in France*, 24 (in translation).

[44]   Corsini MS I.13 (*Il Mago*), I.23 (*L'arme mutate*), I.29 (*Il giardino*), II.60 (*L'amor constante*); Scala, *Il Teatro*, Days 21 (*Il finto negromante*), 29 (*Il fido amico*). *I tappeti, ovvero Colafronio geloso* also features a ladder lazzo in the context of necromancers and spirits (Bartoli, *Scenari inediti*, 282–5). See also Gordon, *Lazzi*, 9–12, 45, 47; Scott, *The commedia dell'arte in Paris*, 211, 304. Capozza, *Tutti i lazzi*, 22–7: nos.35–52; Schmitt, 'Il finto negromante', 310, 320–2.

[45]   Scott, *The commedia dell'arte in Paris*, 203, 204–8, 213, 216.

[46]   *Thomas Platter d.J*, 348–9 (28 January 1599, Barcelona).

[47]   Guarinonius, *Grewel*, 1189, 1256.

soles of his shoes. For his finale, he walked the rope fastened into a sack. He also walked, and executed unusual dances and acrobatics on the rope, with a servant on his shoulders. Platter learned that he was a bachelor and Parisian by birth. Money seemed unimportant to him. He earned what he needed, had no wish to perform every day, had 10,000 crowns earned through his skills invested in France, and was thinking of retiring altogether soon. Whenever he allowed himself to stumble as if he were falling, holding onto the rope only by one arm, hand or foot, a woman (Platter implies that she is a fellow troupe member) would repeatedly scream out that now Buratin would fall to his death. But he always righted himself so adroitly again, without apparent injury, that Platter admitted never having seen the like before. Buratin told Platter that his skills were genuine and attained through long practice, which he was inclined to believe, although noting that many could only explain Buratin's expertise through powerful magic or illusory tricks.

Thomas Platter also records his encounters with several self-proclaimed necromancers. In April 1597, two days after watching attractively costumed young people perform a play in Bagnols-sur-Cèze's town square, the governor, Pierre d'Augier, Provost of Languedoc, invited him to view his curiosity cabinet and plant collection. While they dined alone together, d'Augier regaled Platter with tales of his youth, when he too had studied medicine and travelled overseas before returning home to rise to high office:

> Which had brought him great respect. But just because he professed to unusual knowledge and presented several important people with gold rings in which there was a spirit (*spiritus familiaris*), he was regarded as a magician or necromancer. As I was then told, he was also said to have recently presented a high ranking noblewoman at her request with such a gold ring, in which a secret spirit was trapped. Whenever the woman had a question, this spirit could reveal the complete answer to her. She only had to pay homage to it for two hours every day, as the provost had commanded her to, otherwise she would be in danger of extreme misfortune, which indeed eventually happened. After finding out everything that was said about her and that went on around her, she eventually became so confused and melancholic that she no longer paid the spirit in the ring the homage she had pledged him. So she was possessed by him, and had to end her life miserably, as I was told. I was encouraged to find this more credible by what he did and didn't say, because he spent a good part of dinner discussing evil spirits with me, and how few ceremonies are essential in order to conjure up the abominable Satan.[48]

Despite the efforts of sceptics such as Scot, who scornfully exposes the 'ridiculous coniurations' required 'to enclose a spirit in a christall stone', early modern literature offers a tangible sense of Satan's physical reality.[49] Thomas Platter was

---

[48]   *Thomas Platter d.J*, 212–13 (16 April 1597, Bagnols-sur-Cèze).
[49]   Scot, *Discouerie of Witchcraft*, 411–13, 430.

clearly underwhelmed by the claw-marks allegedly left by the Devil when he got stuck in a fountain Platter was shown at a Marseille church in 1597 ('but as to whether the poor Devil drowned or managed to get away, who can tell?'). But his account of Barcelona inquisition suspects in January 1599 twice emphasizes the devils painted on their robes, and leaves no doubt that even if he questioned the physical reality of devils, many of his contemporaries did not.[50] In 1632, James Howell confirms this inquisition robe as 'the *Sambenito* which is a streight yellow Coat without Sleeves, having the pourtrait of the Devil painted up and down in black'. As late as 1647, Howell ridicules sceptical tendencies in a demonological manuscript[51] lent him by Sir Edward Spencer: 'we read that both *Jews* and *Romans*, with all other Nations of *Christendom*, and our Ancestors here in *Engl.* enacted Laws against *witches*: Sure they were not so silly, as to waste there Brains in making Laws against Chymera's, against *non entia*'.[52]

Platter's account of his evening with d'Augier makes no secret of the fact that he found the loquacious old bachelor tiresome and his tall tales less than credible:

> He got so wrapped up in his discourse that I just wished I was back in my inn. All his speech and conversation was of supernatural arts, evil spirits or beautiful women, in exactly the same way that the comte de Cantecroy of Besançon later regaled me with such talk. I firmly believe that they are inmates of one (*praedicamento*) asylum. At around 11, after finishing the impressive evening meal, he allowed me to be accompanied to my inn by a torchbearer, with the request that I should dine with him and spend time with him every day that I remained in Bagnols. But I excused myself and took my leave of him, saying that I was on the point of leaving. Nevertheless, I stayed on in Bagnols for 17, 18, 19 and 20 April, preparing to take up my professional practice [in nearby Uzès], and not leaving my inn.[53]

His reference to the asylum aligns Thomas Platter with sceptics such as Wier and Scot, who sought medical and mental rather than supernatural explanations for such tales. Felix, who unlike Thomas betrays genuine personal fear of ghosts and spirits,[54] shares his brother's sceptical medical mindset, noting, for example, of

---

[50] *Thomas Platter d.J*, 191 (16 February 1597, Marseille); 351–2 (28 January 1599, Barcelona).

[51] Possibly a prepublication copy of Homes's *Dæmonologie* (1650).

[52] Howell, *Familiar letters*, 219, 425.

[53] *Thomas Platter d.J*, 213 (16 April 1597, Bagnols-sur-Cèze).

[54] *Felix Platter Tagebuch*, 63 (1539, Basle: petrified three-year-old Felix mistook twittering pet birds for the Üllengry, a fearsome spirit said to bite off people's heads. As often, there is a comparable episode in his father's memoir, who, as a young child, mistook hissing geese for the Devil [Platter the Elder, 'Thomas Platters Lebensbeschreibung', 33]); see also *Felix Platter Tagebuch*, 390 (2 December 1562, Belfort: 'the pitiable lamentations of a ghost' terrified Felix and his companions, riding one dark evening through the forested

a mysterious scrap of red cloth appearing from the healed wound of a Mulhouse bow maker, long after he had fallen from a tree and been pierced right through his body by a stake, that: 'many thought it was done by Magick, but it appeared after to be a piece of his Wascoat which he wore when he had the fall'.[55]

Nevertheless, educated early modern physicians clearly considered the concept of black magic itself both real and serious, and routinely treated symptoms allegedly resulting from bewitchment. Felix Platter's case notes record a patient who, because she was unable to relieve the intense, chronic migraine-like pains on the left side of her head with conventional medicines, ascribed them to bewitchment, while he inclined to a psychological, not supernatural, diagnosis: 'She supposed that a Witch had dropt worms into the Ear while she slept.' Felix Platter's trepanation of the most intensely affected area did little to relieve her pain, which finally abated only after she gave birth to a boy some years later, in May 1604.[56] A year before meeting d'Augier, Thomas Platter had carefully sketched a knife in the curiosity cabinet of the late Laurent Joubert, son-in-law and eventual academic successor (on the death of Antoine Saporta) to Felix Platter's former teacher Guillaume Rondelet. Thomas Platter reports, almost certainly on the authority of his host, a younger son of Joubert, that Joubert himself, with his own hands, had pulled the knife from the body of a peasant with terrible internal pains, who had explained during an earlier house call that another peasant had forced him to swallow it under threat of death. Laurent Joubert had treated him only with great reluctance, being 'of the opinion that the Devil, disguised as a peasant (as he thought), must have used sorcery to get it into his body, because it would have been impossible to completely swallow such a long knife by natural means'.[57] The royal surgeon Ambroise Paré's version of this case marginalizes Joubert's involvement, and makes no reference to the supernatural, beyond including his account in the section of his treatise on 'Monsters and prodigies':

> *A knife swallowed, came forth at an abscesse in the groine: Cabrolle* Chirurgian to *Mounsieur,* the Marshall of *Anville,* told mee that *Francis Guillenet* the Chirurgian of *Sommiers,* a small village some eight miles from *Mompelier,* had in cure, and healed a certaine sheepheard, who was forced by theeves to swallow a knife of the length of halfe a foot, with a horne handle of the thickenesse of ones thumbe: he kept it the space of halfe a yeere, yet with great paine, and hee fell much away, but yet was not in a consumption, untill at length an abscesse

---

valley of Valdieu near Mulhouse). Guarinonius dismisses fear of ghosts as a weakness of simple-minded 'women, children and not a few men' (*Grewel*, 305, see also 490, 496).

[55]   Platter, *Obseruationum*, 538–9 (this translation: Plat[t]er, Culpeper and Cole, *Platerus histories*, 355).

[56]   Platter, *Obseruationum*, 347 (this translation: Plat[t]er, Culpeper and Cole, *Platerus histories*, 226); Huber, *Felix Platters 'Observationes'*, 249.

[57]   *Thomas Platter d.J*, 169–70 (9 August 1596, Montpellier).

rising in his groine, with great store of very stinking quitture, the knife was there taken forth in the presence of the Justices, and left with *Joubert* the Physitian of *Mompelier*.[58]

Genuine fear colours Thomas Platter's recollections of his encounters with another necromancer, François Perrenot de Granvelle, comte de Cantecroy. On 8 February 1600, the count showed Platter his outstanding collection of art and antiquities. Later, Dr Jean Chifflet came to the count's palace to take them to a carnival supper party at his house. Chifflet, a graduate of Padua medical school who served his native Besançon as plague doctor, physician and then regent, and was rated by Felix Platter as an 'illustrious and excellent physician [...] and friend',[59] confided to Thomas Platter that he never cared to stay late in the company of Cantecroy, a man with many enemies. Nevertheless, having eaten, and been entertained by 'many masked women', at Chifflet's house, he and his guests accompanied them to other carnival dances and festivities until the early hours, when the count authorized his Moorish torch-bearer to escort them home.[60] The following morning, the count again sent for Platter, impatient to leave for Basle:

and held me up until the midday meal. Spoke repeatedly of the magic arts, which he was extremely interested in using to take the lives of several people. As I was already preparing to leave the city, he sent yet another messenger, requesting me to stay with him until Shrove Tuesday. But I requested him to say that I had already gone. So I rushed off in great haste, because I found his company anything but congenial.[61]

Educated necromancers such as d'Augier and Cantecroy drew heavily on occult traditions recorded in pre-Christian classical literature. The magic and witchcraft featured in early modern drama was informed by elite sorcery of this type, but also by the magic routines developed by stage quacks, and by popular sorcery and white magic of the type practiced by uneducated wise women and cunning-folk, dispensing amulets and charm-based cures and counter-cures. Felix

---

[58] Paré, *The workes*, 999 (original edition: *Deux livres de chirurgie*, Paris 1573); Goulart retells Paré's version (*Admirable and memorable histories*, 80; original edition: *Thrésores d'histoires*, Paris 1600).

[59] Felix Platter praised Chifflet (1550–1602) for transcribing for him the *post-mortem* report on a Burgundian patient Platter treated in September 1599 and early 1600 (*Obseruationum*, 471).

[60] The 'Negre comte Cantecroy' who paid Felix Platter four pounds boarding costs later that year was possibly this or another of the Moorish servants of the count (1550–1607), whose anonymous double portrait with Mlle. Gaille ('La belle verdurière') now hangs in the Louvre (*Felix Platter Tagebuch*, 533; Lötscher (*Felix Platter und seine Familie*, 90).

[61] *Thomas Platter d.J*, 921–2 (29–30 January/8–9 February 1600, Besançon).

Platter, convinced that '*Amulets* also do help, if not by their own virtue, at least waies by imagination', frequently refers to their medicinal use in *Praxis medica*.[62] Guarinonius's vernacular plague treatise of 1612 addresses the widespread medical use of written amulets. It rhetorically asks: 'Whether speaking, blessing, scripts, signs and other similar partly superstitious, partly magical treatments are suitable for the plague?' Identifying them as 'public sins against God, sorcery and idolatry [...] diabolic remedies cursed by God', Guarinonius's caustic reply recalls an itinerant quack sorcerer who devastated the region with bogus magical plague remedies of this type:

> Answer: Of course they are suitable for the plague, in order to inflame it even more, and spread it to regions it has not yet reached [...] In Schwaz, in the twelfth or thirteenth year,[63] one such monstrous person, by training just a stable boy, through his use of such magical scripts, characters, letters and all sorts of magical props, not only poisoned the cities of Innsbruck, Hall and Schwaz, but even more seriously, of almost every village and valley, and bewitched the simpleminded. [...] Is this public disrespect and idolatry against God the Father something that can awaken his anger and encourage the plague? [...] The Bible records God's punishments for those who consult outspoken old whores, or female witches and broomstick riders. If incantations, texts, letters of the alphabet, and signs of the Devil are so effective, and the head sorcerer is sitting in the middle of Schwaz [...], why then does the plague rage more abominably where incantations and sorcery are in greater use? Do you not understand what I am telling you? That superstitious remedies of this type only encourage the plague even more, and inflame God's anger more and more?[64]

Although written amulets were condemned as satanic by prominent churchmen such as Thomas Aquinas or St Augustine,[65] some churchmen also dispensed them. Guarinonius valued one prescribed to his son, whose left leg had become progressively paralysed from the age of eight, by Fra Tommaso da Bergamo:

> During his illness the blessed Brother Thomas visited him, examined him and said "What if the boy were bewitched? Look", he said, "Here's something I'd like to lend you. This is an excellent way of rendering the demonic forces harmless and then, if God pleases, the boy will be cured of this". He handed over a packet the size of a walnut or a large horse chestnut, wrapped in a little cloth and for good measure also sealed. "That", he said, "contains a great deal

---

[62] E.g. Plat[t]er, Cole and Culpeper, *A golden practice*, 4, 17, 25, 36, 43, 75, 77.

[63] The obvious translation for 'im zwölfften oder dreyzehenden Jahr' (as 'around the year 1612 or 1613'), sits uneasily with the treatise's publication date of 1612.

[64] Guarinonius, *Pestilentz Guardien*, 117*–22*. See also Dörrer, 'Guarinoni als Volksschriftsteller', 150.

[65] Bodin, *Demonomanie*, sig.152^{r-v} .

of sacred material as a countermeasure against magic. Fasten it to him and don't lose it before you return it to me". We took it and fastened it to the boy with due reverence. After that the extreme pain stopped and he recovered sufficiently to reach the age of 22, admittedly with the support of a crutch, until he had completed his studies. From Trent he returned home ill, he had a high fever and the growth on his affected foot had recently re-opened. After patiently suffering his many and heavy sorrows, he died at peace with God on Whitsunday, six years after the death of the blessed Brother Thomas [...] By chance we found out after his death: our boy was bewitched at the age of eight by that sorcerer priest from Hall who had been unfrocked and executed in Bressanone. He admitted it under torture.[66]

Even more than men, Guarinonius suspected women, and especially old women, of witchcraft. Declaring that 'almost all old women are full of superstition and useless ideas', he asks: 'Is it at all surprising that through poverty and need, misery and dejection, they often call upon wicked matters, even the wicked enemy, the Devil, and deal with magic?'[67] Thomas Platter's digressions on Villefranche's Catholic peasants afford insights into rural cunning-folk of a type whose quasi-medical activities were often labelled witchcraft:

In their churches, everything they hear is spoken and sung in Latin, which they don't understand. In such mountainous regions there are few sermons, as such people don't regularly attend them, because they often live very far from the churches, and become rough, godless folk easily led astray by the evil spirit, pledging themselves to him and becoming witches or sorcerers, of whom many are to be found in these mountains.[68]

His records of certain superstitious traditions of such 'godless folk' have long been valued by anthropologists and social historians. His account of one of them, ligature, repays examination by literary as well as medical historians, because it brings into sharp focus the occult medical practice central to a Jacobean court scandal widely reflected in English drama. Thomas Platter looked carefully into this sinister, influential black magic for rendering men impotent in 1598, while practicing as a newly-qualified physician in Uzès. Legally referred to as *ligaturas* or *ligare ligulam*, Platter provides French and German terms for it: 'nestel knipfen (de l'aiguillete)'.[69] So feared in Languedoc that few couples dared marry openly, and endemic to coastal Poitou and Normandy, Brantôme's indication that 'an infinity' of marriages was affected by 'this wicked custom in and beyond France' is born

---

[66] Guarinonius, *Thomas von Bergamo*, 61–2.

[67] Guarinonius, *Grewel*, 314, 738.

[68] *Thomas Platter d.J*, 404–5 (25 April 1599, Villefranche).

[69] *Thomas Platter d.J*, 274 (modern French usage: 'nouer l'aiguilette'); Robbins, 'Magical emasculation', 63, 65.

out by its widespread legal acknowledgement.[70] Ligature, branded 'a diabolical enchantment [...] the origin and foundation of all sorcery' by Bodin, was a capital offence punishable by burning.[71] Practiced by female as well as male magicians, and by clergy concerned to divert some of the considerable fees cunning-folk and white witches charged for reversing its effects, it allegedly rendered newlywed men impotent, but only with their own brides.

As late as 1667, the Palermo-based Bavarian Jesuit Kaspar Schott confirms that ligature was so feared that many couples married in private ceremonies the day before their public church wedding.[72] In 1596, before hosting his wedding banquet in Montpellier, Thomas Platter's acquaintance the merchant Roviere had secretly married his bride in a small village, the couple 'going to the church alone and quietly, as is customary in Languedoc, so that their codpiece points would not be knotted'.[73] Noting that similarly private arrangements were made for a wedding in Uzès in July 1598, and realizing that in over three years in Languedoc he himself had seen only 10 weddings, Platter decided to investigate for himself this 'demonic magic, which is nothing less than the work of the Devil'. What he uncovered was the exact procedure whereby occult practitioners knotted a reinforced leather lace ('point'), of the type used to lace up codpieces:

> The whole magic consists only in this. At the same time as the Priest says the words "What therefore God hath joined together, let not man put asunder",[74] the

---

[70]   Brantôme, *Recueil des Dames*, 162. In 1596, the surgeon Eusebio Isorno, from Intra on Lago di Maggiore, was convicted of witchcraft crimes including the use of magical healing to cure impotence (Deutscher, 'The Episcopal Tribunal of Novara', 416). Day provides the medieval Hebrew ('asar') and Swedish ('nalknytning') terms and suggests that Knut was a name chosen by Swedish parents for the boy they hoped would be their last child ('Knots', 246–8). Fuhrmann touches on legal issues relating to ligature in medieval Germany (*Ingelheimer Schöffensprüche*, 93–4).

[71]   Bodin, *Demonomanie*, sig.207[r]. His alternative naming in this passage of ligature practitioners as 'les coupeurs de bourses', an early modern term for cutpurses sometimes also denoting animal castrators, illuminates an iconographic motif popularized by Lucas van Leyden's engraving of 1523, 'The toothdrawer'. Such depictions of cutpurse activity around marketplace quack stages, clearly intended to remind potential patients of the grave medical as well as financial risks of consulting quacks, inform Guarinonius's ironic question to those consulting medical almanacs: 'Can you not also read in them when it is good to cut purses?' (*Grewel*, 1004).

[72]   Browe, *Sexualethik*, 129.

[73]   *Thomas Platter d.J*, 145 (23 March 1596, Montpellier).

[74]   *King James Bible*: 'Mark' 10v.9. Both Bodin and Barclay confirm that the point is knotted while the priest reads a specific passage of the marriage ceremony (*Demonomanie*, sig.207[r]; *Replique*, 114–15). An anonymous French tract of 1599 records an unnamed sorcerer and priest who conferred impotence by modifying the traditional marriage ceremony phrase to 'Quod Diabolus coniunxit Deus non separet' (Clark, *Thinking with demons*, 88). Guazzo's substantial chapter 'Of tying the points' makes no further reference

male or female magician knots a point and says ("Mais bien le diable", en iettant un patac derriere les espaules) "From the Devil", and at the same time throws a penny behind him, saying "Show Devil, take Devil". In this way the penny is lost and the magic is arranged. Following this, the groom is unable to recognize his wife until the point is unknotted again. But they are well able to use their virility with other married and unmarried women, and in this way whoring and divorce ensue [...] Many other variations are also practiced instead of point knotting, on which I prefer to remain silent. The historian Bodin writes that there was a woman who could carry out this magic in 25 different ways.[75]

The notorious passage in *Demonomanie* here referred to summarizes Bodin's discussion of 1567 in Poitiers with his 'innkeeper, a woman of good repute', who personally revealed to him over 50 variations on the practice of ligature to cause magical impotence.[76] It indicates how thoroughly embedded the practice was in France, where it was still performed according to traditional ritual ceremonies continuous with those of medieval Europe. In early modern Britain, this oral medico-magical tradition had been replaced by practices derived from literary sources.

Ligature has ancient roots. Male impotence blamed on sorcery and witchcraft was treated by the Babylonians both therapeutically and with magic incantations, and features in Petronius's *Satyrica*, Virgil's eighth *Eclogue* and poem 3.7 of Ovid's *Amores*, in which the poet considers whether his temporary impotence results from occult spells wrought with wax images.[77] From the sixth century onwards, *Libri Poenitentiales* and manuals of canon law reflect the Christian struggle to contain and suppress traditional superstitious practices such as the amuletic use of magical knots to assign and avert illness and bad fortune. St Theodore of Tarsus, the seventh-century Greek Archbishop of Canterbury, denounced ligature in medieval England, and it was outlawed by Burchard, the sceptical early eleventh-century Bishop of Worms, whose *Decretum* identifies the female enchanters of magically

---

to the laces themselves (*Compendium maleficarum*, 91–5). Another custom relating to laces, the practice known as 'cutting off the laces (nestel abschniden)', was current amongst boisterous young German-speakers immediately after they started addressing each other with the familiar 'Du'. To the distress of the fastidious Felix, many of his silk laces were then indeed cut off by a rowdy new travelling companion (*Felix Platter Tagebuch*, 290: 6 May 1557, Besançon).

[75] *Thomas Platter d.J*, 274–5 (16 July 1598, Uzès). The somewhat different ritual practices Engelbert Kaempfer extracted from 'an old witch' during his late seventeenth-century Near Eastern travels involved cloths and bodily fluids (Bowers and Carrubba, 'Sexual binding spells', 343).

[76] Bodin, *Demonomanie*, sig.58ʳ.

[77] Biggs, 'Medicine in Ancient Mesopotamia', 102–3; McLaren, *Impotence*; 1–2; Entin-Bates, 'Montaigne's remarks', 643.

impotent newlywed husbands as their rejected previous lovers, and condemns both practitioners and believers.[78]

While the notion of magical impotence was little known in England,[79] on mainland Europe it became extremely widespread. Fifteenth-century witchcraft tracts insistently focused on magical impotence include that famous witch-hunting tool of inquisitors, Heinrich Kramer's *Malleus Maleficarum* (1486) and one of its most influential sources, Johannes Nider's *Formicarius* (c.1437). They use the term *maleficium* less to denote the malicious damage caused by black magic in general, than specifically with respect to ligature hindering male consummation of matrimony as defined by canon law.[80] Warning his readers 'do not doubt that [impotence] can be brought about by the power of witchcraft', Kramer explains that witches 'act in the despite of married women, creating every opportunity for adultery when the husband is able to copulate with other women but not with his own wife; and similarly the wife also has to seek other lovers'.[81] Canon law permitted the annulment of marriages permanently rendered barren by magical impotence. Practitioners were punished by excommunication or death, and as late as 1718, the Parliament of Bordeaux condemned a convicted practitioner to be burned at the stake.[82] Seventeenth-century medical professionals increasingly rejected the acceptance of earlier colleagues, such as Ambroise Paré, of witchcraft as the standard explanation for magical impotence. However, its practitioners continued to be vigorously pursued throughout the century, especially by the Spanish Inquisition. Some cases involved incidental disclosure of local variants on the practice during trials, as in 1666, when Aldonza Cardoso de Velasco testified to the Toledo inquisitors that María Román had rendered a man impotent by reciting incantations over knots she had made in his undergarment laces and ritually stamping on the garment itself.[83] Others were high profile, none more so than the long running politically motivated, unsuccessful enquiries to identify the perpetrator of Carlos II's alleged magical impotence.[84]

Rather than female black magic, Felix Platter attributes the impotence of his patients, even those suspecting witchcraft, to male health issues. In a substantial section of his *Observations*, Platter identifies the source of one patient's impotence as coming from 'some internal fault hidden in the Seminal Vessels and not from Witchcraft as the Vulgar suppose, because he was always so. He could not endure

---

[78]   Day, 'Knots', 246; McNeill, 'Folk-paganism', 457, 461, 464; Browe, *Sexualethik*, 122.

[79]   Thomas, *Religion and the decline of magic*, 437.

[80]   Smith, 'The flying phallus', 93.

[81]   Stephens, 'Witches who steal penises', 499, 502, 519, 521 (in translation).

[82]   Browe, *Sexualethik*, 126; Anon., 'Witchcraft', 226.

[83]   Graizbord, *Souls in dispute*, 15.

[84]   Nada [Langdon-Davies], *Carlos the bewitched*. The Spanish Habsburg line ended with Carlos II's (1661–1700) barren marriages to Marie-Louise of France (James VI/I's great-granddaughter) and Maria Anna von Neuburg.

the Shame'; and casts doubt on another patient's suspicions that his impotence stemmed from his wife's witchcraft: 'he confessed seriously that he could not couple with her, and he thought she had bewitched him'.[85] This sceptical viewpoint, pioneered by Wier, was refined by Montaigne. His insight that the controlling factor of magical impotence is not external occult enchantment, but internal psychosexual problems, presented in an essay of the 1570s, is developed in a memorable late essay, exploring tensions between the limits of male potency and female desire.[86] In mid-seventeenth century Paris, leading scientists continued to debate on whether the causes of male impotence were natural or supernatural, while increasingly conceding that: 'the tying of the Codpiece-point is accounted an effect of the Fancy, and is cur'd by curing the Fancy alone'.[87] Long after that, the practice continued to be widely feared. Russian nuns in particular were 'accounted very dextrous both in tying and unravelling the Codpiece Point', and according to Engelbert Kaempfer's treatise of 1712, it was considered 'both usual and proper' to have white witches in attendance at Russian court weddings, to thwart impotence spells.[88] Literary references to this occult ceremony persisted in learned and popular publications decades after contemporary fashion had banished codpieces to the comic stage and rural backwaters.[89]

Rare references to magical impotence in British demonological treatises include Reginald Scot's of 1584, in a list of the 'miraculous actions' of witches, noting that they can 'take awaie mans courage, and the power of generation [...], and depriue men of their priuities, and otherwise of the act and use of venerie'. Recording a wide range of 'popish and magicall cures, for them that are bewitched in their priuities',[90] Scot sceptically comments:

> here againe we maie not forget the inquisitors note, to wit; that manie are so bewitched, that they cannot vse their own wiues: but anie other bodies they

---

[85]   Robbins, 'Magical emasculation', 80, n28; Platter, *Obseruationum*, 231–45 ('In Actvs Venerei defectv Obseruationes': these translations, Plat[t]er, Culpeper and Cole, *Platerus histories*, 152–3); Huber, *Felix Platters 'Observationes'*, 235.

[86]   Montaigne, 'Of the force of imagination' and 'Vpon some verses of Virgill', *Essayes*, 40–5, 471–503; Entin-Bates, 'Montaigne's remarks', 645; Parker, 'Gender ideology', 355.

[87]   Havers and Davies, *Another collection*, 260. See also Havers, *A general collection*, 214–18.

[88]   Collins, *Russia*, 10–11; Crull, *Muscovy*, 158; Bowers and Carrubba, 'Sexual binding spells', 340 (in translation).

[89]   Bergerac, *Satyrical characters*, 1: 'Winter hath tyed the Earth's Codpiece point, & hath made the substance Impotent'; Anon., *The women's petition against coffee*, sig.Aᵛ: 'the continual sipping of this pittiful Drink, is enough to *bewitch* Men of two and twenty, and tie up the *Codpice-point* without a Charm'; Anon., *A merry wedding* (single-leaf broadsheet): 'I'll have his codpis-poynt'.

[90]   Scot, *Discouerie of Witchcraft*, 10, 82.

maie well enough away withall. Which witchcraft is practised among manie bad
husbands, for whom it were a good excuse to saie they were bewitched.[91]

Magical impotence was both practiced and persecuted in early modern England.
It is alluded to in the trial record of Joan Flower and her daughters Margaret and
Phillipa, executed in Lincoln in March 1618 for the death by witchcraft of Francis
and Henry, infant sons of Francis Manners, sixth Earl of Rutland, a favoured
courtier of King James VI/I, and his second wife, Cicely Tufton. Margaret Flower
testified that 'her Mother and shee, and her Sister agreed together to bewitch the
Earle and his Lady, that they might haue no more children'.[92] In 1647, the Jacobean
courtier James Howell recalled of this case that: 'King *James* a great while was
loth to believe there were Witches, but that which happen'd to my Lord *Francis of
Rutlands* Children, convinc'd him'.[93]

The most informed pre-seventeenth-century British reference to magical
impotence is that of King James VI/I himself. In 1597, he sceptically decries it as
'such kinde of Charmes as commonlie dafte wiues vses […] by staying married
folkes, to haue naturallie adoe with other, (by knitting so manie knottes vpon
a poynt at the time of their mariage) And such-like things'.[94] As James VI of
Scotland, he married Anna of Denmark by proxy in 1589, before collecting her by
sea. Possibly encouraged by her, he became increasingly interested in witchcraft,
blamed for the storm that nearly shipwrecked them between Copenhagen and
Edinburgh. Magical interference with weather was a noted speciality of witches.
An insight into this aspect of their activities collected by Thomas Platter, in
London in September 1599, illuminates why, as Austern puts it, 'the historical
English witch was persecuted far less than her continental sisters and brothers':[95]

> a great many witches are found in England because, as I am told, they are not
> punished by execution there because once, when the queen was on the water
> and several witches wanted to use bad weather to destroy her, another witch was
> said to have held up the weather through prayer, as she herself acknowledges.
> That is why, even though it is thought that they are still the cause of much hail,
> thunderstorm &etc, they are still not punished by execution.[96]

Platter's perceived mildness of witch persecution in Elizabethan England contrasts
with its brutality in Europe and in Jacobean Britain, as reflected by trial records

---

[91]   Scot, *Discouerie of Witchcraft*, 79–80.

[92]   Anon., 'The examination of Margaret Flower', *The wonderful discoverie* (unfoliated).

[93]   Howell, *Familiar letters*, 427.

[94]   James VI/I, *Daemonologie*, 11–12. See also: Cowley, *Poems*, 31; Leigh,
Observations, 270 ('Nouer l'esguillette. To tye the point. A Charm which they use to hinder
a man from accompanying with his wife').

[95]   Austern, 'Art to enchant', 200.

[96]   *Thomas Platter d.J*, 824 (25 September 1599, London).

and his own journal.[97] In August 1590, less than a year after Anna of Denmark's arrival in Edinburgh, Jonett Grant and Jonett Clark were burnt at the stake on the city's Castle Hill, for witchcraft practices including one closely related to ligature, the stealing and redistribution of male genitals.[98]

In March 1618, the irrepressible corresponder James Howell reported to his father in Wales on the alleged magical impotence underlying a high profile Jacobean legal case:

> Touching the *News* of the time: [...] the Earl of *Somerset*, hath got a Lease of Ninety Years for his Life, and so hath his *Articulate* Lady, called so for Articling against the Frigidity and Impotence of her former Lord: She was afraid that [Sir Edward] *Cooke* the Lord Chief Justice (who had used extraordinary art and industry in discovering all the circumstances of the Poisoning of *Overbury*) would have made white *Broth* of them, but that the *Prerogative* kept them from the *Pot*: yet the subservient Instruments, the lesser Flies, could not break throw, but lay entangled in the Cobweb; amongst others, Mistress *Turner* [...] was Executed [...] at *Tyburn* [...] Sir *Gervas Elwaies* [...] was Hanged on *Tower-Hill*.[99]

Not a witch trial but the nullity proceedings between two young courtiers whose marriage had allegedly remained unconsummated, this court scandal's literary impact was profound. At its centre was Frances Howard, daughter of the Lord Chamberlain, Thomas Howard, Earl of Suffolk. In 1606 she was married at 13 to her first husband, 14-year-old Robert Devereux, third Earl of Essex, who immediately went to the Netherlands. Howard stayed at court, attracting the attentions of James VI/I's favourite Robert Carr, future Earl of Somerset, and allegedly also of James's heir, Prince Henry whose unexpected, sudden death in 1612, ascribed by some to poisoning,[100] deprived many of England's finest writers of a discriminating and generous patron.[101] In 1609, when Essex returned to England, Howard conspired with quacks and occult practitioners to rid herself of this unwanted husband, and ally herself to Carr. Her confidante, the physician's widow Mrs Anne Turner,

---

[97]   *Thomas Platter d.J*, 769 (15 September 1599, Dunkirk: 'two witches were to be burnt in the city, but because we set off from there early, we did not see the execution'), 882 (12 November 1599, Valenciennes: 'shortly before, many witches had been caught, and burned in the village of Ville Causy, through which we travelled, where we came across seven wooden platforms erected by the main road, on which they had been burnt. And our drover told us that when a peasant had recently wanted to take down one of these platforms for his own use, he had been so terrorized and beaten by the evil spirit that he nearly died, so he left the platform standing there').

[98]   Smith, 'The flying phallus', 94.

[99]   Howell, *Familiar letters*, 3.

[100]   Weldon, *King James*, 77–8.

[101]   Frances Howard (c.1592–1632); Robert Devereux (1591–1646); Robert Carr (c.1585–1645); Prince Henry (1594–1612).

introduced her to the elderly Simon Forman, who contributed materially to the unfolding intrigue before dying in 1611. Ben Jonson's Dauphine likens the notorious occult skills of this unqualified medical practitioner, who has left eyewitness accounts of four Shakespeare plays, to those of 'madame Medea'.[102] Howard also 'sought out and had many conferences with a wise woman', Mary Woods, who 'accuses the Lady of divers straunge questions and propositions, and in conclusion that she dealt with her to make away her Lord'.[103] In April 1613, Carr tricked his secretary and mentor Sir Thomas Overbury, who first supported, then vehemently opposed, his liaison with Howard, into the Tower, where the 32-year-old died under suspicious circumstances on 14 September.

In June 1613, Howard (or, according to rumour, an accomplice), was proclaimed 'a pure virgin' by nine 'auncient Ladies and midwifes expert in those matters'.[104] Later that month, the Globe theatre burned down during an early performance of the play staging Shakespeare's deepest engagement with divorce.[105] *Henry VIII* refers to virgin brides, barren marriages, witchcraft, cuckoldry and the fall of royal favourites. Henry responds to his Archbishop of Canterbury's prophetic panegyric to the infant Princess Elizabeth: 'Thou hast made me now a man!'; the epilogue, barely concealing a dig at the unfortunate Essex, concludes: 'All the best men are ours; for 'tis ill hap / If they hold when their ladies bid 'em clap.'[106] Howard's annulment, dependent on proving her virginity and Essex's impotence, was granted on 25 September 1613 by an ecclesiastical commission. Although its chair, George Abbott, Archbishop of Canterbury, bitterly opposed ascribing Essex's impotence to *maleficium* by witchcraft, James VI/I pressed him to conclude that 'the Earl of Essex, for some secret, incurable, binding impediment, did never carnally know, or was or is able carnally to know the lady Frances Howard'.[107] On 26 December 1613 Carr married Howard, supported by James and fêted with masques and poems by Thomas Campion, George Chapman, John Donne, Ben Jonson and Thomas Middleton. Mounting rumours and popular ditties labelled Howard 'A wight, a witch, a Murdresse & a whore'.[108] In 1615, the apothecary James Franklin confessed to supplying Howard with love potions and poisons. He implicated Anne Turner and Overbury's keepers at the Tower, Sir Gervase Elwes and the medical practitioner Richard Weston. On the testimony of witnesses including Forman's widow, who produced exhibits including Forman's occult, sexually explicit, wax and lead models, all four were tried and hanged for Overbury's murder. Carr and Howard, sentenced to hanging in 1616, were

[102]   Jonson, 'Epicoene', IV.i (*Workes*, 567).
[103]   29 April 1613, John Chamberlain to Sir Dudley Carleton (Sanderson, 'Poems', 58).
[104]   Chamberlain (Sanderson, 'Poems', 59).
[105]   Baillie, 'Henry VIII', 247–8, 258.
[106]   Shakespeare, *Henry VIII*, V.iv.64 (Epilogue, 13–14).
[107]   O'Connor, 'The witch', 1124. See also Thomas, *Religion and the decline of magic*, 576.
[108]   Sanderson, 'Poems', 61.

pardoned by James VI/I. On 18 January 1622, they were released from the Tower and banished to their country estate.[109]

Thomas Campion remarks on the Jacobean fashion for replacing or augmenting '*Satyres, Nymphes*' and other mythological stage characters with 'the persons of Enchaunters & Commaunders of Spirits'.[110] Sixteenth-century occult stage characters were typically male, and one of the earliest female English stage witches is Medusa. A direct borrowing from the Italian stage, her longest scene in *Fidele and Fortunio, or the two Italian gentlemen* (1584), an anonymous adaptation of a play of 1575 by Luigi Pasqualigo, is set in a graveyard, where she conjures love spells with a waxen image.[111] From the 1590s, English playwrights explored the powerful potential of female witch scenes as multimedia spectacle in increasingly creative ways. They produced a flurry of major female witch roles, heralded by Lyly's *Mother Bombie*, Melissa and Medea in Robert Greene's *Orlando Furioso* and *Alphonsus*, and the spectacular occult conjuration scenes of Joan of Arc and Margery Jourdain in Shakespeare's *Henry VI parts I & II*. On the all-male stage and, for as long as witchcraft itself was taken seriously, even after the introduction of actresses, both male and female occult stage roles continued to be played by men. Even so, the music, dancing, acrobatics and special effect of the new, more substantial female witch roles changed perceptions regarding the potential of female theatricality on public stages. A major focus for expectations of early modern stage witchcraft was as agents for the loss of sexual honour. For women, this primarily involved loss of premarital virginity or marital fertility, and for men, loss of potency as a direct medical symptom (impotence) and/or via a third party (cuckoldry). After King James VI of Scotland's accession as King James I of England in 1603, an increasing awareness of magical impotence in Jacobean literary circles, through contemporary, classical and demonological information sources, contributed to a perceptible gathering pace of the gender shift from male stage sorcerers and enchanters to female stage witches and wise women.

Jacobean dramatists influenced by Howard's case include Thomas Middleton. It brought to their attention the unfamiliar practice of ligature, whose details they gradually pieced together from classical and European demonological sources. Parallels between Howard's rumour-ridden virginity test of 1613, and that performed by Beatrice-Joanna on her maid Diaphanta in Middleton and Rowley's *The changeling*, would not have been lost on audiences of 1622.[112] Middleton's *Masque of Cupids* was performed for Howard's second wedding.[113] Her circumstances also marked a play which adapted a love triangle taken from Cyril Tourneur's *The atheist's tragedy* of 1611, Middleton's *The witch* (1616).[114]

---

[109] Simmons, 'Diabolical realism', 161–2.

[110] Campion, *Maske*, sig.A2ʳ.

[111] Herrington, 'Witchcraft and magic', 472.

[112] Simmons, 'Diabolical realism', 137–8, 153–5.

[113] Jones-Davies, Hoenselaars and Jowett, 'Masque of Cupids', 1027.

[114] O'Connor, 'The witch', 1125.

It is set far from London, at the court of Ravenna. Unlike Tourneur, Middleton introduces supernatural characters and spells that provide overtly magical causes for the newlywed husband Antonio's impotence. These supernatural additions are not simply haphazardly derived from demonological treatises such as Scot's, but unmistakably informed by the historical circumstances of Frances Howard's marriages and their cultural impact.[115] In *The changeling*, Hecate is invoked as the leader of 'the witches of the night'.[116] In *The witch*, Hecate takes centre stage as the garrulous chief witch ruling over a flourishing coven including Stadlin and Hoppo,[117] her incestuous son the clown Firestone, and the spirit Malkin. Giving Sebastian charms to render magically impotent his rival Antonio, married to the woman Sebastian loves, Isabella, Hecate assures him that:

> Knit with these charmèd and retentive knots,
> Neither the man begets nor woman breeds,
> No, nor performs the least desires of wedlock.[118]

Hecate first appears in Greek literature as the benign, conventionally-bodied, female goddess central to Hesiod's *Theogony*. By the time she features in Euripides' *Medea*, Hecate has evolved into the terrifying, monstrously conjoined underworld triple-goddess familiar from Virgil's *Æneid*. Associating Hecate with Luna and Diana, late classical literature emphasises her connections to witchcraft and black magic.[119] In Elizabethan literature, this triple Hecate features in translations of classics, and in poems such as George Chapman's 'Hymnus in Cynthiam', but impacts in drama only in invocations.[120] Macbeth invokes her twice, in the only Shakespeare play featuring an onstage Hecate.[121] Around 1616, when he was writing *The witch*, Middleton adapted *Macbeth* for the professional acting troupe, The King's Men. First written in 1606, there is considerable scholarly disagreement concerning the authorship and dating of the first folio's occult scenes. They evidence numerous intertextualities and dramatic overlaps with those of Jonson's *Masque of queenes* and Middleton's *Witch*. Middleton's

---

[115]   Lancashire, 'The witch'; *pace* Lima, *Stages of evil*, 208.

[116]   Middleton, *Collected works*, 1653–4 (III.iii.88–91).

[117]   Witch names featured in Johannes Nider's *Formicarius* of c.1437 (the 'grandis maleficus' Staedlin and his disciple Hoppo), *Malleus Maleficarum* ([Kramer &] Mackay, Hammer, 264, 321, 382) and Scot's *Discoverie of witchcraft* (222).

[118]   Middleton, *Collected works*, 1137 (I.i.156–8).

[119]   Kraus, *Hekate*, 104; Marquardt, 'A portrait of Hecate', 243, 251–2.

[120]   Chapman, *The shadow of night*, sig.C.iv\`. On triple-bodied monsters, see also Chapter 11, this volume.

[121]   Shakespeare: *Macbeth*, II.i.52, III.ii.41, IV.i.39–43 (see also: *Midsummer night's dream*, V.i.384, *1.Henry VI*, III.ii.64, *As you like it*, III.ii.2, *Hamlet*, III.ii.258, *King Lear*, I.i.110).

Hecate meekly submits to being addressed as 'Goody Hag'.[122] Quite different is the imperious Hecate with whom Shakespeare embellishes the 'three women supposing to be the weird sisters or feiries' depicted and described in *Macbeth*'s historical source, Holinshed's *Chronicles*.[123] Notwithstanding these differences, and Macbeth's invocations of Hecate in the first folio, *Macbeth*'s Hecate scenes are widely attributed to Middleton.[124] This is not least because Simon Forman's account of his visit to a performance of *Macbeth* at the Globe on 10 April 1611 makes no reference to Hecate, and his sole, low-key reference to the weird sisters, in their opening scene, echoing Holinshed's wording, identifies them merely as 'three women fairies or nymphs'.[125] *Macbeth*'s Hecate enriches the sisters' profane trinity with complex pre-Christian supernatural associations. She informs their staccato loquacity and the play's strikingly numerous repetitive double and triple utterances.[126] This innovative melding of domestic and classical witchcraft elements significantly expands the role of the female stage witch and her opportunity to sing and dance on the public stage. Hecate's popularity on the Restoration stage was boosted by William Davenant's spectacular 1664 adaptation of *Macbeth*. Samuel Pepys, who watched Davenant's 'excellent' production at least four times at the Duke's House between 1664 and 1667, especially praised its 'divertisement […] a strange perfection in a tragedy, it being most proper here, and suitable'.[127]

Hecate is linked to the role of Æthiopia in Ben Jonson's *Masque of beauty* of 1608,[128] and invoked by the chief witch of his *Masque of queenes* of February 1609:

Dame: […] You, that haue seene me ride, when Hecate
Durst not take chariot; […]

And thouᶜ *three-formed starre*, that, on these nights
Art onely powerfull, to whose triple name
Thus we incline, *once, twice,* and *thrise the same*.[129]

In note c to this passage, Jonson glosses 'thou' as: '*Hecate*, who is called *Trivia*, and *Triformis* […] She was beleeu'd to gouerne in witchcraft; and is remembred in all their inuocations'.

---

122   Middleton, *Collected works*, 1138 (I.ii.197–8).
123   Holinshed, 'Scotlande', 243–4.
124   Or even to some 'wretched […] hack writer' (Rolfe, 'Hecate in "Macbeth"', 602).
125   Taylor and Ewbank, 'The tragedy of Macbeth', 1166.
126   Kranz, 'Supernatural soliciting', 369–70.
127   Pepys, *The concise Pepys*: 307, 478, 481, 611 (5.11.1664, 28.12.1666, 7.1.1667: quoted, 16.10.1667).
128   Orgel and Strong, *Inigo Jones*, 94.
129   Jonson, *Workes*, 953.

Masque of queenes' 12 female queens were danced as silent roles by Queen Anna and 11 female courtiers.[130] Like female stage witches on public stages, the 12 witches are thought to have been grotesquely played by professional adult men, rather than adolescent boys, let alone women.[131] In the anti-masque, they have verbose speeches and choruses, spectacular music and magic routines. In the masque, these 'Hagges', reduced to the status of mute beasts of burden, return in groups of four, to aid three groups of heraldic beasts pull the chariots in which the queens ride in state around the stage.[132] The contrast between the jarring, rowdy spectacle of the garrulous witches emerging 'with strange gestures' to the sound of 'hollow and infernal music' from the hellmouth of their anti-masque, and the masque's silent queens heightens the novel effect of Jonson's 'unprecedented juxtaposition',[133] on any kind of pre-Restoration English stage, of amateur female performers and cross-dressed professional male actors. Jonson's anti-masque creatively extends *Macbeth*'s fruitful exploration of the theatrical potential of female stage witches. Their silent subjugation in the masque eloquently dilutes what some specialists have identified as its enactment of 'female empowerment'.[134]

During the anti-masque of *Masque of queenes*, the coven leader directly refers to the sinister black magic of 'tying the knot', when she enters proclaiming:

> *Dame*: [...] You[a] *Fiends* and *Furies* [...] that haue quak'd to see
> These[b] knots vntied; and shrunke, when we haue charm'd.
> You, that (to arme vs) haue your selues disarm'd.[135]

The second note to this passage rather vaguely explains that 'the vntying of their knots is, when they are going to do some fatall businesse', confirming this as a direct reference to traditional ligature knots of the type described by Platter. There are many indications that the practice had long fallen into disuse in urban England. Jonson's hags proclaim: 'With pictures full, of waxe and of wooll / Their liuers I sticke, with needles quicke'; exhibits produced at Frances Howard's annulment hearing, by Simon Forman's widow, suggest that Forman's attempts to induce Essex into magical impotence involved piercing the genitals of a wax effigy of Essex with a thorn.[136] Neither does Shakespeare refer to traditional magical impotence practices with respect to the threat of *Macbeth*'s First Witch to drain a

---

[130]   Jonson, *Workes*, 964.
[131]   Plank, 'Music and the supernatural', 398; Lewalski, 'Anne of Denmark', 346–7; McFadden, 'Reviews: "O let us howle"', 102.
[132]   Jonson, *Workes*, 963.
[133]   McManus, *Women on the renaissance stage*, 134.
[134]   Tomlinson, *Women on stage in Stuart drama*, 31–5.
[135]   Jonson, *Workes*, 952.
[136]   Jonson, *Workes*, 947.

sailor, whose wife has slighted her, 'dry as hay'; while they resonate only faintly in Macbeth's accusation that they 'untie the winds'.[137]

Among the 11 female courtiers who danced the silent roles of the masque's 12 queens alongside Queen Anna of Denmark in February 1609 was Frances Howard, then still Countess of Essex. Four years later, Anna played a rather less transparent role in one of the masques performed at Howard's second marriage, which, unlike James VI/I, she strongly opposed. Written by Thomas Campion, this masque was performed at Whitehall on the evening of the wedding itself, 26 December 1613. Anna's brief but pivotal contribution, not as a costumed masquer, but in her own persona as spectator and queen consort to the ruling monarch, subverts the court festival ceremonial tradition in which rulers, in person or by proxy, triumph over supernatural magical or monstrous opponents, in a theatrical confrontation Stuart Clark insightfully labels the 'political equivalent of the exorcism'.[138] This subversion hints at the gulf separating popular perception of this foreign female consort's unpredictable, potentially harmful or even occult touch, from the privileged touch of the ruling male monarch, its healing power regularly validated in the public ceremony of the Royal Touch.[139] The disturbing nature of Anna's role is sensitively discussed by specialists, without, however, explicating its direct intertextual references to the magical impotence charm alluded to in Jonson's masque of 1609, or this charm's central relevance to the marital history of the bride, Francis Howard.[140] As Anna plucked a bough from a golden tree brought to her seat of honour in the royal dais, a crowned masquer representing Eternity, directly addressing the queen, sang:

> The Tree of Grace, and Bountie,
> Set it in Bel-Annas eye,
> For she, she, only she
> Can all Knotted spels vnty.[141]

Those versed in ligature knew that only those who cast its knots could easily untie them. Anna's involvement with this masque aggressively suggests her power to summon as well as banish witchcraft, and specifically the occult forces of ligature

---

[137]   Shakespeare, *Macbeth*, I.iii.18, IV.i.52; Biggins, 'Sexuality, witchcraft, and violence', 258–60.

[138]   Clark, *Thinking with demons*, 640. A memorable proxy triumph of this type was staged at the 1616 Stuttgart christening, attended by numerous foreign dignitaries, including the Earls of Derby, Winchester and Pembroke. During one tournament entry, Germania, aided by Virtue and Concordia Invicta, vanquished and slayed their monstrous enemy Discord (see Chapter 11, this volume).

[139]   On which see Chapter 4, this volume.

[140]   Clark, *Thinking with demons*, 644–6; McManus, *Women on the renaissance stage*, 176–7; Lewalski, 'Anne of Denmark', 349.

[141]   Campion, *Maske*, sig.B1[v].

that allegedly destroyed Frances Howard's first marriage and, by implication, increasingly overshadowed her own. In 1613, Campion's masque audaciously conflates negative and positive female power, separately personified by Jonson's witches and queens four years earlier, into Anna's single central transforming role. In an illuminating simplification, some specialists identify the central motivation of institutionalized witch hunting as a power struggle between male and female power systems and strategies, and argue for its 'critical contribution to the "domestication" of women in the early modern period'.[142] No single action theatricalizes this enforced domestication more succinctly than Queen Anna's fleeting involvement in Campion's masque.

Alluded to in *Macbeth*, in *Masque of queenes*, and in *The witch*, ligature is central to Thomas Heywood and Richard Brome's play of 1634, *The late Lancashire witches*.[143] Heywood's researches into the practice, based on a careful reading of Jean Bodin, inform his factual discussion of it, published in 1624 in *Gynaikeion*, the earlier of his two historical treatises on women:

> But of all these diuellish and detestable practises, there is none (saith *Bodinus)* more Heathenish, irreligious, and dangerous, than that so commonly in vse now adayes, and by Witches continually practised, to the iniurie and wrong of new married women; it is commonly called *Ligare ligulam,* or to tye knots vpon a point; which as it is vsuall, so it is not new [...] *Bodinus* further addes, That in the yeere 1567. he then being Procurator in Patauia, the gentlewoman in whose house he soiourned (being it seemes a pregnant scholler in this Art) related vnto him in the presence of one *Iacobus Baunasius* [Jacques de Beauvais], That there were fiftie seuerall wayes of tying this knot, to hinder copulation, either to bind the Husband, or the Wife onely, that one hating the others infirmitie, might the freelyer pollute themselues with Adulteries. Shee said moreouer, the man was often so charmed, the woman seldome, and difficultly: besides, this knot might be tyed for a day, for a yeere, for the present time, or for euer, or whilest the same was vnloosed: That it might be tyed for one to loue the other, and not be againe beloued, or to make a mutuall and ardent loue betwixt them; but when they came to congression, to bite and scratch, and teare one another with their teeth and nayles.[144]

This lengthy passage is of previously unrecognized relevance to the plot of *Lancashire witches*, and to the question of Heywood's shared authorship with Brome. The play focuses on the wedding of a simple country couple, Lawrence and Parnell. Before the ceremony, a jealous former lover, Mal Spencer, presents

---

[142]   Bever, 'Witchcraft, female aggression, and power', 975; Alison Rowlands provides nuanced archive-based counter-arguments ('Witchcraft and old women', 53–4).

[143]   Clark, *Thinking with demons*, 89.

[144]   Heywood, 'Of Witches', *Gynaikeion*, 402, drawing on Bodin, *Demonomanie*, Book 2, Chapter 1 (sigs.51ʳ–59ᵛ).

Lawrence with a knotted codpiece point. This renders him impotent with his new wife. In 1634, an early spectator of the play confirms this as a foreign, specifically French, occult custom, identifying it, in the context of his discussion of the play's magical practices, as: 'the tying of a knott at a mariage (after the French manner) to cassate masculine abilitie'.[145]

In order to protect themselves from contagion from powerful spells such as ligature, local communities sometimes performed another superstitious ceremony featured in Heywood and Brome's play, known on mainland Europe as the charivari, a ritual inversion of solemn ritual[146] with supernatural dimensions, intended to publicly humiliate henpecked or cuckolded husbands. Thomas Platter describes its English variant, the riding or skimmington, at second hand:

> [English] women often beat their husbands, and whenever this becomes known, their nearest neighbour is placed on a cart and, in order to ridicule the beaten man, they parade him around the whole town while proclaiming that this is his punishment for not having come to the aid of his neighbour while his wife was beating him.[147]

A satirical poem by Andrew Marvell confirms that those paraded are the quarelling couple's nearest neighbours, not they themselves.[148] The French charivari often targeted newlywed couples in which the wife was older than the husband. Like the English skimmington, it was habitually accompanied by rough music, mocking laughter, religious parody and heavy-handed allusions to cuckoldry and effeminacy through transvestite clothing and rams'-horns (blown or worn).[149] Charivari was performed by rowdy bands of bachelors whose supernatural demonic roots are traced back to the aerial Wild Horde or Herlichini. This legendary hellish band of damned souls provides a possible source for the Witches' Sabbath, and Hellekin, its devilish leader, inspired the most celebrated early modern stage fool, the commedia dell'arte's Harlequin.[150] According to Platter's lively impression of the practice in Uzès in 1598, charivari groups would disguise themselves in Devil masks and meet up nightly to season new couples' immediate neighbourhoods

---

[145]   16 August 1634, Nathaniel Tomkyns to Sir Robert Phelips (Stokes and Alexander, *Somerset*, I, 416).

[146]   Clark, 'Inversion, misrule and the meaning of witchcraft', 103–4.

[147]   *Thomas Platter d.J*, 814 (25 September 1599, England).

[148]   Marvell, 'The last instructions to a painter', *The third part*, 10. For further examples, see Laroque (*Shakespeare's festive world*, 100–1).

[149]   Davis, 'The reasons of misrule', 45; Ingram, 'Rough music', 82, 99. As Guarinonius explains, the ram, closely associated with the 'horned and hellish face of the Devil' and known as the 'witches' steed', gave its name to the popular Italian phrase for cuckolds: 'becco cornuto' (*Grewel*, 742, 1319).

[150]   Driesen, *Harlekin*, 188; Aker, *Narrenschiff*, 272; Behringer, *Shaman of Oberstdorf*; Katritzky, *The art of commedia*, 102.

with intolerable smells and unsocial noises, through raucous singing, shouting and 'playing' of kitchen implements, disbanding only once the shamed couple bribed them into silence.[151] No attempts at regulation, not even those following charivaris that had led to serious injury or death, had managed to stop this ancient custom in Languedoc. William Prynne's Puritan anti-theatrical treatise of 1633 traces it back to at least 1404, the date of a canon law warning clergy to 'be not present at, nor yet play in the play that is called Charevari, in which they use vizards [masks] in the shape of divels, and horrible things are there committed'.[152]

Petruchio's use of a makeshift horse to remove Katherina from the wedding feast, in Shakespeare's *Taming of the shrew*, has been likened to a skimmington, and Francis Beaumont and John Fletcher's sequel features an actual charivari. In this, a band of formidable women, led by the widowed Petruchio's new wife Maria, rejecting female submission, 'fling main Potlids / like massie rocks, dart ladles, tossing Irons / and tongs like Thunderbolts'.[153] In *Lancashire witches*, Parnell's derision of Lawrence's post-marital sexual prowess is instrumental in having him publicly shamed in a skimmington. After much grief, the newlyweds identify the codpiece point given to Lawrence by Mal as 'an Inchauntment'. They solve their problem by burning it. By Parnell's account, the bewitched object 'spitter'd and spatter'd in the fire like an it were (love blesse us) a laive thing in the faire'. Its destruction restores Lawrence's potency and marital harmony.[154] As late as 1634, Heywood and Brome could still get away with a plot dependent on a rustic bridegroom with a use for codpiece points. They are noticeably absent from Thomas Shadwell's radically updated anti-Catholic version of their play, *The Lancashire-witches*, first published in 1682. After every act, Shadwell offers the reader copious, learned 'notes, wherein I have presented you a great part of the Doctrine of Witchcraft, beleive it who will'.[155] His 'Notes upon the Third Act' reference classical sources, Jonson's unfinished pastoral play of c.1637, *The sad shepherd*, whose witch, Mother Maudlin, casts spells against lovers,[156] the ubiquitous Scot, and the authors cited by the play's dim lawyer, Sir Jeffrey Shacklehead in a misguided attempt to establish his expertise in the field of demonology: '*Bodin, Remigius, Delrio, Nider, Institor, Sprenger, Godelman,* and *More,* and *Malleus Maleficarum,* a great Author, that Writes sweetly about Witches, very sweetly.' This bungling witch hunter blames his own marital impotence on a female neighbour's witchcraft: 'I am sure she is a Witch, and between you and I, last night, when I would have been kind to my Wife, she bewitcht me, I found it

---

[151]   *Thomas Platter d.J*, 275–6 (16 July 1598, Uzès).

[152]   Prynne, *Histrio-mastix*, 600.

[153]   Beaumont and Fletcher, 'The woman's prize or the tamer tamed' II.v (*Comedies and tragedies*, 106); Moisan, 'What's that to you?', 120–3.

[154]   Heywood and Brome, *Late Lancashire witches*, IV and V (ff.H3r, Lr).

[155]   Shadwell, *Lancashire-witches*, 'To the reader'.

[156]   Jonson, *Sad shepherd*, 26.

so.'[157] But neither Shadwell's playtext nor his notes provide any hint of traditional magical impotence procedures. By 1682, the knotty occult European practice of ligature, finally unravelled (so to speak) by English playwrights, was no longer topical on the London stage.[158]

Creative early modern London playwrights drew on an astonishingly wide range of printed and other sources to embrace the opportunities that occult characters offered for introducing stage magic, music, spectacle, novelty and exotic excitement into their performances. They researched classical and contemporary dramatic and witchcraft treatises, trial records, pamphlets and popular print, court gossip, and European demonological literature.[159] There is no simple dichotomy between British and mainland European witchcraft concepts or practices.[160] Cultural exchange was constantly facilitated in England at every level, from the highest London court circles to untravelled rural spectators of the itinerant foreign quack troupes who exported their stage magic across Europe's borders. The accounts of educated travellers have the potential to enhance our understanding of these transregional borrowings. Thomas Platter is rightly recognized for his brief notice of an early performance of *Julius Caesar* at the Globe. His record of ligature in Languedoc highlights the potential relevance to our understanding of early modern drama of certain non-theatrical passages in his journal, and enhances our understanding of the theatricality of the occult, and of representations of magic, medicine and gender on the Jacobean stage.

---

[157] Shadwell, *Lancashire-witches*, I and III (9, 37, 44–6).

[158] The skimmington was considered stageworthy well into the eighteenth century (see for example, Hawker's comic opera, *The country-wedding and skimington*).

[159] Theile, *Staging the occult*, 3.

[160] Simpson, 'Witches and witchbusters', 9.

Chapter 11
Performing Monsters

During its examination of some supernatural practices recorded by the three physicians, the previous chapter touched on Hecate as a Jacobean stage witch. Classical representations of this goddess typically depict her with three conjoined human bodies, complete with three heads and up to 12 limbs.[1] Traditionally, witches were represented with physical abnormalities, and those with abnormal bodies were often 'suspected of witchcraft'.[2] Hecate's anatomical configuration offers an extreme example of the type of supernatural humans examined in this chapter, those with congenitally abnormal bodies. Like all extraordinary natural wonders, such as monstrous animals or plants, prodigious floods or hailstorms, solar or lunar eclipses, comets, volcanic eruptions or earthquakes, such humans were regarded as supernatural omen-bringing messengers, with a perceived 'demonstrative' role. With reference to this, the early modern term for humans and animals born with physical nonconformities was 'monster'.[3] Because of their perceived social and religious significance, the birth of every early modern human with extreme physical nonconformities that came to public attention was recorded as a matter of course. The development of printing provided a cheap, portable and profitable way of spreading news of such humans, through broadsheets reporting on their births and activities, and the prodigy and wonder books and other publications drawing on such ephemera.

Early publications of two of most influential researchers in the field of natural wonders, Lorraine Daston and Katharine Park, endorsed a historical trajectory of changing responses to monstrous human births, with early fear of prodigies being replaced by pleasure in entertainment, then by enlightened scientific and medical enquiry. Since 1998, when they reinvigorated the study of wonders and monsters by rejecting this linear historical progression in favour of three overlapping, coexisting responses: 'horror, pleasure and repugnance', the field has been exceptionally active and productive.[4] However, because recent publications on early modern human monsters predominantly foreground political, religious or medical issues, they serve the categories of 'horror' and 'repugnance' far better than Daston and Park's third category, 'pleasure'. Studies of the monstrous as

---

[1]   Kraus, *Hekate*, 104–5.

[2]   Plank, 'Music and the supernatural', 399.

[3]   The term is here used historically. Cultural historians generally consider anatomically abnormal humans within the context of 'monster' (pre-1800), 'freak' (nineteenth and twentieth centuries) and 'disability' (post-1989) studies.

[4]   Daston and Park, *Wonders*, 176.

spectacle are still largely confined to biographical perspectives. In a rare recent study foregrounding the key role of theatricality in the understanding of early modern human monstrosity, Mark Thornton Burnett identifies the monster show as 'an inspirational resource for theatrical representation', and highlights monstrosity as 'one of the most intriguing and least understood' of all early modern discourses.[5] He considers some of the many exhibition sites in which monsters contributed to theatrical culture. In the marketplace and fairground, they were significant as early modern public media celebrities. Given rulers' aspirations to take human monsters under their personal protection, they were also valuable 'tokens' in the aristocratic gifts-for-patronage exchange economy. Some monsters earned their keep travelling the fairground circuits as independent live performers, or being exhibited or shown by itinerant promoters. Dead or alive, monsters were highly prized by collectors, many entering the curiosity cabinets or service of royal or noble patrons.

The Protestant Platter brothers comment on monstrous humans of many types: legendary, partially or wholly preserved, depicted, performing and performed. Whether because he himself had been the father of triplets, or as Locher suggests, because his medical treatises were predicated on a new perspective on wonders and prodigies based on the astonished scientific gaze of the physician, the Catholic Hippolytus Guarinonius does not; only exceptionally noting any type of wondrous omens.[6] Among the most substantial of these records are the medical and case notes on performing hairy people and parasitic conjoined twins published by Felix Platter and augmented by his English translators. This chapter draws on the three physicians' writings to examine some tensions between science and showmanship raised by exhibiting monsters, and their on and offstage impact on early modern theatre. It also touches on the changing medical framework within which different historic periods select and exhibit their monsters, by revisiting differences and similarities between early modern and modern systems for their classification.

Felix Platter's sensitivity to even slight human physical nonconformity predated his ability to speak. He recalls that being fed porridge from the withered finger of a nurse caused him such distress as an infant that she had to be replaced.[7] As a 14-year-old schoolboy, already a professional musician and music teacher, he was sent to stay with the Gebwiler family, to escape the Basle plague epidemic that claimed his sister Ursel. He noted with interest that a second smaller thumb growing from one thumb gave their youngest son, his lute student Karl, 11 fingers in total.[8] Guarininius too considers one supernumerary finger noteworthy, and one of Platter's *Observations* testifies to the interest with which he examined a similar case as an adult physician: '*More then five Fingers and Toes*: I saw a begger Boy that had six fingers on each hand, one grew to the middle finger. And he had

---

[5]   Burnett, *Constructing 'monsters'*, 4, 28.

[6]   Locher, 'Beglaubigungsstrategien', 144.

[7]   *Felix Platter Tagebuch*, 54 (1530s, Basle).

[8]   *Felix Platter Tagebuch*, 117 (1551, Rötelen).

six Toes on his left Foot and seven on his right, so that in his Hands and Feet, he had twenty five Fingers and Toes.'[9] Platter carefully notes the congenitally inwardly-twisted feet of a female corpse he dissected in 1554, after his first grave-robbing expedition.[10] Eighteen months later, Caspar Fry, a Swiss Companion of St James passing through Montpellier, almost persuaded the young student to join his sixteenth Spanish pilgrimage.[11] Felix Platter does not note whether Fry's one-handedness was congenital, accidental or the result of punitive disfigurement.

In September 1599, at Ghent's Palais des Seigneurs, Thomas Platter viewed 'numerous dried-out human hands, fastened with nails onto the palace gate and in the law or audience hall. They were mostly right hands cut off perjurers or other criminals, and fastened here in everlasting memory'.[12] Two weeks later in London, he clarifies the socially unjust law that fuelled the illiterate uprising coordinated by Shakespeare's Jack Cade, underlying Cade's angry taunting of the clerk of Chatham ('*Smith*: He can write and read and cast accompt. *Cade*: Oh monstrous!'):

> There are many strange laws and customs in England, on which whole books have been written. I just want to report on what I have heard. If one person murders another in anger and the murderer can read, he is shown mercy, and only has his hand cut off. Because he can read, the hope is that he is still able to achieve something positive. If he can't read, he loses his life according to the law.[13]

As a schoolboy, Felix Platter witnessed numerous public executions featuring criminals having limbs removed, or being broken on the wheel, quartered, or beheaded. Punitive disfigurement sometimes went beyond the law. In Montpellier, he:

> often saw a man in a long cloak sitting by the cobbler's shop, he had a hacked off nose and walked miserably on crutches. The reason for which, as I found out, was as follows. He had been a handsome young scribe in Nîmes, where he had had an affair with the wife of a doctor of law who, with several students, all masked, surprised him in bed with the wife of Bigot (that was the doctor's name). They tied him up, sliced off his genitals and nose down to the gristle, and in this pitiable condition dragged him onto the street at night, and left him lying

---

[9]   Guarinonius, *Grewel*, 103; Platter, *Obseruationum*, 551 (this translation: Plat[t]er, Culpeper and Cole, *Platerus histories*, 364).

[10]   *Felix Platter Tagebuch*, 210 (11 December 1554, Montpellier).

[11]   *Felix Platter Tagebuch*, 244 (9 April 1556, Montpellier).

[12]   *Thomas Platter d.J*, 748 (10 September 1599, Ghent).

[13]   Shakespeare, *2 Henry VI*, IV.ii.85–7; *Thomas Platter d.J*, 823 (25 September 1599, London).

there. Much later, when his wounds had healed, he came to Montpellier, where he must drag out the dregs of his pathetic life.[14]

The renowned French physician, poet and humanist Guillaume Bigot (1502–50) was imprisoned for this assault, although he denied taking part. The foremost rhinoplasty surgeon of this time was Gaspare Tagliacozzi (1545–99), one of whose enraged patients, according to Guarinonius, plucked off and hurled to the ground his nose-tip, severed in a fight and replaced by Tagliacozzi, after the surgeon admonished him for alcoholic overindulgence.[15]

Congenital nonconformities were less clearly understood. Prior to refinement of the concepts of intra-species infertility, dominant and recessive inheritable traits and mutant genes, disagreement and confusion impeded understanding of the principles underlying the inheritance of physical characteristics. As well as possessing religious and theatrical dimensions, monsters were subjected to considerable medical scrutiny, as perceived test cases for theories regarding non-inherited pre-natal influences on embryos. The correlation between pre-modern and modern definitions of monstrous humans is imprecise. One major factor was a much less well-defined pre-Enlightenment concept of the human itself, as a zoological phenomenon. There was considerable confusion concerning the border between ape and human.[16] Early modern classification systems also blur the boundaries between human and non-human in less predictable ways, with their generous inclusivity of a wide range of liminal hybrids. Some, like mermaids, attempted to rationalize observable human physical nonconformities. Others, like centaurs, reflected myths, legends or travellers' tales. Felix and Thomas Platter viewed mighty fortresses at Lusignan and Cinq-Mars-la-Pile said to have been homes to the serpent-mermaid Melusina.[17] Well-served by medieval French and German myth and legend, Melusina starred in a romance topping the bestseller lists of 1569, when it sold 158 copies at Frankfurt's Lent book fair.[18] Felix Platter admired a Melusina-like hybrid in the costumed tournament entry of a court wedding: 'The siren they led onto the course was half a beautiful women, naked down to the navel,[19] with breasts and long, blonde hair; from the navel down she

---

[14]   *Felix Platter Tagebuch*, 213 (2 February 1555, Montpellier). This case is summarized in Platter, *Obseruationum*, 56–7.

[15]   Guarinonius, *Grewel*, 603.

[16]   Knowles, 'Can ye not tell a man from a marmoset?', 138–9.

[17]   *Felix Platter Tagebuch*, 273 (17 March 1557, Lusignan); *Thomas Platter d.J*, 491 (26 May 1599, Cinq-Mars-La-Pile); Le Roy Ladurie, *The beggar and the professor*, 246.

[18]   Bücking, *Kultur und Gesellschaft in Tirol*, 100.

[19]   Jakob Frischlin confirms that, as standard for early modern stage costume, this singer's upper half was in fact covered with a skin-coloured nude suit (*Hohenzollerische Hochzeyt*, 231).

was like the lower half of a fish, blue and silvery, big and curved in on herself, just like sea wonders are painted.'[20]

Secondly, numerous early modern categories of the monstrous, such as the horned humans discussed below, have since been largely eliminated through their relatively straightforward response to surgical normalization. Thirdly, early modern concepts of the monstrous include certain categories no longer regarded as physically abnormal, although they may still elicit wonder, notably multiple births. Felix Platter, while regarding multiple births as beyond the 'ordinary', viewed anything up to triplets as 'normal'.[21] While collecting medicinal herbs near Uzès in 1597 with the apothecary Antoine Régis and his son Matthieu, Thomas Platter heard of a local woman who had recently borne one child, then eight days later its twin: 'so that her husband was greatly troubled that in another eight days she would also present him with a third. Which did not, however, happen'.[22] Human multiple births were habitually associated with multiparous animals, and many reports of them refer to parental shame and sorrow. They poignantly colour Guarinonius's references to his own triplet daughters, born three months prematurely on 4 March 1604 to his first wife, Charitas Thaler. All three baptized in the name of Christina, they survived only for an hour, and were commemorated with an inscribed marble plaque in the Tirolean Monastery of Sankt Georgenberg near Schwaz. In defiant opposition to popular superstition suggesting that multiple births were indicative of multiple fathers, and medical theories attributing them to exceptionally frequent sexual intercourse, Guarinonius argues for their greater likelihood with faithful, relatively abstinent couples. His record of the birth of quadruplets to the wife of the Schwaz miner N Schmärl is brief and neutral.[23]

Fynes Moryson's report of a triplet birth of the 1590s is more typical:

> While my selfe soiourned at Leipzige a woman had three Chilldren at a birth, and the hauing of more then one was not thought rare or strange, Yea they haue a Common saying, which may seeme fabulous, but in likelyhood came at first from some rare accident in that kynd, namely that a woman reproching another for hauing many Children at one birth, and being Cursed by her, had herselfe the next yeare so many Children, as for shame shee went to drowne some of them in a Ponde, but being apprehended and punished, the Children that were saued were commonly called Hundskindren that is Dog whelps, because they so hardly scaped the fortune of whelpes to be drowned.[24]

---

[20]   *Felix Platter Tagebuch*, 502 (5 October 1598, Hechingen).

[21]   Platter, *Obseruationum*, 706.

[22]   *Thomas Platter d.J*, 229 (25 June 1597, Montaren).

[23]   Guarinonius, *Grewel*, 876, 1062, 1141; Dörrer, 'Guarinoni als Volksschriftsteller', 152–3.

[24]   Moryson, *Shakespeare's Europe*, 294–5.

In Arles, Thomas Platter heard the 'local' legend of a wealthy woman who bore nine sons, after being cursed by a beggar woman she scolded for bearing as many children as a sow. On the boys' eighth birthday, her husband confronted her with the eight sons he had secretly rescued, after she thought she had drowned all but one at birth in the Rhône.[25] Hippolytus Guarinonius notes 'the Duchess of Hennenberg, who soon after insulting God through her sins, became pregnant with 365 children, all born live at once' and a Lombard queen said to have had her septuplets drowned in a pond at birth.[26] According to Book I, chapter 15 of Paulus Diaconus's *Historia Langobardorum*, these seven brothers, one of whom was rescued from drowning by King Agelmund, were thrown into a fishpond not by a queen but by a prostitute.[27]

A fourth major difference of early modern monster classifications is the absence of any firm concept of multiple conjoinment, a congenital complication whose initial occurrence is limited to the early weeks of gestations involving two or more identical foetuses. It results in abortions and still or live births featuring a wide range of physical abnormalities, ranging from an additional limb to its most recognized subgroup, conjoined twins. Far more than other categories of human monstrosity, early modern conjoined twins strained philosophical concepts of what it means to be human, even the very definition of what was legally, socially and medically admissible as the human. Multiple conjoinment, still neither fully understood nor adequately defined and named as a coherent category by modern medical science, was then only dimly emerging as the most complex and varied type of human anatomical nonconformity. Rather than being perceived as one coherent category, different types of multiple conjoinment were then distributed between separate, arbitrarily-defined monstrous groups with little underlying anatomical rationale, as when Guarinonius variously refers to people born with too many limbs, or with 'two heads, more arms, or various other horrible figures'.[28]

Conjoined twins and triplets made a big impact on early modern emblematic and theatrical culture. Multiple conjoinment, celebrated in the visual arts since prehistoric times, is recorded in many classical representations, including those of Hecate, and profoundly integrated into Christian, Hindu and Buddhist iconography and symbolism. Guarinonius conjured up two multi-faced emblematic figures in a polemic on bloodletting, four-faced Ætas, with the faces of a child, youth, man and

---

[25]   *Thomas Platter d.J*, 134–5 (29 February 1596, Arles). Goulart devotes a whole chapter to this (217–18) and similar stories of 'Many Children borne at one Birth' (*Admirable and memorable histories*, 214–24); Grimm and Grimm record a variant set in Saxony ('Die acht Brunos', *Deutsche Sagen*, II, 366–9, nr.571).

[26]   Guarinonius, *Grewel*, 122, 250.

[27]   Shame features significantly in variants (Goulart, *Admirable and memorable histories*, 218–19; Grimm and Grimm, 'So viel Kinder, als Tag' im Jahr' and 'Der Knabe im Fischteich', *Deutsche Sagen*, II, 374–5, nr.578 and 30, nr.392).

[28]   Guarinonius, *Grewel*, 103, 122.

old man, and two-faced Sexus, with those of a man and woman.[29] A similar type of conjoinment features in a second-century AD 'tricephalus' classical sculpture now at the Museum of Lyon, twice seen by Felix Platter *in situ* at the Nîmes amphitheatre in the 1550s: 'Item an upright statue of a figure with three faces [...] I looked at a statue of a man with a triple figure and many other strange things that can be seen'. In February 1596, 21-year-old Thomas Platter saw it there: 'Item, in one corner there is also a large stone statue of a figure with long hair, I thought it was three people with one body [...] on the other side a threefold *Priapus volans*, on whom a woman sits, riding him with reins'.[30] Days later, 59-year-old Felix set off for a Stuttgart court christening not known from official festival books, one of whose 10 costumed tournament masquerades for the running at the ring represented the Roman God Janus as conjoined twins:

> The fourth parade took the form of Janus. First came two black knights with spears, one in full armour, then two boys playing violins together, one dressed in green, the other in ash-grey, placed back to back, as if they were one double human. Then followed Janus, on horseback, with the same figure, as if two were joined together, one in green, the other in grey. The one behind carried a snowball and had a fountain on his head and two faces. The horse's harness was also green and grey. He was followed by another with two faces.[31]

Twenty years later, in March 1616, the Stuttgart court celebrated the christening of Friedrich, second son of Johann Friedrich, Duke of Württemberg, who comprehensively reorganized his cabinet of curiosities in anticipation of the influx of high-ranking diplomats and courtiers, including Princess Elizabeth Stuart and her husband the Elector Palatine, Friedrich V.[32] Published festival books record a tournament entry sponsored by the former patron of Felix Platter (who had died two years earlier), the Margrave of Baden, featuring two triple-conjoined characters, a male Discordia on foot, and Concordia Invicta, the mounted woman who leads him. Matthaeus Merian's illustration suggests that the iconographic source for both is Andreas Alciatus's 1550 depiction of triple-bodied Geryon as 'Concordia Insuperabilis', an upright male with six arms and legs, perhaps via a later variant (Plate 29).[33] In one of many Catalan toponyms derived from Greek mythology, the Spanish city Gerona took its name from Geryon, the fearsome triple-bodied

---

[29]   Representing Age and Gender. Guarinonius, *Grewel*, 985.

[30]   *Felix Platter Tagebuch*, 143, 200–1 (30 October 1552 and 25 June 1554, Nîmes); *Thomas Platter d.J*, 106 (23 February 1596, Nîmes).

[31]   *Felix Platter Tagebuch*, 474 (9 March 1596, Sigmaringen). On this festival, see Chapter 6, this volume.

[32]   Bujok, *Neue Welten*, 104.

[33]   Henkel and Schöne, *Emblemata*, col.1649; see also Norbrook, 'The masque of truth', 98.

warrior whose cattle was stolen by Hercules in the tenth of his 12 labours.[34] Reflecting the status of preserved conjoined humans as prized collectors' *realia*, a festival book notes that the vanquished, dying 1616 Stuttgart Discordia looked fit to be 'skinned and redisplayed as a monument for esteemed descendants; well-tanned and stuffed, in one or another cabinet of curiosities'.[35]

Thomas Platter regretted that ongoing war in the Spanish Netherlands prevented him from visiting 'the widely famed cabinet of Paludanus [Berend ten Broecke] at Enkhuizen'.[36] Founded too late to be recorded by either Platter brother, the curiosity cabinet of Laurent III Catelan had become eminently noteworthy by the mid-seventeenth century.[37] An anonymous visitor to Montpellier records viewing 'the Cabinet of Monsr. Catelan, the famous late Apothecary' in 1647, and Francis Mortoft noted of it in 1658: 'There is here an Apothecary hath a very Rare Cabinet of all sortes of Fowles, Fishes, and strange beastes and other admirable things, which are worth seeing, and which every stranger that comes into the Towne is desired to see.'[38] In 1596, 14 years after his death, the most distinguished Montpellier cabinet was still that of the late Laurent Joubert, whose younger son showed it to Thomas Platter. Shamelessly plundered by previous visitors, Platter was shocked by its sorry state, but nevertheless delighted to accept from it, as a gift for Felix, some necklaces of 'several small bones threaded onto a cotton thread, which the Americans or Anthropophagi, that is cannibals, make from humans they have eaten, and wear as decoration around their necks and limbs'. The other 25 items he recorded include a monstrous child and conjoined animals:

> For the 10th, I also saw several strange monsters. One was the head of a 14 year-old child, which was extremely large, being four spans in circumference. Item 11, a pig with eight feet, four in the usual places, two in front on its chest, and two on its back. The 12th. A large goat with two heads.[39]

As alleged evidence of monstrosity and a key medicinal ingredient, narwhal horns exhibited as unicorn horns were carefully inspected and measured by Thomas Platter. At Hampton Court, he examined 'a completely round horn of a unicorn, seven spans long. It had been filed down for the benefit of the sick, looked like ivory, but the little black veins where it had been turned still showed. Inside it

---

[34]   Or, according to Thomas Platter, lost a battle against the Egyptian King Osiris (*Thomas Platter d.J*, 331–2: 26 January 1599, Gerona).

[35]   Hulsen et al., *Repræsentatio*, 'Vierdte Relation', 14. See also Watanabe-O'Kelly, 'The iconography of German Protestant tournaments', 57–9, and *Triumphall shews*, 57.

[36]   *Thomas Platter d.J*, 871 (24 October 1599, Calais).

[37]   Dulieu, *La médecine a Montpellier du XIIe au Xxe siècle*, 341–3.

[38]   Mortoft, *His book*, 26.

[39]   He also saw the knife discussed in Chapter 10, this volume. *Thomas Platter d.J*, 165–8 (9 August 1596, Montpellier). Albrecht Dürer's engraving of 1496, *The double pig of Landser*, depicts conjoined pigs of this type. Four spans = 80cm.

was hollow, so that a nerve could go through it'. One at Windsor, a span taller than himself, was said to have been obtained from Arabia by King Henry VIII, while the even longer and heavier one he saw at Saint-Denis was 'valued at one hundred thousand crowns'.[40] Walter Cope's cabinet was a highlight of Platter's London visit. He viewed 50 of its treasures, including: '12. The horn and tail of a rhinoceros, it is a large animal like an elephant', but also '16. The round horn of an Englishwoman, that grew from her forehead'.[41] This latter was no hoax, but a genuine human horn, probably shed by the Welsh widow Mrs Margaret Gryffith, who suffered one of the earliest documented cases of *cornu cutaneum*, an extreme form of benign, pre-malignant or malignant skin lesion. Visitors to Gryffith's public showings in London in 1588 could buy a souvenir pamphlet whose title concisely described her condition, and a reference to her in Thomas Dekker's *Old Fortunatus* suggests that she had died by 1599.[42]

Horned humans, who respond well to modern medical intervention, have become exceedingly rare. Giants and dwarfs, by contrast, still represent universally recognized categories of the anatomically abnormal. Thomas Platter comments on the unusual height of Netherlanders, who:

> male and female, are generally taller and more goodlooking than the Italians, Spanish or French. It is thought this is because their region is damper, especially in the case of those from Holland and Friesland. And numerous bones of giants are still found daily when excavations are made in North Holland.[43]

Repeating the legend that 'long ago, England had many strong giants', he also notes unusual numbers of tall Englishmen. At London's Guildhall, he viewed paintings of the legendary British giants Cuemagot Albionus and Corinaeus Britannus, displayed annually during the Lord Mayor's procession, until their replacement in the early eighteenth century by two wooden sculptures.[44] In the 1580s, the apothecary Renward Cysat viewed 'bones of giants' in Felix Platter's collections 'of whom very large teeth were found [...] they were sent to him from England'.[45] In 1584, Cysat showed Platter some massive prehistoric mammoth bones dug up near Lucerne in 1577. Platter judged them to belong to a five-and-a-half metre tall human giant. He recorded this giant in one of his *Observations*, and commissioned a lifesize portrait of him, for display in Lucerne's city hall, from

---

[40]   *Thomas Platter d.J*, 838, 849, 895 (27 September and 30 November 1599, Hampton Court, Windsor, Saint-Denis).

[41]   *Thomas Platter d.J*, 796–7 (21 September 1599, London).

[42]   Anon., *Myraculous, and Monstrous*; Bondeson, *The two-headed boy*, 122–3; Burnett, *Constructing 'monsters'*, 16.

[43]   *Thomas Platter d.J*, 699–700 (1 September 1599, Louvain).

[44]   *Thomas Platter d.J*, 791, 819 (20 and 25 September 1599, London).

[45]   Lötscher, *Felix Platter und seine Familie*, 133.

the Basle artist Hans Bock, for whom he was then sitting for his own full-length portrait.[46]

Grewel's titlepage illustration prominently features a seven-headed monster symbolizing the seven deadly sins (Plate 6), and Guarinonius introduces a condemnation of early modern alchemists with a description of a legendary Nordic giant's prodigious pyromaniac self-harming.[47] He believed that the Tirol was founded by the 'eminent' giant Haimon, over whose skeleton the monastery at Wilten (to whose archives he donated some of his papers), was said to have been built, and whose monstrous body offers the template for his extended metaphorical account of the Tirol.[48] Guarinonius warns that menstruating girls and women should be kept from young children, and that intercourse during menstruation or over-eating during pregnancy can lead to leprous and monstrous births,[49] and takes an uncompromising stance on giants and other monsters:

> The friendly reader asks: a long time ago there were giants, does that mean that nature has declined? Answer: its production of monsters and the incomplete has declined, because to be a giant does not mean to be complete, but incomplete and outside the rightful proportions of nature. Not that which is too large or too small, but that which is average, is the more complete, so that just as dwarfs are far beneath the correct size, giants and suchlike tall, disproportionate people are far above. So nature becomes more noble and pure, the more it rids itself of this type of vermin, of which we should wish to have less.[50]

An anecdote of the 1590s demonstrates Guarinonius and his fellow medical students' robust attitude to physical abnormalities. At the end of his first lecture,

---

[46]   Platter, *Obseruationum*, 548–9; *Felix Platter Tagebuch*, plate 49.

[47]   Guarinonius, *Grewel*, 1262 (the source of this garbled resumé of the inglorious life and death of Hardbeen is Book 6 of Saxo Grammaticus' 16 volume *Danish History* of 1514).

[48]   Guarinonius, *Grewel*, 471–4; Dörrer, 'Guarinoni als Volksschriftsteller', 150; Hastaba, 'Vom Lied zum Spiel', 273–6.

[49]   Guarinonius, *Grewel*, 771, 932–4: 'because this uncleanliness is poisonous and revolting, and during this time the person no less so. It is known and apparent to many that if touched by women during this time, not only young, but also many larger trees will die and decay. How much more easily can such poison get into food or drink and poison it? A sensible housekeeper should take especially good care to ensure that during this time women do not go into her cellars, let alone near wine casks or have anything to do with drawing wine [...] because it is well known and obvious that many expensive wines have been completely ruined through such abominations. That is why a housekeeper who has her wits about her has extra maids and girls, so that she can swap them around during this time and one can stand in for another. Because although this bloodiness [modern literal meaning: 'stupidity'] may be less poisonous and destructive in one than in another, it is not possible to distinguish between them, and in itself it is as revolting in one as in another'.

[50]   Guarinonius, *Grewel*, 49.

they saluted 'a new professor at Padua, learned but extremely short of stature and small' by parading him on high, still seated at his lecturer's pulpit, chanting 'Viua, Viua, nanino! Long live the little dwarf!'[51]

The professional performers attracted to Basle by the commercial possibilities of its annual fair, and because it was a convenient crossing point for north–south and east–west trade routes, included numerous anatomically abnormal show people. 'The third book of observations by Dr Felix Plater. Observations upon deformity' opens with accounts of three dwarfs. One was in the service of Alessandro Farnese, Duke of Parma, in December 1592 succeeded by his son Ranuccio, whom he had called to Flanders to assist in his military campaigns on behalf of the Spanish Habsburgs (Diagram 2):

> *A Dwarfe.* [...] *An.* 1592 I saw the first Dwarfe called *John Estrix* of *Mechlin*, brought from *Basil* to the Duke of *Parma* in *Flanders*, in *November*. He was thirty five years old, and was but three foot long, and had a long beard. He could not go up a pair of stairs, nor into a chair, but was lifted up by his servant. He had three languages, and was very ingenious and industrious. I once played with him at Dice.[52]

In a later, longer case-study, Felix Platter features three members of the Gonzales family, also in the service of the Farnese family, known as noted collectors of 'monsters':

> *Some Men are very Hairy.* It is vulgarly supposed that there are wild men that have Hair all over their bodies, except the tip of their Nose before, on the Knees, the Buttocks, and Palms of the Hands, and Soles of the Feet, as they are painted. But this is false, for none of the Cosmographers have mentioned any such, though they left not out the most brutish, as the Amazons, Canibals, and Americans, and others that go naked, and yet are not Hairy, but pul out Hairs where they grow. But this is true, that there are many of both Sex, especially men, more hairy then others, on their Thighs, Arms, Belly, Breast and Face, such I have seen. There was one at *Paris* very Gracious with King *Henry* the second, that lived at his Court, who had very long hair all over, except a little under his Eyes, his Eyebrows, and Hair in his Forehead were so long, that he was forced to tye them Back from hindering of his sight. He married a smooth Woman like others, and had by her Hairy Children, which were sent into *Flanders* to the Duke of *Parma*, I saw them in *Basil, An.* 1583. and got their Pictures, when they were to

---

[51] Guarinonius, *Grewel*, 492.

[52] Platter, *Obseruationum*, 545 (this translation: Plat[t]er, Culpeper and Cole, *Platerus histories*, 359–60). See also Diagram 2, and, for Platter's 'third dwarf', Chapter 6, this volume.

go into *Italy* with their Mother, a Son of nine years old, and a Daughter of ten:[53] the Male was more hairy in the Face then the Female, but all her Backbone was full of long bristles. But since (as we showed in Anatomy), there are Hairs in all the Pores of the body, it is no wonder that there are more in some then others, as the Nailes. But this is a greater wonder, that in some places they should grow so orderly, as in the Eyebrows, and in others scarce to be seen. There are Hairs in the Palms of every ones hands as appears by Children, but they are smal and continually worn away, which makes the Hand appear smooth.[54]

Pedro Gonzales was born around the year 1537, on Tenerife in the Canary Islands, then known mainly for exporting excellent sugar.[55] The symptoms of his rare congenital condition, hypertrichosis lanuginosa, are permanently growing hair over widespread areas of the face and body, and during the course of his life, Gonzales was moved between several European courts, most with strong Habsburg connections, as a living wild man. The idea of wild men, covered only with hair, leaves or feathers, caught the early modern imagination. Thomas Platter's journal illustrates Juan Guarin of Montserrat, according to legend chased into the mountains, where he grew a hairy coat, and was hunted down and brought back to court, to be kept like an exotic animal. At Hampton Court, Platter admired Cornelius Ketel's now lost portrait painting of the native American 'wild' family brought live to England by Sir Martin Frobisher in the 1580s, and at Greenwich he saw a salt cellar shaped like a wild man clad in feathers.[56] Pedro Gonzales is first noted in a dispatch of 18 April 1547 to Ercole II d'Este from his envoy to the French court, Giulio Alvarotto. It documents the presentation as a gift to Henri II and Catherina de'Medici on 31 March 1547 of a boy of about 10 years old, hairy all over 'just like wild men of the woods are painted', speaking Spanish and dressed according to Spanish manner, but allegedly found in 'the Indies'.[57] The physician Giulio Cesare Scaligero hints that Pedro may have spent time at the Spanish Habsburg court, perhaps even have been presented to the French king by Charles V, in a Latin treatise first published in Paris in 1557. It noted a hairy Spanish boy nicknamed 'Barbet' (the French term for a shaggy Flemish hunting

---

[53]   This incorrect translation of Platter's original wording of 1614 ('masculum 9. & fœminam 7. annorum [a boy of 9 and a girl of 7 years]') demonstrates the ease with which such inaccuracies are introduced.

[54]   Platter, *Obseruationum*, 553–4 (this translation: Plat[t]er, Culpeper and Cole, *Platerus histories*, 365–6); see also Wiesner-Hanks, *The marvelous hairy girls*, 183–4.

[55]   Guarinonius, *Grewel*, 49, 1161.

[56]   *Thomas Platter d.J*, 360–3 (6 February 1599, Montserrat); 834–5, 863–4 (27 September and 6 October 1599, London).

[57]   Alvarotto's dispatch is in the Archivio di Stato di Modena (Zapperi, *Der wilde Mann von Teneriffa*, 189).

dog, the 'Watterhund'): 'brought from the Indies, or, as some think, born in Spain to parents from the Indies'.[58]

The adult Pedro Gonzales was employed as a French court servant from 1556 to at least 1560, and at an unknown date married to a woman, Catherine, with normal hair distribution, who bore him at least four hairy and three non-hairy children.[59] Possibly, he entered the service of the Farnese family through Margareta of Parma. Illegitimate daughter of Emperor Charles V (an uncle of Archduke Karl of Habsburg and of Wilhelm V of Bavaria's mother Anna of Habsburg), her first husband, Alessandro de'Medici, who died when she was aged 14, had been an illegitimate brother of Henri II's wife, Catherina de'Medici (Diagram 2). A former Regent of the Netherlands herself, Margareta of Parma returned to Italy for the last time in 1583 after supporting her son Alessandro Farnese for several years in this post.[60] Having established that 'Don Pietro Gonzalez Selvaggio' arrived with his wife and at least one child at the Farnese court in Parma in May 1591, Roberto Zapperi attempts to reconcile perceived anomalies in Felix Platter's account of his encounter with members of the Gonzales family by suggesting that Platter incorrectly recalled dates and ages, and in fact saw Catherine Gonzales not, as recorded in his publication of 1614, in 1583 with a 'boy of 9 and a girl of seven years', but eight years later, in early 1591, with her 11-year-old son Henri and eight- or nine-year-old daughter Françoise.[61]

This theory introduces more problems than it solves.[62] Felix Platter's writings bear witness to an exceptional memory for dates and people, and accurate, reliable observations, and in this instance, his facts and figures are fairly exactly supported by independent documentary sources. A passage in Montaigne's essays records a personal meeting between a hairy girl and Archduke Karl, who died in 1590: 'There was also presented vnto *Charles* king of *Bohemia*, an Emperour, a young girle, borne about *Pisa*, all shagd and hairy over and over.'[63] This suggests the presence of at least one hairy Gonzales daughter in the German-speaking regions before 1591, albeit not necessarily the girl seen by Platter. However, during precisely the period Platter claims their physical presence in the German-speaking Alps, the Bavarian and central European Habsburg courts exhibited a quite extraordinary

---

[58]   Scaligero (1484–1558), *Exotericarvm exercitationvm*, 427, 790; Bartels, 'Ueber abnorme Behaarung', 230–1; Bondeson, *The two-headed boy*, 7.

[59]   Zapperi, *Der wilde Mann von Teneriffa*, 46–7, 81–2, 115, 215. The date of birth of the oldest son, Paolo (non-hairy), is unknown. Zapperi suggests birth dates for Madeleine/Maddalena (c.1575, hairy), Henri/Arrigo (c.1580, hairy), Francesca (c.1582) and Antoinetta/Tognina (c.1588, hairy); the youngest sons were born in Parma in 1592 (Orazio, hairy) and 1595 (Ercole).

[60]   Hertel, 'Der rauch man zu Münichen', 174; Zapperi, *Der wilde Mann von Teneriffa*, 200–2.

[61]   Zapperi, *Der wilde Mann von Teneriffa*, 89, 92–3, 115, 196, 214.

[62]   *Pace* Wiesner-Hanks, *The marvelous hairy girls*, 185–6.

[63]   Montaigne, 'Of the force of imagination', *Essayes*, 45.

flurry of interest in the Gonzales family. This generated correspondence and major portrait paintings of the family by several renowned artists based at these courts, some of which are still on display at the former seat of Archduke Karl's brother, Ferdinand of the Tirol, Ambras Castle near Innsbruck.[64] Furthermore, a brief Latin biography of 'Petrvs Gonsalvs' inscribed on the back of the Munich-based court artist Joris Hoefnagel's double portrait of Gonzales and his wife Catherine concludes with the sentence 'He appeared in Munich, Bavaria, in the year 1582'.[65]

Duke Wilhelm V of Bavaria's attempts to acquire a living wild man date back to at least 1571, when Duke Philipp zu Hanau responded to his enquiries with assurances that there were none in his forests.[66] On 3 April 1583, Wilhelm drafted a letter to be sent from Munich to Archduke Karl's wife, his sister Maria, in Vienna:

> Concerning my wild people, I want to have them portrayed full-length to send to you. I've also written to France to enquire everything about his origins, comings and goings. But he himself will know little, as he left when he was very young, and was presented to the king. Apart from that they aren't wild, as they are called. The man is a very refined, modest and polite person, apart from being so shaggy. The little girl is also very refined and wellmannered; if she didn't have the hair in her face, she'd be a pretty little girl. The boy can't speak, he is very foolish and diverting. The old father and mother are not hairy, but like other people, and if I understood correctly, they were Spaniards. I also want to send you a full-length portrait of the old man, I have it lifesize, he is not a tall person.[67]

In a letter he sent a month later, on 10 May 1583, Wilhelm specifies 'his wild people' themselves, as well as their painted portrait, among various commodities he shortly intends to have sent to Maria in Vienna: 'I want to send you and your husband the wild people *and* the painting at the earliest opportunity. I will send the stove to Vienna, to your house.'[68] These letters were sent in response

---

[64]   For texts, see Zapperi, *Der wilde Mann von Teneriffa*, 194–7; for images, see also: Wiesner-Hanks, *The marvelous hairy girls*.

[65]   Zapperi, *Der wilde Mann von Teneriffa*, 57 ('Conparuit Monachij boiorum a[nn]o 1582'), 195–6.

[66]   Munich BHStA, Fürstensachen 426/I: 10 March 1571; Baader, *Der bayerische Renaissancehof*, 74.

[67]   Munich BHStA.GHA, Korr.Akt 606 V, f.212ᵛ (file draft of letter sent); Zapperi, *Der wilde Mann von Teneriffa*, 194–5. Felix Platter possibly, and his senior colleague Dr Heinrich Pantaleon almost certainly, met Duke Wilhelm in person in January 1576, when he stopped off in Basle while, at the request of her father Emperor Maximilian II, escorting the widowed Archduchess Elisabeth back from France to Vienna (Baader, *Der bayerische Renaissancehof*, 201, 242–3; Lietzmann, 'Unbekannten Brief', 87). See also Diagram 2.

[68]   Present author's emphasis. Munich BHStA.GHA, Korr.Akt 606 V, f.214ʳ (a draft of the letter sent, as recorded on the verso in a scribal hand of similar date also providing a

to correspondence of 11 March 1583, in which Archduke Karl warmly thanks Wilhelm for:

> the little panel portraying the hairy man together with his wife and children, which y[our] e[steemed self] sent me via my chamberlain, von Herberstain.[69] This is certainly a thing that is well worth seeing. I would ask y[our] e[xcellency], insofar as it is possible, that y. e. would send me full-length portraits of the two children, *and have the little boy depicted naked, while he is still so young.*[70]

For Zapperi, this correspondence demonstrates that Duke Wilhelm and the Habsburgs never saw members of the Gonzales family in person, and that their sole source of knowledge concerning them was lost correspondence from the Parisian court.[71] But Zapperi neither publishes nor takes into account the concluding phrase of Karl's letter. Revealed by my re-examination of the original documents, it strongly suggests that Karl knew that the growing infant himself was present in person at the Bavarian court. This reading of the evidence supports the accuracy of Platter's factual data. It strengthens the possibility that Pedro and Catherine Gonzales and two of their hairy children were associated with the entourage of Margareta of Parma, journeying from the Netherlands to Italy during late 1582 and early 1583, and that they passed through Basle, and spent time in person at courts of her Munich and Habsburg relatives. Platter published the children's ages and the date at which he saw them only in 1614, 30 years after examining them. If he intended to record the boy's age not as nine years but as nine months, then the two hairy children accompanying Catherine, depicted in the Habsburg portraits and noted in Karl's letter can be identified as Madeleine, aged around seven years in 1583, and her then possibly nine-month-old brother Henri.

Guarinonius refers more than once to people born with too few limbs, and Felix Platter's *Observations* features four armless performers:[72]

---

list of subjects covered in the letter, whose item 'Rauchen leüt und tafln' ('hairy people and pictures') again distinguishes between the people and their portraits).

[69] Perhaps Karl, Baron of Herberstein (1538–90), a longserving Habsburg courtier who died in Vienna.

[70] Munich BHStA.GHA, Korr.Akt 609 III/3, f.61 (present author's emphasis of previously unpublished phrase: 'und weill das buebl noch so klein ist nakater abmallen lassen'); Zapperi, *Der wilde Mann von Teneriffa*, 194.

[71] Zapperi, *Der wilde Mann von Teneriffa*, 68: 'the Gonzalez were never in Munich', 196: 'Duke [Wilhelm] never saw Gonzalez himself in the flesh'; Wiesner-Hanks, *The marvelous hairy girls*, 159: 'there is no evidence that any member of the [Gonzales] family was actually at the Wittelsbach court in Munich'.

[72] Guarinonius, *Grewel*, 103, 966. On armless performers, see also Burnett, *Constructing 'monsters'*, 15; Mueller, 'Touring, women', 66–70.

Men without Arms, and yet famous Artificers. [...] in the Court of *Wittemberg*,
I found a writing engraved excellently by one *Thomas Schwicker* of *Hale* that
wanted both his Arms. And the Prince showed me a paper with divers Characters
in it written by the same man, and his Picture to the life, holding a Pen between
his right great Toe, and his little Toe next to it: and the same Prince shewed me
another writing of an Italian written with his Feet. And at Basil I saw a woman
that spun very Artificially with her Feet and Carded, and the like. And I saw
another that with his head and shoulders would lay hold one things, and cut them
and knock them with Instruments and great force. All these were born without
Arms.[73]

As well as the unidentified woman and man Platter saw himself in Basle, he records
the Italian and German performers he learned of at the Stuttgart court through a
proxy exhibition staged for him by the Duke, in which the monsters were played
by their texts.[74] Souvenirs sold by such performers typically included handicrafts
and specimens of writings created by them during their shows, promotional
broadsheets, and portrait prints. Known portrait prints of Thomas Schweicker,
born in Halle in 1580, include one of 1633 by De Bry, also depicting him writing
with his feet.[75]

In 1599, Thomas Platter was fascinated by an enterprising fully-limbed Spanish
craftsman whose similar performances were a publicity stunt: 'I saw a turner in
Barcelona who, even though perfectly capable of using both his hands, still held
the iron with one foot and turned excellent work, as I often watched him do with
great admiration. And he turned a bone inkhorn for me in this way, which I bought
from him.'[76] Six months later, he records two congenitally armless itinerant show
people who publicly performed various tasks with their feet, a woman he saw in
Paris and a boy he evidently saw after returning to Basle:

On the rue St Jacques, in a public inn, I saw a woman of around 40 years who
was about three feet tall. She could speak English and French, and I believe she
was from Hamburg. She had no arms, and her knees grew from her hips, she had
no thighs above her knees, as I observed when I saw her naked. But she could
thread needles with her feet, and play dice, and also write very neatly and do
many other tasks with her feet, just like a young boy I later saw here in Basle,
who had the same ability to write, play and sew. I was also told that this woman
never had any shortage of suitors at any time. This woman was carried from one
place to another in the city, and through her huge sums of money were collected.

---

[73]   Platter, *Obseruationum*, 556–7 (this translation: Plat[t]er, Culpeper and Cole,
Platerus histories, 366).

[74]   On this role of texts, see also Burnett, *Constructing 'monsters'*, 24.

[75]   Reproduced: Holländer, *Wunder*, 115.

[76]   *Thomas Platter d.J*, 372 (17 February 1599, Barcelona).

Anyone who seeks them out can see large numbers of this type of monster, as well as other skilful shows, throughout the year.[77]

The English edition of *Praxis medica* pads out Felix Platter's brief generic acknowledgment of armless performers in the original edition not with the specific descriptions of Schweicker and three unidentified performers from his *Observations*, but with two anachronistic examples seen by Platter's English editors, at mid seventeenth-century London fairgrounds:

> *The want of parts*. The greatest and most usuall Deformities are in the deficiency of number, as when some Instruments are wanting in the birth: as we have seen some monsters wanting both Arms, who have written and done other things with their Feet instead thereof,[78] as I saw *Anno* 1652. Nov. 29. a Woman born without Arms, which gave her Child suck and carried it like a Nurse, making also divers things with her Feet and with more dexterity then many could do with their hands. Her Name was *Maudlin Rudolphs* of *Thainbut*, in the chief City of *Sweedland* being above forty years of age, and the year after February 20 I saw one that way a crooked Dwarf born without Arms, that exercised all things with his feet which were to be done with hands with dexterity to the admiration of the Beholders, his Name was *Theodorick Stieb* of *Vienna* an Austrian.[79]

Magdalena Rudolfs of Stockholm, born in 1612, toured the fairgrounds with the infant featured in some of the 21 vignettes depicting her activities, surrounding her full-length engraved souvenir portrait of 1651 (Plate 28).[80]

Felix Platter's English translators also augmented *Praxis medica*'s description of performing parasitic conjoined twins with an account of a better documented later example, Lazarus Colloredo, who toured England in the 1640s:

> *A double Body*: Many Deformities are in the Body from number abounding, some come from the Birth which if they are great are called monstrous, as when two bodies are borne knit together in divers parts. I have seen a Man which carried with him another of the same bigness compleate in all his Members, except the Head which was as it were grafted to the Neck into his Breast, and he lived so from his birth a long time in very good health. The like unto which *Stumpfius* in his Helvetian History saith he saw.[81] I also upon the fourteenth of *August Anno* 1645 saw naked in mine own house, another, who had his Brother hanging a little below his left Pap, fastned unto him by his breast, he had a great Head, with

---

[77]   *Thomas Platter d.J*, 587–8 (8 August 1599, Paris).

[78]   The rest of this passage has no equivalent in Platter's original account.

[79]   Platter, *Praxeos*, III, 3 (augmented translation: Plat[t]er, Cole and Culpeper, *A golden practice*, 501).

[80]   Holländer, *Wunder*, 119.

[81]   The rest of this passage has no equivalent in Platter's original account.

much curled Hair, his Eye-brows moved, but never opened, his Mouth was open and alwayes full of stinking slimy Flegm, his hinder part of his Head fell down to his Brothers belly, his Face being upwards his Breast was crooked and the Ribbs plain to be seen, and bent like the Keele of a Ship outward, his Shoulders were very deformed, both his Arms trembled and were bent backwards his left Hand had the three last Fingers; his right, a great Thumb and two Fingers, that next to the Thumb was least and grew thereto, from his left side his left Thigh hung downwards bowed, with a short crooked Foot, and onely four Toes, his Heel being turned outwards, you might plainly have perceived his right Foot to be inclosed in his Brothers left Thigh, as if he had two thigh bones, between the Thighs were the Buttocks and a cleft but not open, his brother cloathed him with a shirt doublet Breeches and Stockings. This Monstrous man, was very active, of good Habit of body, well coloured, witty, long winded, he told me he was Son to a noble Merchant of *Genua*, his Fathers Name was *Baptista Collaredo* and Mothers *Belerina Fraginetta*, of the Family of the *Forum Julianum*; and because his Parents and the Priests saw that he was a double Man, he was baptized by the Name of *Lazarus* and *John Baptist* he was then twenty eight years of Age, when I heard from him and saw these things.[82]

Born in Genoa in 1617, Lazarus Colloredo, together with his 'deaf, blind, dumb' parasitic conjoined twin John Baptist Colloredo, was already by 1634 the subject of learned discussion by Parisian scientists and a sensational fairground attraction who 'travelled to almost every country, and showed himself for money'.[83] The previously unidentified performer seen by Felix Platter himself, and recorded in Johannes Stumpf's *Schwytzer Chronica* (Zurich 1554), can here be identified as the fairground performer Hans Kaltenbrunn. He is recorded at the Basle Fair in 1555, 1556 and 1566, when a souvenir broadsheet gives his age as 40 and depicts him in contemporary dress, jacket open to show his headless naked parasitic conjoined twin hanging down to his knees from his upper chest, and is also the subject of one of Platter's *Observations*:

> *A double Body, one growing to the other without a Beard.* About twenty years since, I saw in this City a man of no great stature, that carried another body whole from the neck by which it grew to his breast. And hnug [*sic*] down to the ground, compleat in all parts but the head, which seemed to be thrust into the other body. It had nails and hair under the Arm-pits, and about the Privities. As often as the man pissed, this pissed, but the Arse-hole was closed up and

---

[82]   Platter, *Praxeos*, III, 2 (augmented translation: Plat[t]er, Cole and Culpeper, *A golden practice*, 501); Holländer, *Wunder*, 103, 105 (souvenir portraits of Colloredo, 1645 and 1646).

[83]   Harsdörffer, *Der grosse Schau-platz*, 243; Havers, *A general collection*, 61–3; Bondeson, *The two-headed boy*, vii–xix; Burnett, *Constructing 'monsters'*, 28.

appeared no where. *Stumpfius* mentions such a double body. And I have heard my Father say that he saw it.[84]

Confusion over Hans Kaltenbrunn's date and place of birth and appearance have led to multiple entries in some early modern wonder books, but despite depicting a very different type of conjoinment, a broadsheet commemorating his birth can here be firmly associated with him. It confirms his date and place of birth as 8 October 1529, in Lutenbach in the parish of Oberkirch, and names his parents as Wolf Kaltenbrunn and his wife, the daughter of Hans Zerser of Grienberg.[85] Many performing monsters developed a fairground 'act', and Iranæus indicates that Hans Kaltenbrunn's took advantage of the supernatural associations of births such as his. It identifies him as a fortune-teller: 'This man spoke of wondrous things that were still to happen in the future. This was a most unnatural and wondrous thing'.[86]

The first two chapters of this section mine the Platter brothers' and Guarinonius's writings for information on English actors and the London theatrical culture, and on the general circumstances of European marketplace performers. The previous and present chapters conclude Part III by reviewing writings of the three physicians illuminating some of the intense negotiations between science and showmanship, witnessed on the multifarious exhibition sites of the supernatural and human monstrosity. These sites represent significant meeting points between early modern medicine and theatre, whose most substantial economic merger is quackery. The time has come to interrogate the specific descriptions of performing quack troupes representing the physicians' most explicit records of overlaps between theatre and medicine. This is the task of Part IV, which starts with a consideration of Thomas Platter's much-cited description of Zan Bragetta's quack troupe based on newly-discovered documentary evidence radically transforming its theatre-historical significance.

---

[84]   Platter, *Obseruationum*, 550 (this translation: Plat[t]er, Culpeper and Cole, *Platerus histories*, 362–3).

[85]   Reproduced: Holländer, *Wunder*, 76; Ewinkel, *De monstris*, 369 (neither of whom make the association with Kaltenbrunn).

[86]   Irenæus, *De monstris*, sig.O4ʳ; see also Katritzky, 'Images of "monsters"', 97–8.

PART IV
Performing Healing:
Commedia dell'Arte Quack Troupes

PART IV

Chapter 12
A New Identification for 'Zan Bragetta':
Giovanni Paulo Alfieri

A growing understanding of the profound extent to which the marketing of medicine informed, and economically underpinned, the rise of professional theatre in early modern Italy, emphasizes the importance of cross-disciplinary approaches. As already touched on in Chapter 9, early modern professional performing troupes had to be capable of performing outdoors as well as indoors, and of accommodating widely varying municipal regulations. For outdoor performances, for which they could not charge an entrance fee, the sale of medical goods and services offered an effective alternative economic strategy. Especially in regions with climates permitting year-round outdoor performances, such troupes often invested considerable efforts into setting themselves up as performing quacks.

The researches presented in this chapter acknowledge the need to move beyond examining the same performing quack troupes independently within the context of two separate academic sub-disciplines, theatre history and medical history, with different agendas and limited contact. Their focus is Thomas Platter's account of the 1598 Avignon season of an Italian quack troupe.[1] This troupe's leader, whose stage name, Zan Bragetta, is provided by Platter, has not previously been identified by his real name, nor linked to any other documented event. With reference to newly-discovered archival documents, this chapter identifies Zan Bragetta as the actor Giovanni Paulo Alfieri, and contextualizes his troupe within the historical record of other documentary evidence of their activities.[2] This suggests that Bragetta impacted not just briefly in Avignon, but for half a century across the length and breadth of France, where at least one shared season with renowned French actors put his troupe at the heart of groundbreaking cross-border theatrical exchanges. Before considering Zan Bragetta's identity, this chapter surveys his troupe's activities in Avignon in 1598 by revisiting Platter's description.

For many reasons, Thomas Platter's original account[3] is an evidential source of exceptional importance in the context of cross-disciplinary investigations into

---

[1]   Basle UL, MS.A λ V.7–8: ff.261ᵛ–265ᵛ; *Thomas Platter d.J*, 305–8 (27 October – 24 December 1598, Avignon); English translation: Chapter 17, this volume.

[2]   Katritzky, 'Zan Bragetta a Jan Potage'.

[3]   Generally noted by English authors with reference to Jennett's considerably shortened translation (*Journal of a younger brother*, 181–3); e.g. by Howarth, *French theatre*, 74–5; Brockliss and Jones, *The medical world of early modern France*, 328; Gentilcore, *Medical charlatanism*, 310, 319–21, 329. See Chapter 17, this volume.

performers and healers. As a physician, Platter possessed relevant expert medical knowledge. His account's contextualization within his factually reliable journal considerably adds to its evidential weight. It describes the commercial and medical strategies of Bragetta's troupe as well as their theatrical repertoire. Platter's longest description of professional entertainers, it situates medicine within the theatrical activities of the public marketplace with unusual clarity. Pre-1700 documentary records of itinerant marketplace troupes only rarely explicitly indicate links between performing and medicine. Platter's own record of Italian travelling actors he saw a few months earlier, in May 1598, notes no medical activity. That day, he lunched at the Carpentras home of Dr Guillaume Albert, after which his host, like him a recent graduate of Montpellier medical school, 'led us to a house, where, in a large room, several foreign Italian comedians played, and performed all sorts of strange acrobatics […] then we came out of the play'.[4] In contrast, Platter's much longer account of Bragetta's troupe brings into sharp focus both their activities as performers, and as traders. He details Bragetta's venues, medical strategies and theatrical repertoire, clarifying key aspects of medical and theatrical interrelations within a specific troupe, on specific stages, integrated into specific sessions of economic activity. His account offers the most informative surviving eyewitness account of the modus operandi of a specific sixteenth-century professional itinerant troupe combining theatrical and medical economic strategies.

Thomas Platter's account records repeatedly visiting, in Avignon, performances by a seven-strong mixed-gender itinerant troupe of Italian comedians who combined commedia dell'arte performances with quack activity: '(*Zan Bragetta*) Hans Latz […] with two women and four men […] Zanni was their leader […] all costumed and neatly masked'.[5] The former papal city's large, wealthy community of military and religious dignitaries seconded from the Vatican represented an especially lucrative destination for Italian professional performers. Platter moved to Avignon for two months in late October 1598, after completing his post-qualification medical practice in nearby Uzès (Plate 3). He describes the main elements of Bragetta's repertoire as plays, musical interludes, and variety spectacle. The troupe's pastoral and comic plays often featured stock commedia dell'arte characters, notably the comic servant–master pair Pantalone and Zanni: 'they also performed (*pastorelle*) shepherd comedies most gracefully, and they could act Pantalone as well as Zanni most skilfully, not only with words, but also with dancing, mime and acrobatics, so that everyone had enough to laugh about, and watched with enjoyment.'[6] He praises their agreeable singing to the lute, harp and viola, and two popular stage routines, involved an actor using a whistle to imitate a large variety of animal noises and bird-song, and the simulated decapitation discussed above (Chapter 10). Platter suggests that while the troupe's indoor performances were free of any

---

4   *Thomas Platter d.J*, 254 (31 May 1598, Carpentras).
5   *Thomas Platter d.J*, 305.
6   *Thomas Platter d.J*, 305–6.

medical or quack activity at all, their outdoor stage focused on the sale of medical stock, adapting their repertoire to frame and support extensive medical activity.

Some specialists have drawn more or less firm lines between the types of entertainment offered by commedia dell'arte troupes and itinerant quacks, doubting whether quacks performed full-length plays of the commedia dell'arte type or pastorals.[7] Even some who draw substantially on Platter's journal strictly distinguish between 'farce players' and 'street entertainers. [..] in most cases [...] attached to some herb dealer or medicine man', and 'indoor actors'.[8] In describing in detail how one and the same itinerant troupe staged both indoor appearances funded by entrance tickets, and outdoor appearances funded by the sale of medical products, Platter's account provides the key to how this dual activity could be combined in practice. Confirmation that less exalted commedia dell'arte troupes routinely combined indoor private commedia dell'arte performances involving no selling, with public outdoor marketplace quackery, in this way, is offered by evidence such as Whetstone's literary description of a quack troupe staging a private performance for an Italian nobleman during Christmas 1580. Whetstone emphasizes the tediousness of an act over reliant on redundant medical quack routines. The troupe he describes consisted of:

> a *Mountebanke*, his necke bechayned with liue Adders, Snakes, Eau'ts, and twentie sundrie kinde of venemous vermines [...] & with him a *Zanni*, and other Actors of pleasure: who presented themselues onelie with a single desire, to recreate Segnior Philoxenus, and his worthie companie: and not with the intent of common *Mountebanckers*, to deceyve the people with some vnprofitable Marchandize.

In which desire they were singularly unsuccessful, since: 'the *Mountibanck*, with discribing the quallities of his Vermin, and the *Zanni* in showing the knavish conditions of his Maister, [...] wasted a good part of the night, and wearyed the moste part of the company'.[9] The combination of medical and theatrical activity in Bragetta's troupe was in no way exceptional, and many celebrated Italian actors of his time had personal experience of medical activity. Although established performers and musicians downplayed any professional connection with marketplace itinerants, commedia dell'arte routines were the staple of Italian quack troupes, which were a significant training ground for commedia dell'arte performers. Nicolò Barbieri, famed in his stage role of Beltrame, in the 1634 edition of his *Supplica* recalls the start of his performing career in il Monferino's quack troupe.[10] Giovanni Rivani, who took the stage name 'Dottor Graziano Campanaccio da Budri', repeatedly risked expulsion from the Fedeli troupe for

---

[7]   Richards and Richards, *The commedia dell'arte*, 17.

[8]   Wiley, *The early public theatre in France*, 69–70.

[9]   Whetstone, *Heptameron*, sigs.Liii^v, Mi^v.

[10]   Barbieri, *La supplica*, 126–7.

quack activities.[11] Alongside his stage career, the respected troupe leader Flaminio Scala operated a flourishing Venice-based perfume business. Domenico Ottonelli describes how members of the Uniti troupe preceded a street performance in Trapani, Sicily, in 1638, with the sale of patent medicines and other merchandise; by 1668 Italian quacks routinely offered plays, as testified by *Emilia*'s classic put-down in *The sullen lovers*: 'your Playes are below the Dignity of a Mountebanks stage. *Salvator Winter* wou'd have refus'd them', evoking a Neapolitan quack whose handbills in the British Library document his presence in England.[12] Such briefer records, like Platter's account, imply a far greater overlap between the repertoires of quacks and early modern professional actors than the protestations of the latter would suggest.

Zan Bragetta's preferred venue option was indoor. His troupe started their 1598 Avignon season by renting an indoor real tennis court, in which they performed on a raised platform stage. Platter discusses the popularity of ball games, dancing and other diversions with the military stationed in Montpellier, which then had seven centrally located indoor tennis courts, and an eighth in the suburbs.[13] Often administered in conjunction with public inns, Thomas Platter used tennis courts as convenient meeting places for social gatherings, as well as for sport. Platter's descriptions of one in Avignon's Palais de Papes complex, as 'an old, very big church which had been converted into the biggest tennis court I ever saw in all my life', and of a short tennis court of unusual breadth at Agde near Montpellier, indicate a considerable flexibility in proportion and size.[14] Often, as in La Rochelle and Bordeaux, optimum ball return was ensured by facing the floor and inside walls with large smooth stone slabs.[15] Amateur performances and school plays were held not in tennis courts but in church, school or municipal halls, as when

---

[11]   Letter of 27 August 1623 from Giovan Paolo Fabri to the Duke of Mantua (Ferrone, *Attori mercanti corsari*, 230–1); Ferrone et al., *Corrispondenze*, I, 120n2.

[12]   Ottonelli, 'Della Cristiana Moderazione del Teatro', 495; Shadwell, *The Sullen Lovers*, 34; London BL, 551.a.32, nos.30, 32.

[13]   *Thomas Platter d.J*, 78 (October 1595, Montpellier). Unusually, Thomas Platter documents a female professional player, whose father was the superintendent of a tennis court on the outskirts of Blois. Hoping to earn her dowry through the game, and despite being hampered by women's clothes, she easily beat him and his fellow-Germans (*Thomas Platter d.J*, 501: 28 May 1599, Blois).

[14]   *Thomas Platter d.J*, 117 (25 February 1596, Avignon), 156 (3 July 1596, Agde).

[15]   *Thomas Platter d.J*, 459 (6 May 1599, La Rochelle). In Saint-Denis in 1557, Felix Platter played tennis at the court of the Moor Inn (*Felix Platter Tagebuch*, 281: April 1557, Paris). By the time of Thomas's visit, Paris and its suburbs were said to have 1,100 courts, although he estimated the number at around half that, all in constant use. Barcelona, by contrast, 'had few tennis courts, they still play with hard leather balls, and prefer the diversion of cards or dice', and Innsbruck and Prague had only two each (*Thomas Platter d.J*, 346: 28 January 1599, Barcelona, 594: 28 July 1599, Paris; Bücking, *Kultur und Gesellschaft in Tirol*, 164).

Thomas Platter notes a room used for the staging of plays in Vienne's city hall.[16] While such halls could be let out to professional performers, indoor tennis courts continued to be in common use by actors even after custom-built theatres became widespread.[17] As large, secure, covered halls, free of central pillars, tennis courts provided excellent indoor venues outside which travelling troupes could collect an entrance fee from spectators, and within which they could accommodate them on raised tiered seating around the sides, and temporary seating on the ground floor, and perform on a temporary raised stage.[18] Two years earlier, for example, on 27 February 1596, after attending a wedding at the Church of Sainte Madeleine in Avignon, Platter:

> went to an indoor tennis court near that same church. Inside we watched a French comedian perform a French play with a woman and a boy, and perform several unusual dances and acrobatic routines, in the manner of street performers. Because there are generally comedians in Avignon, who stage their comedies in the indoor tennis courts, of which there are many.[19]

As Thomas Platter points out, the problem with tennis courts as seemingly ideal performing venues comes only when the income from entrance fees no longer covers the performers' outgoings. When Bragetta's troupe reached this point, after several weeks of performing inside the tennis court, they decided to target a new category of spectator within Avignon. Although it was by now November, they abandoned their raised platform stage inside the tennis court, and set up a more modest benchlike long table in Avignon's main market square:

> When they noticed that not many people were coming to their comedies any more, even though they still had to pay a high rent for the tennis court, they set up a long table in the public square called the Place du Change. After the midday meal, they all stood together on this same table, one next to another [...] and [...] played an amusing comedy on this same table for a couple of hours or so.[20]

In an outdoor environment in which they had to perform their repertoire under the pressure of having to collect money from an audience who could not be charged an

---

[16]   *Thomas Platter d.J*, 46 (3 October 1595, Vienne).

[17]   In London, Gibbons's tennis court in Vere Street was used by William Davenant as a playing venue during the 1650s, and converted into a theatre by London's other theatrical patent holder, Thomas Killigrew in the 1660s, when Davenant converted and played in Lisle's tennis court, in Lincoln's Inn Fields (Highfill, Burnim and Langhans, *A biographical dictionary*, IV, 177, 180 and IX, 11).

[18]   Wiley, *The early public theatre in France*, 158–77 and 'The Hotel de Bourgogne', 29–33.

[19]   *Thomas Platter d.J*, 123 (27 February 1596, Avignon).

[20]   *Thomas Platter d.J*, 306.

entrance fee, the troupe turned to quackery, paying their way by selling medicines and cosmetics. Platter goes into the minutiae of packaging, marketing and transport arrangements. Bragetta's troupe used a 'large locked chest' to transport small tins of ointments and perfumed paper envelopes of powders. Although wicker baskets are sometimes depicted for this purpose in friendship album pictures, they typically show mountebank troupes presenting their wares from a medicine chest in the form of a capacious trunk, its visual impact often enhanced by a painted or ornately carved wooden stand (frontispiece, Plates 5, 33–8). Some are lined or covered with rich crimson leather; most are domed, with metal studs, a lock and handles, and patent medicines and other wares, where visible, generally packaged in small round containers or glass phials. Plate 34 affords an unusually detailed look into the contents of a chest containing an impressive selection of ephemeral printed material and differently packaged wares. Bragetta's troupe attracted potential customers by placing a great locked chest on their table in the market square every afternoon, then mounting it themselves to spend a couple of hours acting a play. Then they unlocked their chest and made their sales pitch, punctuating briskly choreographed selling sessions with theatrical interludes intended to retain the crowd's attention. These featured oratorical skills involving lengthy pseudo-scientific monologues and dialogue comical disputes concerning their wares, as well as the music and singing of their regular indoor routines.

Platter's description identifies the troupe's players as skilled actors, singers and performers, who combined medical quack activity with full-length plays. His account confirms that some Italian quack troupes routinely staged a varied repertoire including pastorals and comedies featuring commedia dell'arte stock roles. Numerous early modern friendship album pictures depict performers in commedia dell'arte costume, some with musical instruments, on quack stages. However, those most easily identified as quack troupe depictions tend to feature troupes in the selling or healing phase of their activities rather than in performance, leaving the precise nature of their stage business open to interpretation. Platter's account is important evidence that performing quacks did not simply mimic actors through their choice of stock roles, and that the theatrical costumes worn by quacks in some pictures are not necessarily borrowed or adapted from the stage or carnival traditions, but intended to represent actual stage costumes of the type used in full-length professional drama (Plates 33–6). In at least some cases, these costumes and roles were depicted in conjunction with quacks because they too staged commedia dell'arte plays. The commedia dell'arte was not the only point of contact in a cultural continuum in which the low farces, acrobatics, clowning and comic stage business of quacks overlapped the repertoire of prestigious acting troupes. At the 'low' end of this continuum, even sought-after actors were involved in short verbal or physical clowning episodes, and at the 'high' end, some charlatan troupes staged comic plays, even pastorals.

According to Platter, for several weeks Zan Bragetta's outdoor performances drew audiences of up to 1000 people.[21] Coryate bears out this, noting that early seventeenth-century Venetian mountebank audiences 'perhaps may consist of a thousand people that flocke together about one of their stages'.[22] When this market too became unprofitable, the troupe knew the time had come to leave: 'when they see that their skills start to count for nothing anymore, they pack up and move on to another city'.[23] Platter provides full details of the troupe's wares. In order to keep up spectators' interest, the troupe would, when playing outdoors, each day encourage purchase of a different product from their merchandise, which included herbs, spices, cosmetics, patent medicines and printed broadsheets, the latter both for sale and for show. Bragetta commonly expected to sell at least a couple of hundred of his day's lead product, and have as much again in stock in case of additional demand. Medical wares were thrown to purchasers in the handkerchiefs or gloves in which they passed their money up to the stage, the takings generally stowed in a wooden box or troupe member's belt purse (Plates 35–6). This standard method by which quacks took payment and distributed wares is confirmed by writers such as Moryson or Jonson, and in many images.[24]

Some authorities required traders to display medical wares with the appropriate licence, or to provide customers with printed handbills detailing medical information (Plate 37).[25] Bragetta's publications do not appear to be of this type. Robert Henke suggests that mountebanks played an important role in the dissemination of humanist literature by selling, performing and even publishing pamphlets and literary anthologies.[26] Quack stock's inclusion of printed material is born out by pictures such as Plate 34. Written records confirm Whetstone's marginal note that the 'mountibanks of Italie, are in a maner, as Englysh Pedlers', by adding newletters, ballad sheets, printed fables, 'historie et cose simili', 'instorie et altre carte stampate', '*Newes out of India*, or *The Original of the Turkishe Empire*, or *Mery Tales*, or *Songes and Ballets*', even 'a world of new-fangled trumperies [...] amorous songs printed, Apothecary drugs, and a Common-weale of other trifles [...] trinkets' or miscellaneous goods such as '*Pinnes, Pointes, Laces, whistles & other such ware*', to their medical stock, which typically included allegedly exotic products with costly ingredients from geographically remote regions.[27]

---

21   *Thomas Platter d.J*, 306.

22   Coryate, *Crudities*, 274.

23   *Thomas Platter d.J*, 308.

24   Jonson, 'Volpone', II.ii (*Workes*, 471); Oxford CCC, MS.CCC94, 600; Katritzky, *Women, medicine and theatre*, frontispiece, plate 26.

25   Gentilcore, 'Itinerant practitioners', 304–05.

26   Henke, 'The Italian mountebank', 13–14.

27   Whetstone, *Heptameron*, sig.Liii^v; *Decreti* conferred on Martinelli in 1599 and 1613 (Ferrone et al., *Corrispondenze*, I, 364–5, 395); Coryate, *Crudities*, 273–5; Rastel, *The third booke*, sig.Aiii^v.

Some quacks used stage names with a geographical component chosen to enhance this exoticism, and their stage and given names were not always appropriate to their origins or wares. Despite his Italian name, Antonio Camilla Mary claimed to hail from Constantinople,[28] and peddled a Turkish balsam, and the Italian Jusepe Balsamo hawked a 'medicinal de germania' around Valencia in 1606.[29] Platter gives the stage name of the troupe leader he saw in Avignon as '(*Zan Bragetta*) Hans Latz', preceding his literal German translation with the parenthesized original Italian.[30] This suggests a stage persona and costume based on a variant of the generic comic manservant, Zanni, and Platter's account implies that an assistant was costumed as a medical doctor. Quack troupe leaders are less often depicted or described wearing Zanni suits themselves, than portrayed as concerned to emphasize their credibility and to keep up appearances accordingly, by leaving comic costume to assistants. Placket, the English equivalent to 'Bragetta' or 'Latz', refers to a gendered item of clothing with suggestive sexual connotations: for men the codpiece, for women a similarly positioned pinafore, bib or flap.[31] Bragetta's prosaic name did not prevent him from emphasizing the expensive, exotic nature of his wares, claiming to have brought his pharmaceuticals to Avignon from as far afield as Venice and Turkey, 'where he had bought precious medicines and learned many secret skills'.

My researches into Zan Bragetta's identity have yielded numerous published references to variants of his stage name.[32] Variously including Bragetta as a stage role, stage name or quack identity, they occur in Italian publications from the 1580s, and in seventeenth-century French publications. Early variants include the Bragato of Bartolomeo Rossi's *Fiammella* (1584) and the title-role comic servant of Giovanni Simone Martini's masked comic play *Bragatto* , published in several editions from 1585.[33] Martini's scripted five-act play, set in Venice, includes the stock comic roles 'the peasant Bragato, servant to Pantalone'. A typical commedia dell'arte servant, he sings (badly), cracks jokes, complains about his master and his beloved, uses offensive language and impenetrable Venetian dialect, guzzles macaroni and wine, and stars in several solo scenes.[34] The role also features

---

[28]   Now Istanbul.

[29]   Terrada, 'Medical pluralism', 228.

[30]   Basle UL, Ms.A λ V.7– 8, f.262; *Thomas Platter d.J*, 305 (Keiser reads 'Ian Bragetta').

[31]   '*Clowne*: […] O Ile tickle the prettie wenches plackets Ile be amongst them ifaith' (Marlowe, *Faustus*, sig.B3ᵛ (I.iv.58–60); 'Scorch their plackets, but beware, that ye singe no maiden-haire' (Herrick, 'Saint Distaffs Day', *Hesperides*, 374); 'Userers purses and woments plackets are never satisfied' (Howell, *Proverbs*, 11).

[32]   Katritzky, *Women, medicine and theatre*, 223.

[33]   Lea, *Italian popular comedy*, I, 114; Pandolfi, *La commedia dell'arte*, V, 439; M S G M, *Bragatto, Comedia*, Venezia 1585.

[34]   The edition consulted dates to 1607 (Sig[nor] GSM[artini], *Bragato, Comedia*, HAB Lk 834 [1]).

in several undated late sixteenth-century Italian ephemeral publications and poems. One, lamenting the death, around 1586, of the actor Tabarino, names 'Zan Braghetta' in a list of 'the whole tribe of Zanni'; another includes several defamatory lines of undated verse suggesting that Bragato fathered four felons hanged for petty thieving.[35] Later plays featuring the role Bragato include Oratio Sorio's *I Forestieri*, published in Verona in 1611.[36] By 1591, Bragetta's stage persona was sufficiently well established to merit illustration in Pietro Bertelli's three-volume costume book (Plate 1). *Bragato* was among 14 plates depicting celebrated actors selected half a century later from this book by a descendant, Franco Bertelli, for inclusion in his influential specialist costume book of 1642, *Carnevale Italiano Mascherato*.[37] Literary and visual evidence of this type suggests that Bragetta's troupe was not led by an otherwise unrecorded quack, but by an established professional actor with a solid reputation in the mainstream of commedia dell'arte tradition.

Further documentary evidence indicates that Bragetta and his troupe did not stray casually into France in 1598, but made a deep and lasting impression on French spectators. Suggesting the longevity of Zan Bragetta's popularity, and his connections with France and the commedia dell'arte, are the character 'Braghetto Francese', in Vergilio Verucci's comedy *Le Schiave* of 1629,[38] and a passage in the posthumously published sayings of Cardinal Perron, who died in 1618. This latter recorded Perron's thoughts concerning the relative merits of the French, Italian and Spanish languages for the stage, with reference to itinerant performers visiting his home town, Langres:

> Il [Cardinal Perron] dit un jour à Monsieur Gillot à Langres, le Broghetta Italien avec sa compagnie l'estant venu visiter, que la langue Françoise ne reüssit pas en Comedie comme faict l'Italienne, & que cela venoit de ce qu'il n'y avoit pas d'accens en nostre langue comme en l'Italienne; la langue Italienne est fort propre pour les choses d'amour, à cause de la quantité de diminutifs, qu'elle possede, & est propre à representer quelque chose plus petite qu'elle n'est: au contraire l'Espagnolle est fort propre pour les rodomontades, & pour representer les choses plus grandes qu'elles ne sont.[39]

---

[35]   *Mariazzo fatto al la pavana in le nozze di Bragato; con vn dialogo de dui containi, vno è chiamò barba Menon nostro consegiero; e l'altro barba Bigolo, e Ruzante scauezacolo, che con la schena scaueze vn bigolo* [c.1595, 4 folios. HAB, 550.12 Quod (6)]; *Stanze della vita e morte di Tabarino Canaglia Milanese* (Schindler, 'Zan Tabarino', 542); *Genologia di Zan Capella* (Pandolfi, *La commedia dell'arte*, I, 255).

[36]   Lea, *Italian popular comedy*, I, 209.

[37]   Bertelli, *Il carnevale italiano mascherato*, plate 18. The borrowings are tabulated in: Katritzky, 'Franco Bertelli', 227.

[38]   Pandolfi, *La commedia dell'arte*, III, 51–2.

[39]   [Perron], *Perroniana*, 192.

Previously interpreted by theatre historians as a garbled reference to the stock commedia dell'arte stage clown Brighella,[40] this passage is here presented as evidence that Bragetta's troupe performed Italian-language plays, witnessed by Perron in pre-1620 Langres. The nineteenth-century theatre historian Édouard Fournier's erroneous, unreferenced assertion that the troupe of Isabella Andreini was engaged by a charlatan named François Braquette, in Lyon in 1621, may refer to a connection between Bragetta and the Fedeli troupe, led by Isabella's son Giambattista Andreini (stage name: 'Lelio').[41]

Leases and other documents signed by G. B. Andreini demonstrate that the Fedeli troupe acted in, and controlled the theatrical use of, the Hôtel de Bourgogne between July and October 1621.[42] After they left France in 1624, no renowned commedia dell'arte troupe played in Paris until Tiberio Fiorillo brought the Italian actors back in the 1640s.[43] Two marriage contracts indicate the extent to which successful Italian quacks and illustrious actors maintained contacts in Paris over this period. One of 1620 records the marriage of the renowned French farce actor Hugues Quéru (stage name: 'Gaultier-Garguille') to Aléonor Salomon.[44] The bride's father had been the late Pompée Salomon, 'distillateur'. Her Italian mother, the actress Vittoria Bianca ('Francisquine'), had remarried the 'opérateur', or quack, Antoine Girard ('Tabarin'). With Antoine's brother, the quack Philippe Girard ('Mondor'), he and Bianca ran the most successful quack troupe in Paris. Its repertoire, published in 1622 as Tabarin's *Recveil*, was heavily influenced by the commedia dell'arte. Well-known actors and quacks served as witnesses on both sides. At the 1647 Paris wedding of the perfumer Giovanni Buzzurui, son of a Palermo 'docteur en médecine' to Françoise Belon, daughter and stepdaughter of court musicians, the list of witnesses provides an even more glittering roll call of performers. It includes dancers, acrobats, musicians, the Roman quack couple Clarice Vitriaria the actress, and her third husband, Cristophe Contugi (stage name: 'l'Orviétan de Rome'), and two great stars of the Comédie Italienne, the actors Tiberio Fiorillo and Domenico Locatelli.[45]

---

[40]   Lebègue identifies him as 'Brighella': 'le Braghetta (*corriger en* Brighella) Italien avec sa compagnie', and [Jacques] Gillot (d.1619) as the politician who co-authored *Satyre Ménippée* ('La Comédie Italienne', 15, 17).

[41]   Rigal, *Alexandre Hardy*, 17 and *Le Théatre Français*, 19 (in the Taylorian Library copy, as if we could forget, an outraged reader has helpfully scrawled a marginalia reminding us that the famous actress died on tour in Lyon in 1604). See also Fournier, *Chansons*, liv; Brun, *Pupazzi et statuettes*, 110.

[42]   Howe, *Le Théâtre professional à Paris*, 261–3 (Documents 187–90); Powell, *Music and theatre*, 167–8.

[43]   Possibly as early as 1641 (Howe, *Le Théâtre professional à Paris*, 164–6).

[44]   Howe, *Le Théâtre professional à Paris*, 80–1, 261, 366–9 (Document 185).

[45]   Howe, *Le Théâtre professional à Paris*, 190–3, 333, 402–5 (Document 432); on Contugi, see also Brockliss and Jones, *The medical world of early modern France*, 240–1.

Molière too has been linked not just to quacks, but specifically to the troupe described by Platter. In the French satire 'La Bastonnade', he is charged with purchasing the papers of a quack troupe in order to plunder their plots for his own plays.[46] Referring to this source only as 'some obscure satire', Gustave Lanson dismissively suggests that 'it would be imprudent to accept as historical truth the account of the relationship between Molière and the quack-doctor'.[47] But however unreliable this farce is with respect to Molière, its identification of Prosper, the quack from whom he bought the papers, as 'the operator Braquette's stage fool', again suggests Bragetta's presence in early seventeenth-century France. Though highly unlikely to have any connection to Bragetta's troupe, the venerable local provenance of a late sixteenth-century painting donated in 1986 from a local collection to Avignon's Musée Calvet offers a further possible indication of commedia dell'arte activity in the region (Plate 32). It is a little known variant of a composition consistently linked to the famous Gelosi troupe, known to theatre historians through versions in Parisian public collections.[48]

Data of this type would amount to little more than hearsay without the backing of archival evidence. Previously uncited documents uncovered by my researches in the Dijon archives provide that evidence. They require interpretation in the light of the considerable regional differences of approach shaping official records of quack activity. Itinerant quack troupes required flexibility to adapt to varying regional attitudes and regulations, both in their petitioning of local authorities, and in balancing the medical and theatrical content of their practice. Some communities, such as Calvinist Zurich, were primarily concerned to suppress performances and keep women off the stage. Many provincial French authorities were relatively relaxed about the theatrical practice of quacks, male or female. Instead, authorities such as those at Dijon prioritized thorough policing of quacks' medical practice. A late seventeenth-century example of these differences, with respect to one and the same troupe, is provided by the case of the performing quack couple Johannes and Anna Gertrud Buhlmeyer. Zurich archival documents record that they petitioned the authorities successfully in 1679 and unsuccessfully in 1687, to stage theatrical entertainments and sell medicines within the city, and that as a widow, Anna Gertrud Buhlmeyerin unsuccessfully petitioned in Zurich again in July 1690, both to practice medicine and to perform.[49] Dijon archival records, by contrast, merely note the official examination of Johannes Buhlmeyer of Leipzig's patent medicines by French apothecaries in 1678, without indicating any theatrical practice, wife, or companions.[50]

---

[46]   Brun, *Pupazzi et statuettes*, 170.

[47]   Lanson, 'Molière and farce', 133–4.

[48]   See Katritzky (*The art of commedia*, plates 61, 188–9) for variants in the Musée Carnavalet, Comédie Française and Drottningholm Museum. The present whereabouts of another variant is unknown (French art market 1965).

[49]   Stichler, 'Reisende Ärzte', 289–90.

[50]   Dijon AM, I.134, Document 13.

The Dijon archives also yielded archival documents concerning a quack named as 'Alfier dit Braguette', thus linking the stage name Braguette with the given name Alfier. As with the Dijon documents for Johannes Buhlmeyer, there is no mention of Alfier's theatrical activity or companions. One document records the granting of permission to distribute his medicines to a travelling 'operator and distiller' whose identity and given name are revealed by his signature: 'Gio[vanni] Paulo Alfieri'.[51] Evaluation of this signed document is complicated by its date, 1639. If it refers to the performer whose medical and theatrical activities of 1598 are described by Thomas Platter, who, according to other documentation presented and reviewed here, appears to have been active by at least the mid-1580s, then it extends the length of Bragetta's career to over half a century. This would be unusual but not unprecedented for a commedia dell'arte performer. In 1613 the poet François de Malherbe ungraciously commented of a French royal command performance starring the then 56-year-old Tristano Martinelli and 76-year-old Giovanni Pellesini, in their famous commedia dell'arte signature roles of Harlequin and Pedrolino, that neither was 'any longer of an age appropriate to the stage'.[52] Despite obvious dating issues regarding an itinerant performer of such unusual longevity, the simplest interpretation of the Dijon document is that it identifies the actor whose stage name was Zan Bragetta as Giovanni Paulo Alfieri.

Alfieri is an Italian commedia dell'arte troupe leader known solely through one brief acting season on the most prestigious stage of early modern France, the Hôtel de Bourgogne, the public theatre through which the Confrères de la Passion administered their legal monopoly on professional theatre in Paris. After lengthy closure during the political unrest of the League, the Hôtel de Bourgogne was leased between tours from 1599 to 1612 by France's foremost troupe leader, Valleran-le-Conte.[53] Giovanni Paulo Alfieri shared this stage with Valleran during his final Paris season, in 1612, when Valleran led a troupe including the actresses Rachel Trépeau, Marie and Colombe Venier, and two apprentices signed on in 1609, Jeanne Crevé and Judith Le Messier.[54] Alfieri's existence has been known to theatre historians since the 1920s, when Fransen discovered his signature on a dated follow-up contract of 9 March 1612.[55] It extends the dates of a lease formalized in two subsequently discovered contracts dated 14 February 1612, recording an agreement between the troupe leaders Alfieri and Valleran-le-Conte to share the Hôtel de Bourgogne during spring 1612, in order to: 'act and present, together and separately, all sorts of comedies, tragic-comedies, pastorals and other performances as permitted by the authorities of the Hôtel de

---

[51]   Dijon AM, I.134, Documents 4–6.

[52]   Baschet, *Les comédiens italiens*, 243–4.

[53]   Rigal, *Hotel de Bourgogne*, 16, 23; Deierkauf-Holsboer, *L'Hotel de Bourgogne*, 36, 49; Wiley, 'The Hotel de Bourgogne', 8–9.

[54]   Deierkauf-Holsboer, *Vie d'Alexandre Hardy* (1972), 69–74, 194–5 and *La mise en scène*, 97–8; Howe, *Le Théâtre professional à Paris*, 233 (Documents 92 and 94).

[55]   Fransen, 'Documents inédits', 325, 336, 352 and *Les comédiens français*, 50.

Bourgogne'.[56] Their specific theatrical responsibilities and financial arrangements are formalized in terms suggesting that Alfieri, identified as the leader of a troupe of Italian comedians, was more financially competent than Valleran. Neither in these contracts, nor elsewhere in archival records relating to Valleran, is there any mention of medical quack activity, and their reference to Alfieri as 'Jehan Paul Hallefier, chevalier de l'empereur' suggests an actor of some renown, whose troupe had played before Emperor Rudolf II.

The most informative eyewitness evidence on Valleran's Parisian performances is again provided by Thomas Platter, who saw them in July 1599, less than a year after watching Alfieri in Avignon. Platter notes that Paris attracted performers and entertainers of every type, including Italian and English comedians who sometimes played at the Hôtel de Bourgogne with Valleran-le-Conte, and had commercial companies concerned with the organization of private banquets who could arrange not only food and drink, but hired rooms, fittings, tapestries, women, professional musicians, even plays.[57] The sixteenth-century French fashion for rounding off a tragedy with a topical farce or comedy, likened by Jean Bodin to serving poisoned food, was as popular in Paris as the fashion for theatrical jigs was in London, and Valleran was their acknowledged star.[58] A contract of 4 January 1599 between Benoist Petit and Valleran stipulates that Petit's responsibility for playbills is conditional on Valleran's participation in the farces.[59] Later that year, Platter's journal confirms that Valleran's troupe habitually staged a verse play followed by a prose farce based on topical satire:

> In (*l'Hostel de Bourgongne*) the Burgundian court, every day after the meal, the King's appointed comedian, called Valleran, stages a diverting play in French verse, and at the end of the same a diverting (*farce*) story. This concerns events in Paris or elsewhere, relating to love affairs, matchmaking, or some other scandalous gossip. He acts these so skilfully with several people, relating everything that happened not in verse, but only in (*prosa oratione*) everyday speech, and punctuating it with such amusing tricks, that you can hardly stop gasping, especially if you already know the story or people it concerns. Because whatever of note happens in Paris, as soon as it becomes public knowledge, it is passed on to Valleran. He turns it into a performance, to which a large crowd of people flock, in order to hear this (*farce*) story, when the play is finished. And he is quite prepared to include all sorts of things in the play. He and his troupe act on a raised stage, hung about with tapestries, in a very large hall, in which the common people, who only pay half to enter, have to stand. But those who

---

[56]   Deierkauf-Holsboer, 'Vie d'Alexandre Hardy' (1947), 351–3, 397–8 and *Vie d'Alexandre Hardy* (1972), 73, 206–8; Howe, *Le Théâtre professional à Paris*, 41, 244 (Documents 130–1).

[57]   *Thomas Platter d.J*, 593 (28 July 1599, Paris).

[58]   Lancaster, *French dramatic literature*, I, 145.

[59]   Deierkauf-Holsboer, *Vie d'Alexandre Hardy* (1972), 177 and *La mise en scène*, 113.

pay double are allowed to go up to several galleries, where they can sit, stand, or prop themselves up on their arms in the galleries, and can see everything really well. This is also where the womenfolk like to be. And every day, in this court, a large crowd of folk listens to the plays, which last into the night, so that they often have to use (*torches*) nightlights to conclude them. Apart from this there are also many other actors, acrobats, (*ingenieurs*) performers, musicians, and those who can show wonderful spectacles or skilful things in this city of Paris. Such people move from one street to another. For a day or several they are in one (*quartier*) part of the city, where they put up their placards and take money. Then when they think the locals have paid (*contribuieret*) what they can, they move to another part of the city, until they have got together a large sum of money. And I watched and listened to huge numbers of suchlike in Paris. And because the Parisians are so keen on wondrous sights that they are called (*badauts*) gawpers, and always, as noted above, such huge crowds of people assemble there; everyone who can do or show anything unusual makes a point of getting themselves there and making some money once they have arrived there. Among others, Italian and English comedians very often go there, and they sometimes compete with the King's comedians, and at the same time act with them. Sometimes they rent separate stages, and I have indeed also heard and seen them elsewhere.[60]

Platter's reference to French actors sharing the stage of the Hôtel de Bourgogne, with visiting Italian or English players, refers to a tradition founded by the great French actor and troupe leader Agnan Sarat. A significant body of visual and textual evidence suggests that Sarat, one of whose stock comic roles was that of a lecherous pedant, staged co-productions with Italian commedia dell'arte actors in Paris, notably Tristano Martinelli's troupe, shortly after Martinelli created the iconic role of Harlequin in the mid-1580s. Harlequin features in two, and Sarat himself in five, of six stylistically homogenous woodcuts in Stockholm's well-known *Recueil Fossard* collection of early commedia dell'arte images, each depicting between three and five figures identified by name or role in accompanying captions and verse.[61] Although there is no textual evidence that Sarat collaborated with quacks, the considerable medical content of his repertoire is indicated by representations of him onstage with actors playing healers, including a doctor and an itinerant toothdrawer.[62]

Possible indications of Alfieri's presence in Paris further to the contracts of 1612 include references to a troupe of Italian comedians performing at the French

---

[60]   *Thomas Platter d.J*, 585–7 (28 July 1599, Paris). Other translations include: Powell, *Music and theatre*, 10; Howarth, *French theatre*, 45.

[61]   Beijer and Duchartre, *Recueil*, 29–30; Katritzky, *The art of commedia*, plate 10.

[62]   Katritzky, *Women, medicine and theatre*, 194–201.

court on 16 and 17 May 1612, tentatively identified as Alfieri's.[63] They are briefly recorded in the manuscript journal of Jean Héroard, personal physician to the then 11-year-old French Regent, Louis XIII. As well as commedia dell'arte, Louis XIII's Italian mother Marie de'Medici evidently enjoyed quack farces. The Girard brothers, Mondor and Tabarin, were rewarded with 900 livres by Marie de'Medici for farces and comedies performed by their Franco-Italian quack troupe at court during the winter of 1618–19.[64] A passage in a French pamphlet of 1612 accuses Parisian women of chattering: 'like people who want to divert themselves at the Hôtel de Bourgogne by watching the performance of the street entertainers of Valleran and Laporte'.[65] Underlining the improvised, spectacular nature of the Italians' repertoire, this is another possible reference to Alfieri's troupe. Cardinal Perron's suggestion that Alfieri performed comedies in the Italian language in early seventeenth-century Langres is quoted above. But Platter's account of Alfieri's Avignon season indicates that already by 1598, his performances made some onstage use of the local language. Platter's description of Valleran's 1599 Paris season, on the strength of which Valleran has been called the Dario Fo of his time,[66] reliably outlines his repertoire and collaborations with foreign troupes. From around 1598 to 1613, Valleran's longtime playwright Alexandre Hardy wrote hundreds of plays for his troupe.[67] Unaware of Platter's account, Deierkauf-Holsboer reconstructs a repertoire of nightly 'bilingual' double bills, each comprising an unvaryingly divided programme, in which one of Alexandre Hardy's tragedies, tragi-comedies or pastorals, played in French by Valleran's troupe, is followed by an Italian-language improvised commedia dell'arte play performed by Alfieri's troupe.[68] Without necessarily suggesting that Valleran, like Sarat, acted together with the Italians in the same plays, Platter's account does indicate a less rigid allocation of the two troupes' activities. Awareness of it might have weakened Deierkauf-Holsboer's opposition to suggestions that Hardy wrote farces as well as the tragedies, tragi-comedies and pastorals of his few surviving published works, and the lost comedies evidenced by archival records.[69] Platter's journal suggests that Hardy was involved in the writing of farces for Valleran, who would not have been prepared to relinquish his involvement in farce for a whole season lightly to Alfieri's troupe.

Jean de Gaufreteau's *Chronique Bordeloise* and German supplications testify to the impact made on provincial audiences of the 1590s by Valleran-le-Conte's

---

[63]   Lough, 'French actors in Paris', 226n10 and *Paris theatre audiences*, 35; Wiley, 'A royal child learns to like plays', 144.

[64]   Lancaster, *French dramatic literature*, I, 220; Lough, *Paris theatre audiences*, 42.

[65]   Rigal, *Le Théatre Français*, 53–4.

[66]   Kröll, 'Spectacles de foire', 256.

[67]   Deierkauf-Holsboer, *Vie d'Alexandre Hardy* (1972), 39–41.

[68]   Deierkauf-Holsboer, 'Les représentations bilingues', 'La vie théâtrale', 11 and *Vie d'Alexandre Hardy* (1972), 70; Pagani (Bibiena, *La nouvelle Italie*, 1).

[69]   Deierkauf-Holsboer, *Vie d'Alexandre Hardy* (1972), 53, 140–4.

actors and actresses, and their popularity with audiences, if not always with municipal authorities, even beyond France.[70] The response of Frankfurt town councillors to Valleran's supplication of 1593, underlined his tendency to topical farce and satire. They permitted him to play in the city provided his troupe 'stage nothing controversial, and play in such a manner that no-one is ridiculed by them'.[71] Platter, who saw Valleran's troupe in 1599 at the peak of their success with Parisian audiences, refers to collaborations with English and Italian actors. In 1600, they shared their spring season at the Hôtel de Bourgogne with Saulo Donati and Giulio Rizi's Italian troupe.[72] By 1612, Valleran's theatrical activities were compromised by serious financial problems. His season with Alfieri, his final attempt to carry on the tradition of cross-border cooperation between French and Italian speaking troupes, was a commercial failure. Forced out of Paris by debt, in 1613 Valleran led a newly recruited young troupe to the Low Countries. Possibly, they performed at the festivities in The Hague for the formal entry of James VI/I and Anna's daughter, the future Queen of Bohemia, Elizabeth Stuart, in May 1613. Valleran was back at the Hôtel de Bourgogne by 1615.[73]

In October 1613, Tristano Martinelli leased the Hôtel de Bourgogne for eight months, and thereafter no Italian troupes performed there or at the French court until Martinelli himself returned to Paris, in 1620.[74] Deierkauf-Holsboer's thorough Parisian archival researches produced no evidence of Alfieri or his troupe before or after 1612, when 'Alfieri and his troupe disappeared again and it has proved impossible for us to find any further trace of them'.[75] Alfieri's stage name, Bragetta, occurs in a broad range of early modern literary texts. His given name is so far known only through official documents, those of 1612, and the newly-discovered Dijon documents of 1639. Alfieri and Bragetta have always been regarded as separate performers, each leaving only one recognized historical footprint: Bragetta's quack Avignon season of 1598 and Alfieri's commedia dell'arte Paris season of 1612. The documents of 1639 suggest that Bragetta and Alfieri are one and the same performer, also active as a quack in Dijon in 1639, allowing several groups of documents, some well-known, others still unpublished, to be brought together here to contribute to knowledge of this performer's career. This pooling of evidence from contrasting regions and groups of documents, archival and literary, represents a major step in the rehabilitation of an Italian commedia dell'arte quack troupe leader who collaborated with the most celebrated

---

[70]   Lancaster, *French dramatic literature*, I, 16–17; Trautmann, 'Französische Schauspieler', 201–2, 206, 291–2.

[71]   Frankfurt StA.BMB 1592, f.212ʳ (27 March 1593).

[72]   Deierkauf-Holsboer, *Vie d'Alexandre Hardy* (1972), 183–4.

[73]   Fransen, *Les comédiens français*, 45–52; Deierkauf-Holsboer, *Vie d'Alexandre Hardy* (1972), 76–8; Hoppe, 'La circulation comique', 166; Howe, *Le Théâtre professional à Paris*, 69, 256 (Document 167).

[74]   Fransen, 'Documents inédits', 326.

[75]   Deierkauf-Holsboer, *Vie d'Alexandre Hardy* (1972), 74.

French performers of his age, and whose theatrical and medical activity impacted across early modern France for over four decades. It illuminates the mechanisms of cross-border theatrical and medical exchange, and early modern links between medical and theatrical practice by one and the same itinerant quack troupe, and underlines the significance of Thomas Platter's status as a qualified physician to his interest in, and records of, theatrical events.

Chapter 13
Quack Performances in Guarinonius's *Grewel*

Thomas Platter's description of Zan Bragetta's quack troupe, the subject of the previous chapter, offers compelling insights into ways in which medicine and performance could be combined on the stages of Italian quacks, and a comprehensive account of the medical retailing strategies of one particular troupe. It is less informative concerning the particulars of their stage repertoire, for the most part providing little more than broad indications. Some three dozen descriptions of lazzi, or professional stage business involving stock commedia dell'arte characters, in Hippolytus Guarinonius's medical treatise *Grewel*, provide considerable detail concerning the actual stage business of quack troupes, confirming Thomas Platter's indications that some based their repertoire on the commedia dell'arte. Twenty-three of these descriptions are listed under the term 'Zani', in *Grewel*'s index, of which five were pirated in another publication as early as 1615.[1] Most were known to nineteenth-century literary historians, and Jürgen Bücking and Jean-Marie Valentin respectively acknowledged their cultural and theatrical significance, in the 1960s and 1980s.[2] However, these 23 indexed lazzi by no means exhaust *Grewel*'s theatrical content. More recently identified passages on the theatre include 12 additional commedia dell'arte-related episodes, boosting its total known lazzi to 35.[3] Twelve lazzi have been identified in the treatise's fourth book, nine in each of the second and sixth books, five in the fifth book, and none in its introduction or in Books 1, 3 or 7.[4] This chapter contextualizes an assessment of the theatre-historical significance of Guarinonius's commedia

---

[1]   Albertinus, *Gusman von Alfarche*, 452–60 ('Capvt LIV. Gusman wirdt auß einem Bergknappen ein *Comediant*, und erzehlt ettliche artliche Possen die er gerissen').

[2]   Bücking, *Kultur und Gesellschaft in Tirol*, 95–7; Valentin, 'Herr Pantalon', 206–16, 'Bouffons ou religieux?' and *Theatrum Catholicum*, 19–48.

[3]   Here referred to as lazzi nos.1–35 (for English translations and bibliographic references to the printed and manuscript versions of *Grewel*, see Chapter 18, this volume). Eleven of the new lazzi were first published by the present author in 1999 (Katritzky, 'Hippolytus Guarinonius' descriptions', 71–2, 104–23), and a twelfth by Alberto Martino in 2003 (Martino, 'Fonti tedesche degli anni 1585–1615', 684). See also Katritzky, 'Comic stage routines' and 'Guarinonius' lazzi'.

[4]   1. On God; 2. On the human mind; 3. On air; 4. On food and drink; 5. On physical elimination; 6. On exercise; 7. On sleep.

dell-arte-related descriptions within an overview of relevant evidential sources and scholarly resources, including further theatrical references in *Grewel*.

Although Guarinonius does not link individual theatrical descriptions to a medical or commercial context, the connection between quacks and the Italian comedy is made, for example, in the passage containing his sole brief mention of the English players (discussed in Chapter 8, this volume). This confirms his personal experience of professional performances staged in the context of quack activities, by itinerant Italian troupes, whom he compares with the English players as follows:

> Similar plays and spectacles can now be seen in Germany, and their actors, as I myself have seen, are from Netherlandish and English cities. They travel around, from one town to another, performing their amusing farces and acrobatics (but without unseemliness) to a considerable extent, as far as they can, in German and with the use of mime, in exchange for payment by those who wish to watch and hear them. Just like those comical buffoons, who in almost all Italian cities, but especially Venice, sell their bars of soap and suchlike every evening in the squares, and entertain the people for several hours there with their antics. Called *Ziarlatani* in Italian, after Ziärlare, namely chattering, they are generally two, three or more people, including a *Magnificus*, or Venetian citizen, otherwise known as Master Pantalone, who is the master, and *Zane* his servant. They present their comical tricks, speeches, gestures and suchlike, at which one has to laugh whether one wishes to, or regrets doing so.[5]

Here, Guarinonius's qualification of non-Italian performances as being without unseemliness indicates that, in his perception, the stages of Italian quack troupes were not free of obscenities. In elsewhere likening fashionable men to professional 'acrobats and stage fools or actors', he dismisses stage players as itinerant entertainers of the lowest status.[6] His enthusiasm for Italian itinerants is heavily qualified by his lively sense of their potential for moral corruption, through their inherent immodesty and folly. Repeatedly emphasizing health-threatening aspects of their activities, he warns against joining the volatile, unpredictable, dangerous audiences of the 'charlatans or comedians' who 'perform their tricks on every Italian square' in a discussion of the sin of inquisitiveness with regard to 'unnecessary, useless and frivolous spectacles'.[7] He points out that such quacks give pleasure only to the young or irresponsible, because their performances generally deal with nothing more than frivolous love, lechery and suchlike matters, which offer little

---

[5]   Guarinonius, *Grewel*, 214 (manuscript version: Innsbruck UL, Cod.110, I, f.308ᵛ).

[6]   Guarinonius, *Grewel*, 66.

[7]   Guarinonius, *Grewel*, 373. A further discussion of this passage concludes Chapter 14, this volume.

to please the ears of those who are old, discerning, honest, cultivated and pure in spirit, or above all of priests and monks, and perhaps more to offend them.[8]

However, Guarinonius also provides a less negative assessment of quack troupes with respect to health and safety issues. Specifically including the Italian comedy of quack drama, he identifies the therapeutic effects of theatrical performances as a powerful *antidotum melancholiae*, viewing comedies, tragedies and plays as:

> the most powerful and effective means of raising the human spirits, because the ears of the spectators are wonderfully entertained and nourished not only by the delightful music which almost always accompanies them, but also through the varied and entertaining dialogue, and their eyes are wonderfully diverted and captivated by looking at things which are simultaneously represented and performed with skill in speech, in gestures and in everything. These plays are nothing less than *tableaux vivants*, especially those that are attractive and worthwhile, and in which everybody is suitably costumed.[9]

This passage continues by noting that Aristotle confirms the venerable tradition of this lovely delight for the senses, which is still practiced in many countries, notably in Italy, in whose principal cities such plays are performed almost every day throughout summer and autumn, and also at other times of the year, in the late afternoon or evening. Unlike Thomas Platter's account of Bragetta's troupe, and some other types of spectacle described by Guarinonius, his Italian comedy descriptions are never characterized as having been recently seen, or identified as specific performances by named performers, in a given place and time. Even so, it is clear that Guarinonius, like Platter, draws extensively on eyewitness experience of live performances. His recognition of the healing power of theatre is firmly based on his observations of commedia dell'arte performances, as a medical student at the University of Padua during the 1590s, when he was plagued with *melancholia*.

Then associated with academic genius, *melancholia* was a common early modern diagnosis for mentally troubled scholars.[10] Guarinonius's medical professors in Padua, Alessandro Massaria, Albertino Bottoni and Emilio Campolongo, struggled to find an effective cure for him.[11] Anti-melancholic therapies based on dramatic or musical diversions were commonly recommended

---

[8]   Guarinonius, *Grewel*, 214.

[9]   Guarinonius, *Grewel*, 213. See also Locher, 'Von der Bewegung', 94–5.

[10]   Gowland, 'Melancholy', 114–16.

[11]   Massaria (d.1598), Bottoni (d.1596), Campolongo (1550–1604). Others include Ercole Sassonia (1551–1607), Horatio Eugenio (1527–1603) and Hieronymo Acquapendente (1537–1619). Guarinonius, *Grewel*, 598; Innsbruck UL, Cod.110, IV, f.515^v).

by early modern physicians.[12] At last, they advised Guarinonius to benefit from the therapeutic effects of drama by attending the plays staged in Padua's market squares, by Italian quacks performing and peddling their patent medicines (Plates 4–5). On doing so, he was completely cured of his debilitating *melancholia* within four months.[13] This experience enabled him to observe, closely and critically, the activities of marketplace quacks of the type described in *Grewel*, and to familiarize himself with the healing effect of their plays, which, he claims, revitalized spectators by dispersing troubled feelings accumulated throughout a day of heavy responsibilities and tensions. While Guarinonius's piety inclined him to strong disapproval of quacks' robust antics, he confesses that however little inclined he was towards laughing at them while watching them perform, he was no more able to withstand laughter than any other member of the audience, deploring his reaction of involuntary laughter to the entertaining Zanniesque acrobatics of the Italian comedies. This healing laughter opened his heart and cured his affliction, an outcome which, he notes, accorded excellently with the teachings of Galen, who wrote that he had healed many patients purely by raising their spirits.[14]

Most of *Grewel*'s references to the Italian comedy describe specific *lazzi*. These improvised verbal and physical set pieces were the trademark skill of the professional Italian stage, pre-rehearsed transferable self-contained units of improvised stage business of central importance to early modern commedia dell'arte performances. Some already known to literary historians of the nineteenth century, at least one not identified until the twenty-first, *Grewel*'s three dozen *lazzi* descriptions represent the most substantial textual source of documentary information concerning early modern *lazzi* outside the writings of the commedia dell'arte actors themselves, and a potent indication of the substantial overlap between medical and theatrical activities on their stages. Featuring particular combinations of stock characters, *lazzi* were designed for use in different plays with minimal modification, in longer or shorter form, in response to positive or negative audience reaction. Actors recycled successful *lazzi* in different dramatic contexts, in order to contribute to plot development, comment on plots, provide quasi-independent interludes showcasing their own skills, cover for scene-

---

[12]   And supported by churchmen such as Martin Luther (Neuber, 'Vom Grewel deβ Trawrens', 76). See also Burton, *The anatomy of melancholy*, Part II.ii, 372–5: 'Musicke a remedy'; Marston, *Iacke Drums entertainment*, sig.H4ᵛ; 'C', *The two merry milke-maids*, sig. I2ᵛ: 'O you speake musicke to the melancholly, Health to the sicke'; Barbieri, *La supplica*, 1628, 35; Fischart, *Geschichtklitterung*, 14–15. Church music relieved Felix Platter's melancholy homesickness en route to Montpellier (*Felix Platter Tagebuch*, 142: 28 October 1552, Avignon).

[13]   Despite claiming that he continued to remain in good spirits to the time of writing (Guarinonius, *Grewel*, 213: this section written 1606 and revised 1608), his 'melancholy nature' was evidently chronic. He refers to a recent lengthy bout in a manuscript of 1643 (Guarinonius, *Thomas von Bergamo*, 70).

[14]   Guarinonius, *Grewel*, 213–14, 942.

changes, or serve some other non-narrative function. Predominantly associated with the comic and acrobatic stage business of the commedia dell'arte's masked menservants and masters, certain lazzi were also played by unmasked and serious roles, notably verbose military captains' tirades and inamoratas' showpiece madness scenes. Some of these latter were monologues, others involved more than one inamorata, or even a combination of comic and serious roles, as in the penultimate scene of a seventeenth-century scenario, a madness scene in which a magician restores to sanity the lovers Ardelia and Aurelio, and the comic servants Ulivetta and Stoppino.[15]

Grewel's very first lazzi description, occurring in a part of the treatise written in 1606, features a Zanni on an outdoor Paduan stage, 'in an Italian comedy' who, performing 'at that time in the public square', wishes that his neck could be stretched 'from Padua to Constantinople' (lazzo no.1). This suggests that it describes a marketplace commedia dell'arte performance staged in Padua well before the time of writing, which could, like many of Guarinonius's lazzi descriptions, recall a quack routine he saw as a student. As confirmed by Thomas Platter's account of Zan Bragetta, travelling troupes also acted indoors, often on portable trestle stages set up in rented covered tennis halls. Guarinonius, like Platter a great enthusiastic of the game, notes that Padua had five tennis courts in the 1590s, without situating any of his lazzi in specifically indoor settings.[16] Probably outdoor stages feature in lazzi recording that Pantalone was 'running up and down the stage with fright', Zanni 'lay quite motionless on the stage on his bed', or the old Venetian Pantalone, his shoulders encumbered by weights which Zanni has persuaded him to carry, 'staggered around the stage for a good while' (lazzi nos.22, 27, 32). One lazzo notes a routine intended by the comedians to provoke laughter, and others refer specifically to great or hearty audience laughter (lazzi nos.5, 16, 22, 27). In lazzo no.35, Zanni addresses the audience directly.

The importance of Guarinonius's lazzi is brought into focus by considering the relative paucity of previously identified documentary sources for lazzi. The commedia dell'arte was based on pre-rehearsed improvisation, and its actors, concerned to protect the repertoires through which they earned their livelihoods, typically recorded their plays not as fully-scripted texts, but as compact plot summaries or scenari, of which over 800 manuscript and published examples are extant.[17] As vehicles for providing succinct overviews of whole performances, scenari seldom made space for more than perfunctory indications of individual lazzi. Detailed written records of pre-eighteenth-century lazzi are rare, and many lazzi are now lost, or exist only in name. Troupes jealously guarded their repertoires and scenari against competitors. Often, a scenario merely notes that a particular character is to perform 'his' or 'her' lazzi, with no further specification, or just provides a title whose significance is no longer apparent. The only collection of

---

[15]   Bartoli, *Scenari inediti*, 210 (*I quattro pazzi*).

[16]   Guarinonius, *Grewel*, 1210.

[17]   For major primary sources, see Heck, *Commedia dell'arte: a guide*, 14–16, 332–56.

scenari published during the early modern period, that of the great troupe leader and actor Flaminio Scala, appeared in 1611, postdating *Grewel* by a year.[18] The travel writer Joseph Baretti evokes its enigmatic obscurity, confessing that on reading Scala's 'scenario's, or skeletons', he 'could not make much of any of his plots, which are not easily unravelled but by comedians long accustomed to catch their recriprocal hints'.[19] Equally unintelligible scenes in the manuscript Corsini collection include one from its scenario *La trappolaria*, specifying without further description that Zanni performs 'il lazzo delli scartoccietti, del confetto, della frittata'.[20] Precise knowledge of what early modern actors actually did and said on stage during their lazzi has largely vanished, even though entire scenes in some scenari are taken up by them. Typically, another such scene, in the seventeenth-century Florentine scenario *La spada fatale*, enigmatically reads: '*Scena IX. Pulcinella e Bari, e Cola.* Lazzo del Mondo Nuovo, e finisce l'Atto 2°.[21]

The Luccan priest Don. Placido Adriani is generally identified as the earliest collector of lazzi in significant numbers. The 800 quarto pages of his dated manuscript 'Zibaldone di concetti comici' or miscellany of 1734 include 22 scenari, and a numbered list of 42 lazzi, with generally two- or three-sentence long descriptions.[22] Domenico Biancolelli's detailed lazzi descriptions represent another significant resource. They are to some extent limited in all involving his own stage character, Harlequin, and compromised by surviving only through Thomas-Simon Gueullette's French translations after Biancolelli's lost Italian manuscript of the 1660s, which came into Gueullette's possession only after the death of Biancolelli's son, in 1734.[23] Fully scripted plays and other writings by professional actors and their amateur imitators have also been extensively investigated, in order to augment the information on lazzi available in scenari and *zibaldone*. Primarily motivated by a desire to draw on the Italian comedy for independent artistic ends, they were scrutinized for accurate information on improvised stage practice. Bartoli's analysis of a scripted play of 1630 is an early example of this approach. It was prompted by his belief that it was written after its

---

[18]   Scala, *Il Teatro*.

[19]   Baretti, *Customs of Italy*, I, 174–5.

[20]   Corsini MS I.28 (transcribed in Brouwer, 'Due scenari inediti', 290).

[21]   Bartoli, *Scenari inediti*, 231. Capozza classifies this 'Lazzo del Mondo Nuovo' with 'Lazzi di bastonatura e rabbia: mondo nuovo', together with a similarly named, more amply described lazzo from a Neapolitan scenari collection of c.1700 featuring Coviello, the Dottore, Orazio and Celia, which possibly throws light on its content (*Tutti i lazzi*, 229, nos.1212–13).

[22]   MS della Biblioteca Comunale di Perugia, segnatura A-20. On which, see: Del Cerro, 'Lazzi inediti', 591; Lea, 'Bibliography', 15–16; Pandolfi, *La commedia dell'arte*, IV, 263–74; Hallar, *Teaterspil og Tegnsprog*, 212–25; Garfein and Gordon, 'The Adriani Lazzi', 8–12.

[23]   Spada, *Domenico Biancolelli*; Scott, *The commedia dell'arte in Paris*; Gambelli, *Arlecchino a Parigi*, II–III.

author, the famous commedia dell'arte actor and former quack performer Nicolò Barbieri, had taken part in improvised performances based on its plot, and that its dialogue and lazzi closely reflected those of the improvised stage.[24] Lea, for whom fully-scripted plays written and published by commedia dell'arte actors are 'as truly documents of the *commedia dell'arte* as the miscellanies', notes that they share many of the lazzi of the scenari, and also draws attention to the plays of amateur academicians inspired by the professionals.[25] Rejecting the validity of this approach, Campos identifies Raparini's *L'Arlichino*, a lengthy three-act poem published in 1718, as 'a compendium of lazzi'. Ignoring Guarinonius's descriptions, she describes *L'Arlichino* as 'the only document which permits genuine insights into what really constituted improvisation, the only one which offers examples of the actors' genial skills, including their lazzi', and contrasts the modesty of its lazzi with the 'disgusting vulgarity' of Adriani's.[26]

Each of these sources has limitations as documentary evidence. Selecting from them, but never featuring Guarinonius's lazzi, scholars have variously sought to classify lazzi. In the vanguard of this work was Ludovico Zorzi. His comprehensive researches into lazzi, based on coordinated and systematic archival researches of individual collections of commedia dell'arte scenari with successive generations of his graduate students at the University of Florence, remained unpublished at his death. Royce divides the lazzi of the unillustrated Correr manuscript into the four categories of bargaining, bantering, focusing audience attention, and servants making fun of masters.[27] More substantial lazzi classifications are published by McDowell, Hallar, Gordon and Capozza.[28] Hallar divides lazzi into four categories: pantomime, wordplay, episode and practical joke. Chosen primarily to facilitate access for the modern practitioner, the 12 thematic categories into which Gordon divides some 206 early modern lazzi are of limited use in classifying Guarinonius's comic episodes, with which they have little overlap. For Capozza, the only admissible lazzi sources are commedia dell'arte scenari, and the miscellanies or *zibaldone* in which actors collected useful passages and quotations.

---

[24]   Bartoli, *Scenari inediti*, XCVI ff. (*L'Inavvertito overo Scappino disturbato e Mezzettino travagliato*).

[25]   Lea, 'Bibliography', 23–4.

[26]   Campos, 'L'Arlichino', 174–5, 203. Neither Campos nor Pandolfi (*La commedia dell'arte*, IV, 212) could trace the anonymously published first edition of Raparini's *L'Arlichino*. Discovered by the present author in Milan's Scala Library (CR.U.119), its virtually unchanged 1,147 lines are greatly augmented by the much longer 1718 second edition. Some scholars recognize it as a significant lazzi source (e.g. Gambelli, by whom it is repeatedly cited: *Arlecchino a Parigi*), others do not (it is not cited in Capozza's *Tutti i lazzi*).

[27]   Royce, 'The Venetian commedia', 82.

[28]   McDowell, *An iconographical study*, part I, chapter IV: 'Stage business and lazzi', 120–46; Hallar, *Teaterspil og Tegnsprog*, 'Lazzi', 76–142; Gordon, *Lazzi*; Capozza, *Tutti i lazzi*.

Using Gordon's classification system as a point of departure, but without referring to McDowell or Hallar's work or to visual evidence, her compendium classifies around 1,200 lazzi descriptions into 17 thematic categories.[29]

Debate surrounds the status of Guarinonius's lazzi. In particular, this has focused on whether the quack troupes he observed in the 1590s and describes in his treatise of 1610 were full-sized professional acting troupes (typically with around a dozen players), performing full-length commedia dell'arte plays, or smaller troupes of perhaps only three or four quacks, staging loosely connected brief 'highlights' and comic routines pirated from professional actors. Inclining to this latter view, Valentin suggests that Guarinonius deliberately shrunk his Italian troupe to focus on the archaic servant–master duo Zanni and Magnificus, allowing Zanni and Magnificus to stand for all the stock characters of the professional players. In his view, in order to characterize what he sees as the pre-Christian, heathen origins of the commedia dell'arte, Guarinonius's episodes deliberately reflect already old-fashioned stage practice. In short, he believes that Guarinonius's lazzi describe 'primitive' street theatre with a minimum of performers offering brief essentially self-contained routines, rather than 'genuine' full-length commedia dell'arte performances. Sprengel is likewise unable to determine any indication, in the 23 indexed commedia dell'arte episodes, of the multiplicity of characters and intrigues characterizing Flamino Scala's scenari. He suggests that, rather than consciously archaizing the commedia dell'arte, they reflect popularized and truncated street-theatre variants, and (unconvincingly) attempts to demonstrate that they bridge the gap between Italian comedy and German farce by conflating Zanni with a clown popular on the German eighteenth-century stage, Hanswurst.[30] Martino also identifies Guarinonius's troupe as a 'micro-company' of perhaps only two or three actors, presenting a prototypical 'genetic nucleus' of the commedia dell'arte rather than its fully-developed form.[31] However, he agrees with the present author in viewing these descriptions as professional commedia dell'arte lazzi, of the type which Guarinonius could as easily have seen embedded in full-length plays as in short routines.

Rather than a clear-cut binary divide between 'full-sized' acting troupes staging 'full-length' plays and 'micro-companies' staging brief comic 'quack' routines, my reading of Guarinonius and Platter's accounts of quack performances indicates a less easily categorizable situation: fluid gradations in size of troupe as well as length of performance, with only imperfect correlation between the two. Many quack troupes drew on a portfolio of commercial strategies. They did not invariably incorporate quack activities into their stage routines, and their quack activities

---

[29]   Capozza, *Tutti i lazzi*, 10, 15. Numerous uncrossreferenced duplicate entries, bulking this publication out to 1,830 sections, compromise its usefulness as a scholarly resource.

[30]   Valentin, 'Herr Pantalon', 202–3, *Theatrum Catholicum*, 43 and *Französischer 'Roman comique'*, 26; Sprengel, 'Herr Pantalon', 13.

[31]   Martino, 'Fonti tedesche degli anni 1585–1615', 676, 691, 707.

were not invariably supported by full-length plays. Indisputably, the main focus of *Grewel*'s lazzi is the servant–master duo.[32] Many of the supporting characters are offstage or play minor roles, and there is little mention of key commedia dell'arte stock characters known to have limited involvement with lazzi, such as the lovers. Each of Guarinonius's lazzi typically involves few players, and onstage women rarely feature. But this is in line with standard early modern stage practice, and close scrutiny of all 35 lazzi reveals a more complex picture.

The comic manservant, invariably identified by Guarinonius as Zanni, has a variety of masters in these lazzi. Most commonly, he is an old Venetian Pantalone or Magnificus.[33] In lazzo no.5, Guarinonius notes that, by the time of writing, the popularity of the lecherous old man has established him as a stock character of the commedia dell'arte. Where there is no indication of the master's age,[34] he is by no means invariably from an older generation than his servant. In lazzo no.4, Zanni serves a lovesick young master, and in lazzo no.7, a wealthy student. The wife of Zanni or his master each feature only once, and never when the Zanni–master pair are together. In lazzo no.2, a slothful and angry Zanni terrorizes his pregnant wife. Lazzo no.26 refers to a 'cuckolded Venetian Pantalone' and his whorish wife. Wives of old masters rarely feature in sixteenth-century scenari, and were only exceptionally an important onstage presence in commedia dell'arte plots, whose central trio was the comic threesome of servant, master and whatever woman happened to be the master's current love interest. References in lazzo no.22 to the master's sweethearts and mistresses confirm that several women, of contrasting social status, could occupy this position simultaneously. Sometimes, the master's offstage beloved is referred to only indirectly, by describing him as lovesick (lazzi nos.4 and 5). More often, she is specifically referred to in passing, as in lazzo no.3, where Magnificus relates to Zanni how he had seen his beloved and her maid; or firmly integrated into the plot, as where Zanni acts as go-between for his master and his beloved (lazzi nos.9 and 21), or advises his master on how best to impress his beloved (lazzi nos.32 and 33). Occasionally, the onstage appearance of a woman, either Zanni's wife or the master's beloved herself, or another woman mistaken for her, is crucial to the plot (lazzi nos.2, 22, 28).

In Guarinonius's lazzi, as well as the object of the master's lust, the supporting cast to the servant–master duo may include a maid (lazzo no.3) or old bawd (lazzo no.28), tradesmen such as a cobbler (lazzo no.6), vengeance-seeking enemies of Zanni's master (lazzo no.7), unspecified servants and extras (lazzi nos.8, 13), his master's friends or rival in love (lazzi nos.10, 32), and a horse or donkey (lazzi nos.33, 35). Donkeys feature in the Scala and Corsini scenari, and early modern

---

[32] For whose typical costume, see Plates 14–19.

[33] Magnificus (lazzo nos.3 ['Venetian' in manuscript version only: Innsbruck UL, Cod.110, 1, f.416^v], 28); lovesick old fool (lazzo no.5); Venetian Pantalone (lazzi nos.14, 22–6, 29, 31–3, 35).

[34] Unspecified master (lazzi nos.9–13, 20, 27, 30); nobleman (lazzo no.6); infatuated fool (lazzo no.21).

depictions of comedians performing onstage with live or pantomime horses are known.[35] In addition to the lazzi with their wives, others featuring only one of the servant–master duo are those where a lecherous old master (lazzo no.5) or a Zanni (lazzi nos.1, 18) are alone; or Zanni is with two ghosts, a young Devil, and unspecified rescuers (lazzo no.8), or with a parasite and unspecified rescuers (lazzo no.16). The 'Italian sponging glutton and comedian' of lazzo no.34 is a thinly disguised Zanni. Lazzi featuring neither the servant nor his master include a brief generic quote from an unidentified 'Italian comedian' (lazzo no.17) and references to two military captains, the *tedesco* or German mercenary, and Spanish *Grandes* (lazzi nos.15, 19). Taken as a whole, the 23 indexed Zanni episodes and 12 more recently identified lazzi indicate a broad dramatic framework, peopled by a mixed-gender troupe with authentic professional commedia skills, offering a rich selection from the verbal and physical repertoire of the late sixteenth-century comic stage. In terms of the sheer quantity of lazzi described, and the unprecedented detail, for this early date, with which several of them are recorded, Guarinonius's descriptions collectively challenge the commonly held assumption that 'our knowledge of the structure of individual lazzi is limited to brief descriptions'.[36] Through their number, detail and early date, they deserve recognition as a major record of the early commedia dell'arte, and a valuable guide to the theatrical repertoire of quack troupes.

Despite being cited at first,[37] second,[38] and even third hand[39] from Guarinonius's original treatise, these lazzi descriptions still await incorporation into the mainstream of early modern theatre history. Several factors contribute to their significance. Guarinonius's main source for them is his eyewitness recollections of the professional Italian stage at a precisely defined time and place, Padua in the mid-1590s. Representing the most substantial and informative early modern German-language source for lazzi descriptions, the authority and authenticity

---

[35] For example, Scala, *Il Teatro*, Day 43 ('L'Alvida'); Pandolfi, *La commedia dell'arte*, V, 256–7 (the Corsini titlepage illustration to *La mula grande* (I.20) depicts a live mule); Katritzky, *The art of commedia*, plates 42, 48, 70 (pantomime horses).

[36] Moro, 'Lazzi', 66.

[37] Albertinus, *Gusman von Alfarche* [=AA]; Meissner, *Die englischen Comoedianten* [=JMe], 4–10; Bücking, *Kultur und Gesellschaft in Tirol*, 95–8; Valentin, 'Bouffons ou religieux?', *Theatrum Catholicum*, 19–48 and 'Herr Pantalon' [=J-MV]; Katritzky, 'Hippolytus Guarinonius' descriptions' and 'Comic stage routines'; Martino, 'Fonti tedesche degli anni 1585–1615', 670–706.

[38] Trautmann, 'Italienische Schauspieler', 232 [via JMe]; Reinhardstöttner, 'Aegidius Albertinus' [via AA]; Trautmann, 'Deutsche Schauspieler', 386 [via AA, JMe]; Rausse [=HR], *Zur Geschichte des spanischen Schelmenromanes* [via AA]; Morris, 'A Hapsburg letter', 17n8 [via JMe]; Limon [=JL], *Gentlemen of a company*, 120 [via JMe]; Sprengel [PS], 'Herr Pantalon', 11–15 [via J-MV]; Schindler 'Mio compadre Imperatore', 128n85 [via J-MV, PS].

[39] Hansen, *Formen der commedia dell'arte*, 10 [via JMi, HR]; Balme, 'Cultural anthropology', 50n44 [via JL].

of *Grewel*'s lazzi are further enhanced by their author's medical expertise. Guarinonius's lazzi range in length from brief allusions in a single phrase or sentence, to several paragraphs of densely observed insights clarifying the structure, dialogue, presentation, reception and context of discrete units of comic stage business. With their wealth of references to this broad range of characters, these episodes make less dramatic sense as brief isolated stage routines than as professionally-performed lazzi. Guarinonius has selectively quarried them from his memories of the full-length mixed-gender commedia dell'arte plays in which they were embedded. Originally staged as a medical marketing strategy, in Guarinonius's most substantial medical treatise their inclusion is motivated by didactic and literary, but also therapeutic aims, by an author concerned to promote the health and well-being of his own readers through healing laughter.

Chapter 14

Marketing Medicine, Exemplifying Folly: Lazzi and the Deadly Sins

Hippolytus Guarinonius's medical treatise *Grewel* situates descriptions of lazzi, or popular commedia dell'arte stage routines, within a framework of health-threatening sins and vices. This is the context in which they are examined in this chapter. Guarinonius perceived human sins as being quite literally 'deadly'. For him, they represented potentially fatal pathways to spiritual, mental and physical breakdown, against whose symptoms it was his highest professional duty as a physician to warn his patients, as when he blames Prague's high death rate neither on nature nor on its geographical situation, 'but on the sloth and sinfullness of its people', explaining that:

> if some cities and places have all the good and healthy gifts and virtues of nature, but there are still plagues and other illnesses there, it is a sure sign that their inhabitants themselves have disgraced and defiled these places through one or more sins.[1]

Central to the concept and title of *Grewel*, the term 'sins' provides an alternative gloss for its key title word, more usually translated as 'abominations'. The close links between the two words are emphasized by Thomas Platter's reference to abominable sins,[2] or by Guarinonius himself, in one of many rhetorical dialogues with the 'friendly reader':

> *Reader*: You must indeed be a merciful doctor. But as yet, I have been able to discern little of your mercy in this your book, in which you mercilessly attack, expose, damn and ban the abominations and sins.

> *Doctor*: I am merciless in this respect so that I can warn everyone against becoming dependent on medicines and doctors. Because if I were merciful in this respect, I would willingly allow them the medicines. But he who diligently takes heed of such abominations can avoid all medicines.[3]

---

[1] Guarinonius, *Grewel*, 419, 429.
[2] *Thomas Platter d.J*, 643 (16 August 1599, Arras): 'greülichen sünden'.
[3] Guarinonius, *Grewel*, 969.

Guarinonius's lazzi are carefully crafted to emphasize didactic points in *Grewel*, regarding the attainment of physical, mental and spiritual health and well-being. Rather than recollecting complete performances, they are intended to evoke theatrical episodes in just enough detail to support specific points. In this context, Valentin helpfully defines them as dramatic *exempla* of moralizing intent focusing on specific sins, notably gluttony.[4] Human follies, vices and sins are a major focus of renaissance drama.[5] *Das Narrenschneyden*, one of many mid-sixteenth-century Shrovetide plays by Hans Sachs inspired by the merchant scenes of religious plays, stages a surgical operation in which a loquacious quack heals a patient by extracting from within his body seven miniature fools personifying the sins. The harangues of this stage quack, linked by some modern critics to Martin Luther, provide a vehicle for anti-Papist propaganda intended to spiritually heal the play's spectators.[6] Devoutly Catholic Guarinonius likens Protestant preachers in their pulpits to 'alchemists or toothdrawers haranguing the crowds from their horses in the public square'; false healers respectively of soul and body, who promote rather than prevent the sinful and unhealthy behaviour of their congregations or patients.[7]

Sins are central to Guarinonius's blending of medical advice and didactic moralizing, and almost all of *Grewel*'s 35 lazzi can be associated with one or more of those which became commonly identified as the seven deadly sins.[8] By the time Guarinonius was writing, as the first scene of Act 2 of Marlowe's *Faustus* famously demonstrates, the seven deadly sins had become commonly identified as pride, avarice, lechery, envy, gluttony, wrath and sloth.[9] Early schema varied the number as well as identification of the 'deadly' sins. Some authorities included, for example, *melancholia* or its spiritual equivalent, *tristitia* (either with or in place of *acedia*),[10] *inepta laetitia* or *vana gloria* (eventually subsumed under *superbia*). As well as both vainglory and pride, St Bernard's list of deadly sins includes loquacity, and a failing condemned by many as a lesser sin, namely inquisitiveness or curiosity.[11] Guarinonius, concerned to expose the medical use of astrology as a dangerous and blasphemous superstition, offers his own schema of sins, based on the seven planets and the 12 astrological signs, in which *curiositas*, assigned to the

---

[4]   Valentin, 'Herr Pantalon', 197.

[5]   Happé, 'The vice and the folk-drama'.

[6]   Schade, *German comedy*, 76–9; Remshardt, 'Hans Sachs and "Das Narren-Schneyden"', 71–3, 77.

[7]   Guarinonius, *Grewel*, 1163.

[8]   Gemert, 'Tridentinische Geistigkeit', 48, 61; Valentin, 'Herr Pantalon', 197.

[9]   Not least through Thomas Aquinas's popularization of a handy mnemonic, 'Dat septem vicia dictio *saligia* [=**S**uperbia /**A**varitia /**L**uxuria /**I**nvidia /**G**ula /**I**ra /**A**cedia]' (Gothein, 'Die Todsünden', 457). Marlowe, *Faustus* sigs.C3ᵛ–Dʳ (II.i.104–75).

[10]   Neuber, 'Vom Grewel deß Trawrens', 75.

[11]   Gothein, 'Die Todsünden', 439, 450, 454; Wenzel, 'The seven deadly sins', 11; Little, 'Pride goes before avarice', 23; Brüggemann, *Die Angst vor dem Bösen*, 213–19.

sign of Virgo, ranks high, being the main focus of one of his lazzi, and featuring in conjunction with one or more of the deadly sins in several more.[12]

Gluttony, sloth and lechery are the sins typically associated with the commedia dell'arte's central comic trio, the master, his manservant Zanni and his maid. In Guarinonius's lazzi, only one of the remaining four deadly sins (anger, pride, envy and avarice), is encountered independently of the dominant three. This is pride, in lazzo no.6, describing a proud aristocrat out in public basking in his reputation and boasting of his refinement, when his cobbler approaches and requests payment for a credit note. He refuses, and is put on the spot by the persistent cobbler until Zanni arrives and saves his master's pride by getting rid of the cobbler with excuses. The much briefer pre-revised manuscript version, related by Guarinonius in the manner of an eyewitnessed everyday event, raises the possibility that he saw it in the street rather than at the theatre. Commedia dell'arte stock characters are named only in the published version, augmented with a manuscript *addendum*. Here, comparison of the published and manuscript versions offers insights into Guarinonius's strategy for presenting apparently dramatic events in *Grewel*; suggesting that not all its commedia dell'arte descriptions can be taken at face value, as straightforward documentary evidence for stage practice. The sin of avarice, according to Montaigne 'the most ridiculous of all humane follies', receives even shorter shrift than pride from Guarinonius.[13] Labelling the avaricious 'gold fools' and 'money fools', he accuses them of being created in the shape not of God but of the Devil, and nominates this 'demonic' sin as the greatest and most uncouth of all, neither human nor even bestial, but 'devilish'. However, although Guarinonius repeatedly identifies it as the sin of old age, lazzo no.22 relegates avarice to Pantalone's pleasure of third choice, after lechery and gluttony, and it otherwise hardly features in his lazzi.[14] Envy and anger, respectively discussed in chapters 35 and 36 of *Grewel*'s Book 2, feature in several lazzi exemplifying more than one sin. The underlying sins of three acrobatic lazzi slotting less easily into this schema are here identified as anger or sloth (lazzi nos.29, 30, 31).

Unsurprisingly, given its status as a leading motivator for comic stage business involving commedia dell'arte masters and their servants, the dominating sin of these lazzi is gluttony. While reporting with awe and respect on the saintly anorexics Brother Nicolao of Switzerland who fasted for 20 years, and Magdalena Felsinger, a nun in his own convent at Hall who drank nothing for eight years, Guarinonius warns 'certain mad and tyrannical parents' against the dangers of encouraging anorexic daughters purely to raise their chances of advantageous marriages.[15] But he has no sympathy for obese patients. Castigating them as 'lazy, fat [...] belly fools' and 'meat fools', he highlights drunkenness and gluttony-

---

[12]   Guarinonius, *Grewel*, 1030–3.

[13]   Montaigne, *Essayes*, 136; Guarinonius, *Grewel*, 320–45 (Book 2, Chapter 34).

[14]   Guarinonius, *Grewel*, 168, 282–3, 324.

[15]   Guarinonius, *Grewel*, 139, 547, 593. Nicolas de Flue (1417–87), also known as Nicolaus Helvetius Undervaldensis or Bruder Klaus, whose only food for the final 20 years

induced incontinence as foolish, shameful symptoms of ill-health resulting from overindulgence.[16] Gluttony, drunkenness and incontinence dominate some two-thirds of his lazzi. The five lazzi concerned with bodily incontinence include two of his lengthiest, describing involuntary incontinence in the contexts of sloth (lazzo no.27) and lechery (lazzo no.22). Three shorter lazzi feature spitting or flatulence. Table manners dominated court etiquette, occupying, for example, 15 of the 24 pages of Duke Heinrich Julius's court ordinance of 1589, confirming domestic regulations for his courtiers. They stipulated that, when seated in Wolfenbüttel's ducal banqueting hall, courtiers refrain from precisely the sort of uncouth and foolish laughter, impolite gestures, whistling, swearing, loud conversation and similar social transgressions representing the routine stock in trade of court and stage fools.[17] Having outlined guidelines concerning spitting and gargling, Guarinonius uses lazzo no.25 to contrast refined courtly etiquette, strictly vetoing their practice during meals, with Zanni's uncouth attempts at politeness. In lazzo no.25, Zanni interrrupts a conversation with Pantalone to warn him of his sudden urgent need to spit.

Audible flatulence, the punchline of lazzo no.23, was openly mocked at court, as in Guarinonius's anecdote about noblewomen laughing at the nervous envoy who passed wind when finally granted an audience with their duke.[18] In lazzo no.23, Zanni and Pantalone march to war kitted out for battle. This firm favourite of the commedia dell'arte repertoire already features in the Munich court wedding performance of 1568. As Massimo Troiano reports, this lazzo provided comic actors with ample opportunities to ridicule commoners' ignorance of the chivalric etiquette expected of every educated nobleman: 'Pantalone appeared in full armour, but not properly fastened, and Zanni with two arquebuses over his shoulder, eight daggers in his belt, a sword and buckler in his hands, and a completely rusty helmet on his head.'[19] In Guarinonius's lazzo, the situation is again used to develop the subject of bodily incontinence, with the cowardly Zanni fainting when he mistakes Pantalone's flatulence for cannon shots. Guarinonius's remark that such flatulence always has its origins in windy food immediately introduces a second flatulence lazzo. In this, Zanni stumps his master, Pantalone, with the question: 'Which food delights nature most?', justifying his solution that it is the radish, by pointing out that no other food is so lavishly honoured with drumming, piping and cannon salutes (lazzo no.24). Such sounds typically

---

of his life was the Eucharist every eight days, was canonized in 1947 (Collins, *Reforming saints*, 99–122).

[16]   Guarinonius, *Grewel*, 758–764 (Book 4, Chapter 51: 'On the abomination of the determined, portly, fat and bestial fattening of the body').

[17]   Wolfenbüttel HAB, A:57.8 Pol (24), *Fürstliche Braunschweigische Hoff-Ordnung* (26 October 1589), sig.b(iv); Schade, *German comedy*, 139–40; Midelfort, *A history of madness*, 265.

[18]   Guarinonius, *Grewel*, 306.

[19]   Troiano, *Dialoghi*, sig.151ᵛ. On this wedding, see also Chapter 7, this volume.

heralded early modern entries into cities, at every level from the highest royalty to informal private journeys. Felix Platter witnessed numerous cannon salutes in honour of Emperor Ferdinand I, during his formally celebrated entry into Basle in 1563, but also records firing a private two-shot gun salute to celebrate his own re-entry into Basle from his years away from his home town.[20] The well-worn joke of likening such salutes to noisy flatulence was rolled out as late as 1681, when a character in a novel by Johann Beer maintains that it is healthier to punctuate an alcoholic drinking bout with great belches than to have it accompanied by 25 gun salutes.[21] In an early seventeenth-century Roman lazzo, a comic servant bursts pig bladders, announcing that cannons are heralding his arrival.[22] This aural pun is revived in the 1658 production of *Il convitato di pietra*, by the Italian comedians in Paris, whose Harlequin, played by Biancolelli, celebrates surviving a shipwreck by clinging to inflated bladders: 'I do the lazzi of breaking one of the bladders by falling on it. That makes a noise which I say is from a cannon I've fired, rejoicing that we have been saved.'[23] Flatulence lazzi were a staple of the repertory of the Italian comedy in Paris, and Biancolelli even records one he played with two actresses, Eularia and Aurelia, in the scenario 'Il regalo delle damme'.[24]

Generally, in Guarinonius's hunger lazzi, Zanni's primarily food-orientated gluttony is appeased at the expense of his elderly master. However, in two lazzi which, exceptionally for those in *Grewel*, feature neither of the master–servant duo, sinful, unhealthy gluttony of this type is exhibited by military captains. This stock role ultimately draws on the *miles gloriosus* of Roman comic drama typified by Terence's *Eunuchus*. The commedia dell'arte's military captains were Spanish and Italian captains, predominantly associated with romantic wooing and cowardly loquacity, and the foolish Germanic *tedesco* or mercenary foot-soldier, who shared more characteristics with comic servants than serious lovers. Above all, the *tedesco* was noted for prodigiously gluttonous consumption of alcohol. Early modern travellers of all nationalities commented on German drinking habits. Felix Platter, who 'saw few drunks in Montpellier apart from us Germans', occasionally proved quite capable of alcoholic overindulgence himself as, to his evident disapprobation, did his father-in-law.[25] Visiting Germans provided the impetus for numerous alcoholic festivities for Platter and his fellow German medical students. They fêted friends, but also complete strangers such as Hans Brombach and Hans Pfriendt, two *tedeschi* or Swiss guards in the service of the King of Navarre, stopping off in Montpellier on their way home to Basle. Having

---

[20]   *Felix Platter Tagebuch*, 293, 395 (May 1557 and January 1563, Basle).

[21]   Beer, 'Narrenspital [1681]', *Sämtliche Werke*, V, 170; Battafarano, 'Literarische Skatologie', 192–3.

[22]   Gordon, *Lazzi*, 29.

[23]   Scott, *The commedia dell'arte in Paris*, 72 (in translation).

[24]   Capozza, *Tutti i lazzi*, 131 no.769.

[25]   As, in his student years, did Guarinonius (*Grewel*, 627). *Felix Platter Tagebuch*, 166, 228 (May 1553 and 20 September 155, Montpellier), 404–5 (8–9 June 1563, Valais).

treated them to a liberal evening meal, and escorted them out of the city gates in the morning, they saw them off with a final drinking session, during which they 'christened them with a glass of wine, poured down onto their heads'.[26]

Memorably bibulous Germans recalled by Felix Platter include Christoph von Grüt, Abbot of Muri, who during the evening Platter spent at his venerable monastery, renowned for its medieval Passion play, progressed steadily from 'fairly tipsy' to 'comprehensively drunk'.[27] Fynes Moryson notes that Germans have: 'no shame […] if they drincke till they vomitt, and make water vnder the table, and till they sleepe'.[28] Thomas Platter considers Netherlandish men:

> much greater alcoholics than the Germans. They enjoy sitting at their beer, with which they get themselves so drunk that they don't know what they are doing. Wine, which is extremely expensive for them […] is even more popular than beer with them. They don't just get drunk at home but also, and indeed very heavily, on their journeys when they should be seeing to their business. […] On their feast days, after their guests have left, they stay at their tables for five or six hours, or even until midnight, toasting each other with their beer mugs until they are all blind drunk. […] The women are extremely sober, the men, as noted above, very given to drinking […] and to buying rounds of wine at the inns […] its a sure way for someone to get through their money, unless they stay away from drinking any wine at all. Itinerant musicians usually come there too, who then also empty one's purses.[29]

Of the French he writes: 'they don't regard whoring and adultery as any more sinful than we regard drunkenness, which in turn they are so against that anyone who is inclined to it can no longer be appointed to high office. The greatest insult you can make against anyone [French] is to call them a drunkard'.[30] Warning that strong drink turns men to beasts and fools, Guarinonius confirms that alcohol abuse was widely regarded as the 'national sin' of the Germans. When pressed to characterize Germans with a single adjective, he picks 'drunken', admitting that even German physicians are not immune from this sin, and agreeing with the Italians that 'we Germans have the reputation of heavy drinkers, as is indeed actually the case'. While conceding that 'whereas wine makes the Italians and others enraged and angry, it makes Germans merry and good-natured', he abhors the buying of rounds and drinking of toasts.[31] Alcohol abuse and the superiority of water over wine were themes of such importance to him that, referring to Galen's teachings, and identifying water as the 'theriac' of wine, he expanded *Grewel*'s

---

26   *Felix Platter Tagebuch*, 196–7 (18–19 April 1554, Montpellier).
27   *Felix Platter Tagebuch*, 375 (1561, Muri).
28   Moryson, *Shakespeare's Europe*, 342.
29   *Thomas Platter d.J*, 700–1 (1 September 1599, Louvain).
30   *Thomas Platter d.J*, 593 (28 July 1599, Paris).
31   Guarinonius, *Grewel*, 49, 93, 363, 548, 622, 709.

suggestions regarding the moderate and watered-down consumption of wine in a Latin treatise of 1640.[32]

Popular on the sixteenth-century comic stage, the *tedesco* was increasingly ousted after 1600 by Spanish military captains. His colourful costume was based on that of the Swiss mercenaries who formed the Papal Guard, and were the fashionable guards of choice at many early modern French and Italian courts. The *tedesco* was generally depicted with a weapon and military instrument, and some symbol of his prodigious drinking habits, such as a wine-glass or beer barrel.[33] A rare documented lazzo alluding to *tedeschi*, placing them firmly in the context of alcohol consumption, involves Celia and Coviello disguised as *tedeschi*, surrounded by bottles and wine-glasses, drinking at an inn.[34] In lazzo no.15, expressing deep regret that the great German nation's drunks are a comic target for actors, Guarinonius features the *tedesco* in a brief allusion to the Italian comedy noting that, although when the Italian comedians represent German drunks they act like drunk brutes, the actors themselves remain sober.

Felix Platter's journal reports several tall tales reminiscent of the bombastic bragging of conquests and feats of strength with which the military stage role is typically associated. The elderly Swiss guard in the service of Claude de Savoie, Comte de Tende, who showed him around Marseille, claimed that he was nicknamed 'chasse diable' after a fight in which he overcame the Devil himself, and Fritz of Zurich, a Swiss guard to the King of Navarre, told him of a fight with a lion and a bull, in which the bull had gored him so deeply below the navel that it punctured his back.[35] Platter's retelling of this latter in his *Observations* testifies to the care with which he investigated and documented such cases:

> *Flux of Urin, from a Wound in the Loyns.* When I was at *Narbo* in *France*, it hapned that when there were Sights and Bear-baitings, that among the rest a Lyon did fight with a Bull, and the Bull was running, but a Helvetian of *Tigur*, one of the Guard to the King of *Navarre* opposed him, and the Bull gored him with his horns, and thrust one in the pectin cross the Bladder, and the Urin came out at the Loyns. A Chirurgion of *Montpelior* cured him without any inconvenience, and he lived long after.[36]

---

[32] Guarinonius, *Grewel*, 664–8 (Book 4, chapter 34: 'On the abomination of unwatered wine'); Guarinonius, *Hydroenogamia trivmphpans*; see also Mayr, 'Volksnahrung', 125–8.

[33] Katritzky, *The art of commedia*, 217–18.

[34] Casamarciano II.57: 'Naufraggio di lieto fine' (quoted in Capozza, *Tutti i lazzi*, 125, no.733).

[35] *Felix Platter Tagebuch*, 192 (26 January 1554, Montpellier), 227 (20 September 1555, Marseille).

[36] Platter, *Obseruationum*, 798 (this translation: Plat[t]er, Culpeper and Cole, *Platerus histories*, 520–1).

Platter witnessed Pauli Füerer's resignation as Basle's municipal hangman, on 9 September 1559, immediately after bungling his public execution of the child rapist Felix Hemmig, by requiring a second blow from his sword of office to behead him. Later, as his patient, Füerer told Platter another of these military tall tales, namely that in a battle of 1525 he had used this same mighty thirteenth-century two-hander (now on display in Basle's Historical Museum), to decapitate over 500 opponents.[37] The Spanish *Grandes* of lazzo no.19, however, does not speak at all. Standing outside a kitchen window, he concentrates all his efforts into using the delicious smells wafting out, of someone else's roast dinner, to satisfy his gluttonous impulses, by making his own meal, a piece of stale bread, more palatable.

Overwhelmingly in *Grewel*'s lazzi, as in the commedia dell'arte in general, comic business featuring gluttony concerns stage servants. As perceptively discussed by Robert Henke, such lazzi are less about food than about hunger.[38] In lazzo no.17, Zanni is the probable subject of an aside highlighting how easily people can slide unthinkingly into gluttony, in a comparison of German eating and drinking habits with those of the fictional 'Schlaraffenland', the German Land of Cockaigne. Cuccagna, the Italian Cockaigne, whose 'world upside down' is explicitly linked to the commedia dell'arte and carnival in popular prints, is the focus of lazzi in many Italian and French scenari.[39] Lazzo no.34 also offers a short aside on gluttony and sloth, in which Guarinonius quotes an 'Italian sponging glutton and comedian' (surely a stage Zanni) reassuringly addressing his fat paunch. In lazzo no.1, Zanni attempts to prolong his gluttonous enjoyment of the pasta he is swallowing by retaining it in his gullet for as long as possible. In lazzo no.18 he adopts the opposite tactic, repeatedly grasping his neck to keep his gullet clear, so that he can illicitly devour noodles not meant for him as quickly as possible. The steaming bowl of pasta, a popular lazzi prop from at least 1568, when Massimo Troiano's Munich commedia dell'arte performance description alludes to it, plays a prominent part in lazzo no.27.[40] Pasta again features in lazzo no.11, where Zanni's master puts a delicious dish of macaroni in front of him, who, suggesting that it might be a health risk, offers to eat it all himself in order to protect his master.

Lazzo no.13 also concerns the theme of Zanni disguising his rampant gluttony with transparently suspect selflessness. Mistaking a dish of lampreys, an eel-like

[37]   *Felix Platter Tagebuch*, 354–5 (9 September 1559, Basle).

[38]   Henke, 'Representations of poverty'. On such lazzi, see also Gordon, *Lazzi*, 21–3: 'Food lazzi'; Capozza, *Tutti i lazzi*, 268–79: 'Lazzi di fame'.

[39]   Such as Scala, *Il Teatro*, Day 4 ('Le burle d'Isabella'); Biancolelli, 'Le voyage de Scaramouche et d'Arlequin aux Indes', 1676. See also Scott, *The commedia dell'arte in Paris*, 206; Capozza, *Tutti i lazzi*, 278–9: 'Lazzi del paese di Cuccagna'; Katritzky, 'Italian comedians in renaissance prints'.

[40]   Troiano, *Dialoghi*, sig.149ᵛ.

Lenten fish speciality enjoyed by Felix Platter,[41] for young adders, Zanni thought they had been brought to poison his master. But seeing his master's enjoyment on eating them, Zanni, in a suspicious display of loyalty, grabbed the bowl from him and finished them up himself, declaring that even though he would shortly die, at least the poison tasted good. In lazzo no.14, Zanni again gets the better of his master. When asked to help Pantalone decide whether it would be easier to do without food or without drink, far from concerning himself with his master's learned enquiry into the relative merits of liquid and solid nourishment, the sly servant exploits the situation's opportunity to indulge in gluttony. Having tricked Pantalone into lavishly providing both food and drink, he smugly pronounces himself well content with results of his experiment. In lazzo no.12, Zanni encapsulates this life philosophy, advising his master that as you never know if a meal is going to be your last, you should eat as much as you can at every meal, so that when death does come, you can at least fight it with a well-nourished body. Gordon subdivides food lazzi into those with real onstage food and those miming its presence.[42] In lazzo no.10, of this latter type, Zanni is distracted from his unwilling task of carrying a heavy bundle by his master's discussion of well-roasted capons and similar delicacies with a friend. Whenever he hears a particular food or delicacy mentioned, he makes a big, long, deep swallowing gesture, as if he is not simply hearing about the food, but actually savouring it in his mouth.

Lazzo no.16, in which the servant Zanni's stage partner is identified not as his master, but as an unnamed carnivorous parasite, features another perspective on gluttony and hunger. Guarinonius, a strong supporter of vegetarianism, here targets the health dangers of overindulging in meat. His case for supporting, on health grounds, a diet based on bread, for him 'the most delicious food on earth', far above one based on meat, openly criticizes lowland Protestant Germany communities not observing the frequent and regular abstentions from meat imposed by Catholic fast days: 'the plague rages more strongly where a lot of meat is eaten, and especially where there is not a single day of abstention observed in the entire year, let alone the quarterly Ember Days, or weekly fast days'.[43] Discussing the health risks of eating meat, Guarinonius recalls Galen's anecdote concerning an innkeeper who got away with serving his unwitting guests human meat until one of them found a fingertip in his soup, noting that 'this, which has also happened, and continues to happen, in our own times, is something that need neither be feared nor regretted with other foods'.[44]

In the pre-revised manuscript version of lazzo no.16, Zanni, hearing a gluttonous parasite list various types of meat he has feasted on, goes into shock and then faints right away. Two manuscript *addenda* incorporated into the published version add a cannibalistic slant. In the first, wanting to help, the parasite runs towards the

---

[41]   *Felix Platter Tagebuch*, 272 (11 March 1557, Bordeaux).

[42]   Gordon, *Lazzi*, 21, 41.

[43]   Guarinonius, *Grewel*, 747, 750, 801.

[44]   Guarinonius, *Grewel*, 748.

unconscious Zanni, who screams for help until people come running up, in whose presence he soon revives. The second rounds off the lazzo, by noting that this seemed not unreasonable, and speculating on Zanni's hypothetical reaction to two legendary classical gluttons. Locatelli records a lazzo featuring cannibalistically gluttonous reactions to unidentified meat, and lazzi of physical fear were popular and widespread. A terrified Pantalone and a fainting Zanni respectively feature in lazzi nos.22 and 23. Guarinonius's observations in these lazzi supplement those in his chapter 'On the abomination of frivolous fear and fright', adding valuable contextual and physiological details to the sparse early modern records on the significant theme of stage manifestations of symptoms of extreme terror, of a type featured in lazzi of fear indicated by Scala and Locatelli, and refined in Paris, where Biancolelli's 'lazzis de frayeur' became a popular speciality.[45]

Several of Guarinonius's lazzi feature a second deadly sin, sloth, often linked to other sins or vices, such as anger. Sometimes stage servants' dealings with their masters betray suppressed anger at their more comfortable status, and lazzi of beatings and anger involving the servant–master duo were popular.[46] In lazzo no.31, concerned with exploring ways in which Zanni can get away with expressing his anger, Pantalone gives him the task of catching midges. Instead of successfully completing the task in hand, Zanni jumps around, waving his arms and hands in the air and performing contortions which Guarinonius likens to the grotesquely exaggerated movements of German fencing masters, and ends up punching his master on the nose with his fist. Here Guarinonius provides the earliest known description of an iconic lazzo of the Comedie Italienne. This 'lazzo of the fly' was made famous by Biancolelli, who as Harlequin could count on bringing the house down trying to kill a fly which has settled on the face of his master Don Juan. Laconically recorded by him as 'je fais le lazzy d'attraper une mouche', one variation of this lazzo achieved the distinction of being depicted in a painting formerly attributed to Antoine Watteau.[47]

Underlying anger between servant and master is sometimes expressed in the aggressive horseplay of acrobatic physical routines. Lazzo no.29 ends with Zanni being punished for tripping up his master by having to carry him on his back,

---

[45]   Guarinonius, *Grewel*, 304–11 (Book 2, Chapter 32); Scala, *Il Teatro*, Day 22 ('Il creduto morto'); Locatelli I.32, II.4 ('Il finto marito', 'La pazzia di Filandro'); Bartoli, *Scenari inediti*, 266 ('Le disgrazie e fortune di Pandolfo'); Biancolelli: 'I morti vivi', 'Il convitato di pietra', 'Grotta nuova', 'La magia naturale' (Gambelli, *Arlecchino a Parigi*, II, 107–8, 300, 357–8, III, 774). See also Scott, *The commedia dell'arte in Paris*, 72–3; Capozza, *Tutti i lazzi*, 244–58: 'Lazzi di paura'.

[46]   Gordon, *Lazzi*, 14–19: 'Comic violence/sadistic behavior'; Capozza, *Tutti i lazzi*, 215–43: 'Lazzi di bastonatura e rabbia'.

[47]   *Pantaloon* [*sic*: actually a Pierrot] *catching a fly*, oil on canvas, Art Institute of Chicago (Bequest of Mrs Sterling Morton 1969.333). Scott, *The commedia dell'arte in Paris*, 74 ('Il convitato di pietra', c.1658,); Capozza, *Tutti i lazzi*, 40–1: 'Lazzi della mosca'; Speaight, 'A commedia dell'arte "Lazzo"'.

and lazzo no.30 with Zanni refusing to come down from Pantalone's shoulders. In contrast to the typically vague indications of comic routines involving dance and acrobatics in most textual[48] and visual documentation (Plates 7, 13, 15–19), these two lazzi provide detailed insights into the actual physical routines of early modern acrobatic lazzi. Unlike Guarinonius's descriptions of lazzi involving bodily incontinence in the form of defecation, urination and flatulence, these step-by-step acutely observed descriptions of specific acrobatic lazzi involving Zanni and Pantalone have attracted little theatre-historical attention.[49] Lazzi of this type were already well-established by the time of the 1568 Munich wedding performance, when the court goldsmith, Giovanni Battista Scolari, as Zanni, gave the leader of the Bavarian court musicians, Orlando di Lasso, playing the role of Pantalone:

> a hefty push. Over which they got into a fight, finally recognized each other, and in his great joy, Zanni invited his master onto his shoulders, spun him around like a millstone, and carried him around the whole stage. And then Pantalone did the same with Zanni, and finally both of them fell to the ground.[50]

Similar acrobatic horseplay features in pictures such as Plate 13, depicting a Pantalone on the shoulders of a Zanni standing on a grassy hummock. They are engaged in a comic routine with obscene as well as acrobatic content, as a second Zanni holds Pantalone's cloak aside with one hand, in order to expose his backside to a mirror which he holds in the other.

The Zanni of lazzo no.2 behaves like those 'enraged fools who instantly want grown-up, wellbred, educated and intelligent children, without doing any of the things needed to achieve this'. Fearing the pressures of imminent fatherhood, the sins of sloth and anger lead Zanni to bombard his pregnant wife with unrealistic expectations regarding their awaited child, by demanding that she does not allow the young Zanni into the world until he can look after and clothe himself. Although sloth is primarily the province of the servant, lazzo no.35 is another example of stage business in which his master's sloth is the butt of the joke. Criticizing the increasing reliance on forms of transport other than walking for being lazy and unhealthy, Guarinonius here quotes Zanni's cheerful cry on seeing his master Pantalone riding towards him on a donkey: 'Look here, good people: see how my master approaches on bestial feet'. He comments that Zanni wants to draw attention to the fact that his master would be safer relying on the feet of a rational human, than trusting his body to an irresponsible dumb beast.

---

[48]   Gordon, *Lazzi*, 9–13: 'Acrobatic and mimic lazzi'; Capozza, *Tutti i lazzi*, 16–41: 'Lazzi acrobatici'.

[49]   Grass notes them, but not their theatrical content ('Ein Vorkämpfer', 62); Katritzky, 'Hippolytus Guarinonius' descriptions', 90–1 and 'Comic stage routines', 223.

[50]   Troiano, *Dialoghi*, sig.149ᵛ.

In lazzo no.20, Zanni's inherent slothfulness, which makes him wish to be free of his duties as a servant, is framed in the context of an agreement with his master that while he eats, his master should not make demands of him or address him. Biancolelli records a lazzo on this theme in which comic servants attempt to avoid their duties by feigning sleep, and in a Parisian lazzo of the 1660s, a comic servant's preoccupation with eating prevents him from responding to his master's enquiries in a way appropriate to his status as servant.[51] Lazzo no.7 offers a more drastic version of the theme of the slothful Zanni who envies his master's freedom from servile chores and status. In it, Zanni is overcome by three sins, the third an *addendum* to the pre-revised manuscript version: slothfulness, curiosity to know what it would be like to be a master, and envy of his master's status.[52] This leads to a variation on the theme of the 'world upside down', resulting in cross-dressed servant–master role swapping of a type recorded by Guarinonius in a personal encounter he likens to 'a comedy or play'. It took place at a country inn: 'where I was unknown and taken for a priest, which pleased me greatly. When we sat down for the meal, the innkeeper came to me, asking "Will your Honour have some water?", because he was well aware that churchmen take precedence'.[53] In sharing the delight and mocking laughter of his fellow diners when, during this same meal, the true, lowly status of a rank-pulling, pretentious servant masquerading as his noble master was revealed, to his public shame and embarrassment, Guarinonius ridicules and condemns a comparable deception without drawing parallels with his own. In lazzo no.7, to Zanni's great pleasure, the student who is his master agrees to fulfil his wish to exchange clothes with him.[54] When Zanni struts out, his master's enemies approach, and mistaking him for the student, beat him up until he is half dead. When they refused to admit to the injustice of their behaviour even after realizing their mistake, Zanni has had more than enough of the status of being a master, and longs to reclaim his old clothes, job and position.

Lazzo no.27 combines four sins: Zanni's gluttony, sloth and envy for his master's status, and the anger of his master. They enter a pact whereby Zanni is completely freed of any work or exercise for a period of eight days, and permitted to rest his body and limbs totally, albeit with the proviso that, should he as much as move a single limb, his master will beat him black and blue. His master distracts the dozing Zanni by having a delicious bowl of macaroni brought to his bedside, but beats Zanni, forcing him back to his bed, when he tries to reach them. He continues to beat Zanni every time he breaks their pact again by trying to speak,

---

[51]   Gordon, *Lazzi*, 12, 55.

[52]   Innsbruck UL, Cod.110, I, f.514ᵛ.

[53]   Guarinonius, *Grewel*, 317. Eighteen years after *Grewel*'s publication, Daniel Zenn, Bishop of Brixen, formally granted Guarinonius permission to become a lay preacher to the young, in the mountain villages of the Tirol (Bücking, *Kultur und Gesellschaft in Tirol*, 9; Klaar, *Dr Hippolytus Guarinoni*, 38).

[54]   Another favourite lazzo, already represented in the 1568 Munich wedding performance (Troiano, *Dialoghi*, sig.149ᵛ–150ᵛ).

smell or see, and refuses to release him from the pact he regrets so naively entering. Zanni's frustrated attempts to satisfy his desire for this bowl of macaroni recall a Scala lazzo in which two comic servants are tied up and bound back-to-back. Every time one bends down to try and eat a tempting dish of ricotta cheese placed at their feet, the other is violently lifted into the air.[55] Later lazzi on this theme staged in Paris include one in which Scaramouche is continually frustrated in his attempts to satisfy his gluttony, at a magnificent table loaded with delicious food, and another in which a comic servant is unable to enjoy his status as king, because every time a dish of food is passed to him, his doctor confiscates it on health grounds.[56] Lazzo no.27 continues with, two hours later, Zanni being gripped by another basic physical need, forcing him to try to rise to relieve himself, despite continuous beatings to keep him down from his master. Only when, overcome by double incontinence,[57] he releases the contents of his bowels and bladder into his breeches, does his master finally release him from their pact, and his enforced rest. Plate 14 depicts a realistic indoor setting untypical of the comic stage, with an elaborate window and numerous props, including a live cat, and is linked with a proverb quoted in several Latin and vernacular versions by Guarinonius, admonishing the reader not to put off contemplating his last hours.[58] Although its inscription is primarily of allegorical rather than dramatic significance, its bedridden Zanni and attendant elderly master wear stock stage costume. They are engaged in a scatological encounter involving an overflowing chamber-pot which may draw on or reflect stage routines like lazzo no.27, which Guarinonius rounds off with a precise description of Zanni's discomfort and embarrassment at his soiled breeches, and the hearty laughter with which his spectators responded as he gingerly negotiated his way offstage.

Whether it befalls an injured servant, his elderly professor of medicine Jean Schyron in mid-lecture, two young German noblemen who ruin their fashionable outfits in a drunken stupor, or his friend and colleague Dr Jacob Myconius on a horseback journey after overindulging in unfermented wine, Felix Platter's approach to loss of bladder and bowel control is always that of the medical

---

[55]   Scala, *Il Teatro*, Day 42 ('Gli avvenimenti comici, pastorali e tragici'). See also Capozza, *Tutti i lazzi*, 272.

[56]   Biancolelli, 'La Rosaura imperatrice di Constantinopoli', 1658, 'La proprietà o Arlecchino re di Tripoli' (Gambelli, *Arlecchino a Parigi*, III, 739; Scott, *The commedia dell'arte in Paris*, 68); Capozza, *Tutti i lazzi*, 270–1. A similar lazzo involves two desperately hungry Zanni tied together in such a manner that they can only reach a bowl of food by diving between each other's legs. Having enlisted the present author's help with unravelling its mechanics at a delightful dinner party hosted in Venice by Virginia Scott, Rob Henke, aided by our chair Eric Nicholson, demonstrated it to great acclaim during the RSA 2010 panel presented by the four of us the following morning.

[57]   Elsewhere identified by Guarinonius as symptomatic of extreme fear (*Grewel*, 310).

[58]   Guarinonius, *Grewel*, 7, 223, 280, 1160; Maley, 'Hippolyt Guarinoni als Dichter', 330–1. 'Quidquid agas prudenter agas respice finem'.

professional.[59] He relates its occurrence as a routine symptom, whose status as a favoured source of early modern humour is implicit rather than openly acknowledged, as in his account of an incident involving his servant boy, Pierre Bonet, during a family journey to the Alpine spa town of Leukerbad:

> He had trodden on a nail, was limping, and so much sand and dirt had got into his little wound that he could hardly walk any more. I and my wife led him to the water, where he took off his hose, and I dug around in his little wound with my pocket knife, got out the sand and dirt. My wife watched us, and as he fainted away, my wife came up to us, wanting to support him so that he wouldn't fall. Then in his fear he shat himself, and the mess overflowed from his clothes onto my wife's blue apron. She ran from him, leaving the filthy mess lying there. When he regained consciousness and recovered from fainting, he wiped himself in the stream, immediately realizing that while I had dug around his small hole, he had purged himself through his big hole.[60]

Thomas Platter's rarer descriptions of public incontinence foreground comic effect over medical symptoms or cures, as when he describes his gluttonously intoxicated carriage-driver's ill-judged reaction to an encounter with a noble retinue on the road just outside Edingen in the Spanish Netherlands:

> When we were within about two pistol shots of the town, the Marquis d'Havré rode out of the town with several carriages to meet a great lord, accompanied by many horses. They rode past us on the road in a wide column. And because our drover had clients in almost all the villages and inns at which we had stopped on our way, he was always brought a draft of beer, of which he had drained so many that he was quite drunk. As the said marquis hastened past us, our carriage-driver, not wanting to be showed up, headed towards the town at full speed. This made his guts shake up in his body so much on horseback, that in front of everyone he had to dismount and clean himself with his shirt, causing great laughter.[61]

Grewel also contains autobiographical passages involving incontinence, such as a childhood memory of a game during which a six year-old who lost control of his bowels was shamed by an older boy.[62] While these are related in a factual style close to that of Felix Platter, Guarinonius's robust and explicit dramatic scatological episodes explicate the comic and ridiculous element much more

---

[59]   *Felix Platter Tagebuch*, 162, 228 (Spring 1553 and 20 September 1555, Montpellier), 347 (Autumn 1558, Thann).

[60]   *Felix Platter Tagebuch*, 403 (3 June 1563, Balsthal).

[61]   *Thomas Platter d.J*, 655–6 (20 August 1599, Edingen).

[62]   Guarinonius, *Grewel*, 883.

harshly than Thomas Platter, suggesting to some modern critics a response of 'shame, indignation or pity'.[63]

In marked contrast to Guarinonius's forthright approach to onstage incontinence, although his treatise vigorously condemns wanton dress, lewd speech and lecherous behaviour in everyday life and in the visual and dramatic arts, and they are stock elements of the Italian comedy, the nine or so of his lazzi concerned with the sin of lechery only vaguely allude to lascivious stage business. Lecherous goings on between stock commedia dell'arte characters, abundantly depicted in the visual record, are rarely explicated in detail in the surviving lazzi descriptions.[64] While discussing the health hazards of excessive carnal congress, within or outside marriage, Guarinonius emphasizes the bestiality of lust by constant reference to 'Venus fools', even 'Venus asses'.[65] Lechery in his lazzi is mostly that of Zanni's elderly or young master, sometimes combined with pride or gluttony. Lazzi nos.4 and 22 predictably pair the master's lechery with the servant's gluttony. In lazzo no.4, Zanni makes fun of his young master for letting his lovesickness render him incapable of enjoying food, drink or sleep, and expresses his appreciation that this situation allows him to enjoy many tasty meals he rejects. Lazzo no.22 is a detailed description of an elaborate scatological lazzo involving Zanni and Pantalone, and the sins of lechery, gluttony, incontinence, avarice, inquisitiveness and wrath, in which the standard contrast of lecherous master and gluttonous servant is temporarily imbalanced when Zanni engages his elderly master Pantalone in an animated discussion concerning identification of 'the greatest of all physical pleasures on earth'. Zanni ridicules all three of Pantalone's suggestions, namely the favours of his mistresses, delicious food and wine, or bags of ducats. Zanni points out that Pantalone's current riches benefit no one, because only fools gain pleasure from money, and it even drives some to hang themselves. He then reveals that his own very greatest pleasure is to vigorously unload his bowels after lengthy suppression of this need. While Zanni enlarges on his theme in graphic detail, his master is overcome by curiosity, and Zanni encourages him to delay his bowel movements for over two hours by walking and wriggling around on stage.

Plates 16a and 17, in which an anxious-looking Pantalone squats on the ground, his right hand supporting himself on his knee, his left hand holding his cloak clear of his backside, while Zanni towers imperiously above him, hands on hips, may reflect a scatological lazzo of this type. Several friendship albums include variants of this popular composition, all dating to around 1580, and perhaps from the same workshop.[66] This image is one of many compositions featuring scatological,

---

[63]   Sprengel, 'Herr Pantalon', 15.

[64]   Gordon, *Lazzi*, 32–5: 'Sexual/scatological lazzi'; Capozza, *Tutti i lazzi*, 91–123: 'Lazzi erotici'.

[65]   Guarinonius, *Grewel*, 1133–42 (Book 5, Chapter 69).

[66]   Variously accompanied by inscriptions to the effect that 'He who possesses neither virtue nor money is worthless in this world', 'It is better to be alone than in bad company'

obscene and erotic routines, involving characters wearing stock costumes of the early Italian comedy, whose exact relation to professional stage practice remains elusive, because it is unclear whether it is directly based on stage business, or depicts it at second-hand, reflected through the carnival revelry of costumed non-actors. The archetypally foolish 'ship of fools' used to transport the comic pair in Plate 16b foregrounds even more sharply the interpretative challenges of such pictures.[67] Although their costumes are clearly borrowed from the stage, such props may have allegorical rather than theatrical origins. Theatrical friendship album depictions were not always produced or bought simply as carefree reminders of Italian tourist attractions. Iain Brown notes of the 'Mascherata venetiana' and other Venetian costume pictures in Sir Michael Balfour's Scottish friendship album of around 1600: 'Venice was depicted as sin personified: sin in the guise of opulently dressed, aristocratic ladies with the most elaborate of coiffures, shameless courtesans with revealing costumes [...] and wicked happenings in a gondola'.[68] Early modern *ars apodemica* strongly associated Italy with 'unruly sexuality', and could 'admit the possibility of Italian pleasures only in order to warn the reader against them'.[69] Such associations inform the outlook of Guarinonius, illegitimate son of an Italian mother who contributed little to his upbringing, and a father whose profession positioned him at the very heart of the German Habsburg courts. He sharply reminded a 20-year-old Bavarian nobleman who claimed that his Italian studies taught him more in a month than he could learn in a year from the Munich Jesuits that Italian universities taught 'villainy not discipline and virtue, learning and art', and rhetorically asks his readers: 'Why is it that you wish to follow the Italians in all their follies, and ape all their clothing, gestures, and other matters like a monkey?'[70] Early modern German-speaking purchasers of friendship album costume images, Catholic as well as Protestant, did not simply view them as visually appealing souvenirs. In the context of stage and carnival, significant religious and political implications invested their images of masked stock characters of the Italian comedy with intensely negative undertones of decadent excess, deception, wanton folly and sinfulness.

Lazzo no.22 continues by describing how, urged on by Zanni, the old man fights for control. The physician Guarinonius notes that the actor walked up and down the stage simulating the symptoms of extreme alarm, by breathing rapidly, rolling his eyes, sticking out his tongue and screaming for help. Meanwhile, Zanni secretly summons out his master's mistress, and the old man, unexpectedly

---

or 'the tricks of Zannis and fools are fine words and wretched deeds' (see also Katritzky, *The art of commedia*, plate 250 and 'Comic stage routines', figure 7).

[67]   On Jacob Praun's friendship album, the source of plates 16, 19 and 34, see Schnabel, Die Stammbücher, 39–44. My profound thanks to Dr Werner Wilhelm Schnabel for drawing these pictures to my attention.

[68]   Brown, 'Water, windows and women', 15 and figs. 1, 5–10.

[69]   Craik, 'Reading *Coryats Crudities* 1611', 87–8.

[70]   Guarinonius, *Grewel*, 211, 671.

becoming aware of her presence, is shocked into relieving himself, with loud screams, into his breeches. Guarinonius notes that the woman was assaulted by a mighty smell – indicating an exaggeratedly negative mimed or spoken reaction by the actress – and that Zanni and the spectators reacted with hearty laughter. Ægidius Albertinus primarily derived his comparable stage descriptions, discussed in the following chapter, not from the stage, but directly from *Grewel*.[71] The scatological lazzi catalogued by Gordon are mainly variations on the theme of urination, and none of the defecation lazzi identified by Capozza provide anything comparable to the detail and clarity evoked in Guarinonius's treatise.[72] Rare examples of recorded lazzi involving stage simulations of incontinence symptoms include one in a Scala scenario. In this, the unsuspecting, elderly Pantalone's beautiful young wife facilitates a meeting with a young lover by pretending to need privacy to relieve herself, in order to mislead Pantalone into misinterpreting her obvious signs of physical exertion when she finally rejoins him.[73] More closely related to Guarinonius's scatological stage business than these sparse surviving commedia dell'arte records, are extended scatological stage dialogues in Ruzante's 'La Pastoral', or in traditional German Shrovetide comedies, of the type in which inarticulate, diarrhoea-ridden German peasants are interminably interrogated by incomprehending Italian-speaking quacks.[74] Regardless of whether Guarinonius's commedia dell'arte accounts were directly influenced by this German literary tradition, or relied only on memories of Italian performances, lazzi nos.22 and 27 offer unprecedented insights into the stage practice of scatological lazzi, and their enthusiastic audience response.

Lazzi nos.9[75] and 21 are variants on the popular theme of Zanni's duties as runner of errands and go-between for his master's love messages. Plate 12 is one of many images featuring the comic servant in this messenger role. It depicts a city street scene, in which a Zanni with a wicker shopping basket approaches a shop staffed by two traders, while a second Zanni, whose traditional white suit is complemented by a green cloak and black hat, dallies at the shop's entrance with a young woman. Like the Zanni, she wears a full-face mask. A second woman looks out from an open window above the shop front.[76] This and other pictures in the

---

[71]   Albertinus, *Gusman von Alfarche*, 452–60.

[72]   Gordon, *Lazzi*, 32–5: 'Sexual/scatological lazzi'; Capozza, *Tutti i lazzi*, 127–32: 'Lazzi scatologici'. For a Parisian defecation lazzo of 1672, see Scott, *The commedia dell'arte in Paris*, 203 (*Le collier de perle*).

[73]   Scala, *Il Teatro*, Day 6, *Il vecchio geloso*; see also Capozza 124, no.728.

[74]   On similar scenes in Vigil Raber, 'Der scheissend' (1516), see Siller, 'Der scheissennd', 153. Others of this genre include Peter Probst 'Ein kurtzweillich fasnacht Spil von krancken Baurn vnd einem doctor sambt seinem knecht' (1553); Hans Folz, 'Ein Faßnachtspil von einem Artzt vnd einem Krancken'.

[75]   The source for Albertinus' fifth lazzo, on which see Chapter 15, this volume.

[76]   The far right-hand of three windows, of which no more than their bases can be seen in reproduction, because the top of the picture is bound too tightly into the album's spine to

same album, also featuring characters in stock commedia dell'arte costumes, may be intended to represent genuine street scenes with masked carnival revellers, or actors on stage sets.[77] In lazzo no.21, Zanni succeeds in indulging his gluttony by exploiting his old master's lust. He deliberately delays delivering a message from his master's mistress until his master is seated at table and about to eat a delicious tart. Then, as if only just remembering it, Zanni gives his master the news that his mistress is urgently expecting him. No sooner has the old man hurried off to his beloved, than Zanni devours the tart.

Lechery is combined with pride in lazzo no.32, in which Pantalone, anxious to win a contest against a rival for his mistress, asks Zanni for advice. Zanni makes a fool of his lustful old master, by loading impossibly heavy weights onto his shoulders, then disappearing offstage, while Pantalone, thus burdened, is eventually forced to the ground by the weights even without any rival. Lazzo no.33 also concerns the theme of the lustful old master made a fool of by his servant, while trying to impress his mistress. Under the guise of teaching him to ride in a 'chivalrous' way that will be more impressive to his beloved, Zanni persuades Pantalone to mount his donkey 'backwards, with its tail in his hands for reins, lifting both legs as high as possible' and pointing them straight out on either side, thus adopting the ridiculous riding posture forced on quacks who are ridden out of town.[78] Elsewhere, Guarinonius explains that correct posture is very different to that of professional performers: 'not voluptuous, not frivolous, not shameless, not indecent, nor with fantastical or lascivious gestures of the body or limbs, as with itinerant entertainers, from all of which defective exercises, personal or physical damage can result'.[79]

In lazzo no.3, Zanni mocks his master Magnificus for woefully misinterpreting a friendly gesture from his beloved to her maid, by extravagantly celebrating it as a sign of her favour to him. Guarinonius offers this as an example of how love robs many of their wits, by distorting their interpretation of the evidence of their senses. In lazzo no.28, Zanni fiddles, while his old master Magnificus dances for joy at seeing his beloved at her window. After a while, Magnificus realizes that the woman over whom he is making a public fool of himself is not his beloved, but the gruesome 80-year-old bawd. In a comparable case of mistaken identity in the Locatelli scenari, the Captain beats an old woman after mistakenly courting her, while in another Locatelli lazzo, Zanni deliberately utilizes his delivery of a message to the bawd as an opportunity to flirt with the old woman.[80] Plate 7 depicts Zanni, holding an unsheathed dagger, and his lute-playing master, in an even less unequivocally joyful dance. Paulus Schuth signed the accompanying

---

allow photography without damaging the album: clear evidence that it was painted before being bound into the album.

[77]   See also Kurras, *Zu gutem Gedenken*, figs. 36 (1575), 37 (1574).
[78]   On which see Chapter 9, this volume.
[79]   Guarinonius, *Grewel*, 1161.
[80]   Gordon, *Lazzi*, 17, 52.

inscription not at the Venetian carnival, during the peak half-century of popularity for commedia dell'arte depictions in friendship albums (from around 1570 to 1620), but in Nürnberg, in October 1648. His chosen motto: 'Permanent merriness is impossible', also quoted in *Grewel*, refers to the sin of *inepta laetitia*, or inappropriate merriment, the subject of lazzo no.28. Chapter 23 of *Grewel*'s second book warns of grave health risks associated with indulging in this sin, including the danger of triggering fatal choking fits and heart attacks through excessive laughter.[81]

Grewel's lazzi also provide two briefer allusions to the theme of elderly lechery on the comic stage. Lazzo no.5 notes that the lecherous old man has become a stock character in the Italian comedy, because he gives the actors their most effective way of making their audiences laugh, and that it ill becomes old men to take part in war or love, because age should bring wisdom, not provide a bad example for the young. An unpublished phrase in the pre-revised manuscript adds that while diverting to read about, such behaviour is tiresome to watch.[82] Guarinonius dismisses mineral springs and public baths as places for those who foolishly try to save the few coins they would be better off paying a qualified physician for proper medical advice, 'houses of disgrace' into which no honest man should allow his wife unless he wants to be crowned with cuckolds' horns.[83] Lazzo no.26 unfavourably compares the folly of husbands who allow their wives to frequent mineral springs with that of the 'cuckolded Venetian Pantalone', shown up in comedies as 'a blind fool' partnered by a wife who is 'a vulgar strumpet', because errant wives use springs as a convenient meeting-place for 'their gallants and lovers, or the nearest sturdy young lumberjack from the surrounding forests'. Remarkably open comments in Felix Platter's journal confirm such goings on. During his 1563 visit to the Valais, to take his wife to Leukerbad, he recalls being the recipient of always unsought, but not invariably repelled, alcohol-fuelled lecherous attentions, shamelessly pressed on him by more than one adulterously-minded woman.[84]

The Platter brothers often visited mineral springs for professional reasons. During his first week in Montpellier, Thomas Platter joined 20 medical students collecting local medicinal plants and herbs, led by François Ranchin to the medicinal hot springs of Balaruc, a walled village of around 90 households, some 16 miles south-west of Montpellier. Despite poor facilities, the perceived powerful properties of Balaruc's waters attracted wealthy patients from the region, and especially from neighbouring Montpellier, whose physicians had the sole right to

---

[81]   Guarinonius, *Grewel*, 172, 239–42.

[82]   Innsbruck UL, Cod.110, I, f.417ᵛ.

[83]   Guarinonius, *Grewel*, 250, 948, 956.

[84]   *Felix Platter Tagebuch*, 408, 416–17, 421 (June 1563, Sion, Visp, Leukerbad). In 1553, his mother visited Bad Lostorf for its sulphurous waters, renowned for gout and rheumatism (185: September 1553, Montpellier). Lötscher, *Felix Platter und seine Familie*, 114–15; Le Roy Ladurie, *The beggar and the professor*, 7.

prescribe and profit from its waters. There were few bathing booths and the warm, salty and soupy waters were more revered for their medicinal than for their healing properties. Patients were typically advised to drink between six and 12 glasses a day, and take coastal walks to aid their purgative effects. According to Platter, due to the absence of trees or bushes, the resulting evacuations could be observed by all. Platter's description of his return in May 1596 evokes the fairground-like atmosphere of mineral spring resorts in high season, at a time when they offered a significant economic forum for both performing and healing. He bought sea shells from one of the numerous merchants, including an apothecary, trading from temporary booths, and compares the diversity of performances and spectacles on offer to what he was used to from saints' days' fairs.[85]

An eighth sin, *curiositas* or inquisitiveness, indexed 22 times in *Grewel*, plays a significant part in lazzi nos.9 and 22, and dominates in lazzo no.8. Shocked by the relative lack of censure attracted by this sin, Guarinonius denounced it as the most widespread, and one of the greatest, of all sins. None of the seven 'deadly' sins plays a prominent role in lazzo no.8. Featuring a Zanni who gets into trouble when he cannot resist investigating his sighting of ghosts and a Devil, it targets 'inquisitiveness in looking at forbidden things', a type of excessively prying impertinent curiosity sharply differentiated from the 'positive' masculine pursuits of knowledge-led scientific collecting and investigation throughout the early modern period and beyond.[86] Warning that it gravely threatens the bodies and souls of those who succumb to it, Guarinonius leaves his readers in no doubt of its sinful nature. Although lazzo no.8 specifies no actresses, the sin of curiosity is specifically linked to women in *Grewel*, where Guarinonius's consideration of it affords him opportunities for extended misogynist passages on 'female folly'.[87] A discussion of 'unnecessary, useless and frivolous spectacles' indicates some dangers threatening over-inquisitive male and female spectators at public quack stages. The impersonal published account replaces a longer eyewitness account of a commedia dell'arte performance in Padua, deleted but still partially legible in the pre-revised manuscript version, revealing *curiositas* as a sin to which even Guarinonius was not immune. In this latter he describes in the first person how, while watching charlatans perform their farces in Padua's Piazza dei Signori (as one is depicted doing more than 70 years later in Plate 5), his cloak and hat were stolen in a crush of spectators so great that he could hardly breathe.[88]

Thomas Platter lists the practice of stealing hats and coats off people in large public gatherings among typical crimes of rowdy Toulouse students.[89]

---

[85]   *Thomas Platter d.J*, 85–7, 149–50 (13–14 October 1595 and 25–27 May 1596, Balaruc).

[86]   Benedict, *Curiosity*, 118.

[87]   Guarinonius, *Grewel*, 65–9, 368–79 (Book 2, Chapter 37: 'On the abomination of inquisitiveness'); Innsbruck UL, Cod.110, I, f.541^v ('Fürwitz').

[88]   Innsbruck UL, Cod.110, I, ff.540–4.

[89]   *Thomas Platter d.J*, 415 (27 April 1599, Toulouse).

Guarinonius's cloak and hat both reappeared a few days later, sported by an Italian promenading up and down the Piazza dei Signori, prompting him to regret his idle inquisitiveness, and to relief that he lost items of clothing rather than his health or life. The published version excludes all traces of the physician's disarming admission that he too is susceptible to the sin of curiosity. It replaces his first person account with a brief impersonal report on conflicts caused by the charlatans' ability to turn the prying curiosity of the uneducated to their advantage, by attracting huge crowds, identified as a major civic safety hazard:

> Charlatans or comedians perform their tricks on every Italian square. And because the crowds run to them in such numbers to watch their foolery, longstanding disputes often unexpectedly flare up. When unsheathed weapons gleam everywhere, the crowd takes fright. In the ensuing crush to escape one loses a hat, another a coat or purse, some even leave behind their hand, a foot, or even their life. Even pregnant women cannot protect themselves in such an inquisitive crush, so these disorderly events put them and their unborn children in great danger.[90]

This passage again demonstrates that while *Grewel*'s strong polemical slant is not incompatible with the broadly factual presentation of its commedia dell'arte episodes, they cannot be taken at face value, as literal, unadorned descriptions of the stage business of quacks. Comparison of *Grewel*'s manuscript, and its *addenda* and *corrigenda*, with the published treatise, suggests that several of Guarinonius's lazzi have non-theatrical origins.

Guarinonius's revisions significantly lengthen lazzo no.16, and boost the Italian comedy content of the surviving manuscript texts to 21 lazzi, by adding several completely new lazzi, and adapting lazzo no.6 from a short autobiographical account of an actual event unrelated to the stage, to a longer episode involving stock commedia dell'arte characters.[91] The theatricality of his autobiographical interpolations has been taken by some as a possible reflection of techniques absorbed from the commedia dell'arte.[92] Less speculative is that, for the most part, his lazzi genuinely seem to be drawn from his own first-hand experiences, and that their theatrical content may be taken to represent a reasonably undistorted reflection of actual stage practice. As such, their interpretation is little affected by a problem common to much of the documentary material associated with the commedia dell'arte, namely that of establishing the degree of influence of earlier visual or textual documentations of stage practice. However, any attempt to evaluate the significance of these episodes for the early modern stage has

---

[90]   Guarinonius, *Grewel*, 373.

[91]   Innsbruck UL, Cod.110, I, ff.545ʳ; 547ʳ; II, ff.253ʳ, 266ᵛ, 274ʳ, 462ʳ, 512ᵛ–513ʳ. The manuscript includes lazzi nos.1–21 (of which lazzi nos.8, 9, 12–15 are added at revision stage).

[92]   Kemp, 'Hippolytus Guarinonuis als Schriftsteller', 17.

to address another challenge. Each of them has to be located on a very broad spectrum, ranging from accurately observed stage business, right through to material which may have had little or no connection with the stage, prior to heavy editing, to fit in with Guarinonius's employment of the literary device of using the stage fools of the Italian comedy as potent symbols of folly and sinful behaviour, in his medical treatise. Even the selection and presentation of lazzi based solely on stage business is distorted by Guarinonius's concern to contrast the sinful folly of the stage fools of the Italian comedy with the wise behaviour of devout German Catholics responsibly promoting their own health and well-being. His revisions reflect a conscious stylistic decision on his part, to maximize the impact of the commedia dell'arte content of his treatise. The following chapter examines some motivations and receptions of Guarinonius's theatrical inclusions.

Chapter 15
Physical, Mental and Spiritual Health: Stage Fools in a Medical Treatise

Written in the vernacular, *Grewel* deliberately targeted a wide lay and medical readership. Even within Guarinonius's own lifetime, many of his readers failed to understand why a learned medical treatise addressing devout Catholic males should contain any descriptions of secular professional stage business at all, let alone so many, and so scatological in content. His judgment in including this theatrical material was challenged. Few of his readers appreciated the extent to which its inclusion, or the comprehensive programme of changes Guarinonius undertook to enhance it while revising his manuscript, were influenced by the conventions of the late medieval literary genre of moral satire sometimes referred to as folly literature ('Narrenliteratur'). Inaugurated by Sebastian Brant in 1494, Desiderius Erasmus, Thomas Murner and François Rabelais were among those who contributed major works to this ethically-motivated literary genre. At this time, increasing tensions between canon and civil law precipitated unprecedented literary interest in sin, and popular fear of the Devil as the supernatural, satanic, personification of evil prompted Heinrich Kramer's *Malleus Maleficarum* (1486) and the Spanish Inquisition. Folly literature shifted responsibility for malevolent evil and its consequences away from external demons, and towards internal human sins and folly. Variously equating folly with carnival excess, amorality, ugliness and mental instability, the genre camouflages radical social criticism with satirical censure of specific sins.[1] Physicians were drawn to folly literature's healing dimension, its refinement of an influential literary convention dating back to Lucretius, whereby authors drew on quack rhetoric and theories of laughter therapy to present their writings as a literal cure in themselves. This concluding chapter of these investigations into the writings of Guarinonius and the Platter brothers features folly literature in this context.

Some critics of *Grewel* were sufficiently outraged by Guarinonius's detailed descriptions of the reviled itinerant quack troupes' lazzi to openly attack his reputation as a respected court physician and public health officer. The present chapter revisits these concerns in the light of early modern literary responses to them, not least Guarinonius's own. His tentatively acknowledged anticipations of such misgivings in *Grewel* itself suggest that he gravely underestimated the degree of their severity. *Grewel*'s introduction ends with repeated references to its comical and diverting passages, while its closing chapter disingenuously claims

---

[1]   Brüggemann, *Die Angst vor dem Bösen*, 20–7, 209–19, 283.

no further agenda to its inclusion of comic dramatic episodes, than to leaven its serious content, by mixing in 'diverting and amusing tricks, because, to tell the truth, my nature does not incline me to melancholic tedium'.[2] Indisputably, one major function of Guarinonius's comic theatrical episodes or lazzi is anecdotal, complementing and leavening medical points made in his lengthy treatise. But his ambitions were more complex. He viewed his patients' physical bodies as only one aspect of his responsibilities as a physician. Considering the world and humanity 'immeasurably enlightened and wiser through the true Roman Catholic Faith', he regarded humans as 'half angel and half beast', the sum of 'two quite separate and contrasting components, one, incorruptible and immortal, being the intelligent soul, the second, mortal and subject to decomposition, the body'.[3]

As he reiterates in his plague treatise of 1612, Guarinonius wrote *Grewel* to serve and glorify God.[4] Its structure, placing God both firmly above the six Hippocratic non-naturals, and at the centre of Guarinonius's health agenda, is summarized in 'Gesondt', the acrostic for the word 'health' he devised to showcase the word 'God' and summarize his medical approach.[5] For him, the two greatest gifts of mankind, 'a pure and sin free soul and good health', were inextricably connected. His medical agenda is based on the premise that virtuous living and a clear conscience are the most essential 'theriac', or medicine, for a healthy body and life.[6] Far from being random, his choice of lazzi from the Italian comedy was dictated by the tightly planned didactic agenda intimated in *Grewel*'s dedicatory prefaces, to the Virgin Mary and Emperor Rudolf II. Proclaiming that 'it has almost universally come to that most deceitful, ignoble and materialistic blindness, that while most people make the effort to inform themselves concerning temporary and physical health, they ignore their spiritual and permanent health', Guarinonius likens this approach to that of the short-sighted craftsman who invests effort into using real gold to set a worthless imitation jewel, and brands the Reformation the greatest threat to German souls.[7] Readings of *Grewel* which view his counter-Reformational strategy as either dictating or being dominated by his medical aims are less productive than those which accept that his holistic view of the human body, mind, and soul is based on his conviction that spiritual and physical health indivisibly depend on each other.

---

2   Guarinonius, *Grewel*, 4, 1330.

3   Guarinonius, *Grewel*, 9, 48, 167.

4   Guarinonius, *Pestilentz Guardien*, 164–6.

5   Guarinonius, *Grewel*, 110, 142: 'G-e-s-o-n-d-T' (G[ott /God] E[ssen vnd trincken /food and drink] S[chlafen vnd wachen /sleeping and waking] O[ede oder Ringerung deß Uberfluß /elimination of waste] N[utzung oder Ubung deß Leibs /exercise] D[auglich Lufft /air] T[rost deß Gemühts /solace of the soul]). See also p.40, this volume.

6   Guarinonius, *Grewel*, 108, 311.

7   Guarinonius, *Grewel*, 'Dedicatio' [Aviᵛ].

Guarinonius and Albertinus

A context suggesting that the moralizing and didactic intent of Guarinonius's lazzi descriptions was both understood and admired by contemporary German Catholics, and in which their significance has long been widely recognized by literary historians, occurs in a fictional account published only five years after *Grewel*. Its author, the Munich courtier and Netherlandish Catholic convert Ægidius Albertinus, copied long passages from five of Guarinonius's lazzi almost word-for-word into his free German translation of an unauthorized sequel[8] to Mateo Alemán's Spanish picaresque novel *Guzmán de Alfarache*.[9] A year later, in 1616, Albertinus extensively explored the seven deadly sins in a late contribution to folly literature entitled *Lucifers Königreich und Seelengejaidt oder Narrenhatz*. His five derivative interpolations in *Gusman von Alfarche* were linked with Guarinonius by 1889, but it took another century to formally identify the exact passages in *Grewel* on which they were based.[10] They occur in a chapter in Albertinus's book, the first German-language picaresque novel, entitled 'Gusman changes from a miner to a comedian, and relates several comical diversions which he acted'.[11] This describes how the itinerant hero Gusman joins a troupe of nine wandering players whom, significantly for the chapter's Tirolean source, he meets in 'the widely famed city of Innsbruck'. Later references trace this fictional troupe's wanderings through Germany, the Netherlands and France to Spain. Here they present 'a comedy and tragedy' at the very wedding festival Thomas Platter so regretted missing in 1599, when it was relocated from Barcelona to Valencia, that of King Philip III.[12]

Valentin's comparative publication of all but one paragraph of Albertinus's chapter 54, and relevant sections from *Grewel*, clearly demonstrates how closely the lazzi descriptions of Albertinus, writing in 1615, follow those of Guarinonius's treatise of 1610.[13] A key paragraph, directly following one which outlines plays whose representations of pious Christian lives have inspired 'some Godless people who have been led astray' to return to the path of virtue, reveals that the comedies staged by Gusman's troupe are not of this type:

> By contrast, you can find other comedians, who as well as acting good historical plays also present comical farces and acrobatics with them, and stage diverting tricks, and travel from one place to another. Just such comedians were these, and

---

[8]   Written and pseudonymously published in 1602 by Juan Marti.

[9]   Albertinus, *Gusman von Alfarche*, 452–60; Valentin, *Theatrum Catholicum*, 22–8 and *Französischer 'Roman comique'*, 9–10.

[10]   Trautmann, 'Deutsche Schauspieler', 386n205; Gemert, 'Übersetzung und Kompilation', 142.

[11]   On miners as performers, see Chapter 6, this volume.

[12]   Albertinus, *Gusman von Alfarche*, 489.

[13]   Valentin references the pagination of the first, 1615, edition, but spelling of the 1618 edition (*Theatrum Catholicum*, 34–41).

with them I travelled throughout the whole of Germany and the Netherlands. I was extremely happy being with them, and became very popular through my skilful drolleries, for soon I was also representing and acting a servant of an old Master who was in love, by the name of Pantaleon, and I was called Gusmändl.[14]

This paragraph introduces the five lazzi descriptions with which Albertinus concludes the chapter, of which the first four closely follow the spirit and wording of four of Guarinonius's episodes (lazzi nos.22, 23, 21, 12).

Albertinus's version of lazzo no.22, some 40 per cent shorter than Guarinonius's original, is almost the same length as the remaining four episodes, and all five are related in the first person by Albertinus's fictional hero, Gusman, as typical scenes between himself and Pantalone, from plays staged by their troupe, rather than in the third person, used by Guarinonius. This and certain other minor deviations from Guarinonius in Albertinus's versions of lazzi nos.22, 23 and 12, contribute to their heightened effect of obscene physicality. They include, in Albertinus's versions of lazzi nos.22 and 23, the naming of Pantalone's backside, the specific body part on which these two lazzi focus; and in his version of lazzo no.12, that the servant, rather than simply advising his master to eat as much as he can, exhorts him to stuff and swill himself to choking point. In the fifth and final lazzo, with which Albertinus concludes this chapter, the heightening of obscene physicality achieved in his first four lazzi is taken much further, in an episode twice as long as the original source, lazzo no.9. Like lazzo no.21, a variation on the popular theme of the comic servant delivering a love message, in lazzo no.9, Zanni is led to the radical action of eating his master's token of affection for his beloved. Guarinonius identifies the vice concerned not as gluttony, but as inquisitiveness. It features Zanni delivering a pie, a popular lazzi plot in few of whose many variations the pie was ever consumed by the intended recipient.[15] In order to keep it as far as possible out of temptation's way, he had been instructed to carry it to his master's mistress on his head. Prompted to uncontrollable salivation by its delicious smell, Zanni became increasingly unable to resist succumbing to the temptations of the sin of curiosity. This led him first to investigate what he was carrying, then what was in it, furthermore, to speculate on how it tasted, and what it would be like to have the experience of stilling his hunger by eating it. In this way, his excessive curiosity led him to polish the pie off completely. Whereupon he felt encouraged to return

---

[14]   Albertinus, *Gusman von Alfarche*, 454. This paragraph, omitted by Valentin (*Theatrum Catholicum*, 34, 37), links '[…] Leben an sich zunemmen' with 'Einsmals fragte ich […]'.

[15]   Capozza, *Tutti i lazzi*, 268–72: nos.1447–8, 1451, 1462. Never suspecting the possibility of a leg-pulling hoax of the type practiced by Montaigne's 'Gentleman' (in 'Of the force of imagination', *Essayes*, 44), Felix Platter was 'not best pleased by the deception' of being told that the 'rabbit' pie served to him at a final farewell supper, arranged in his honour by fellow medical students, was made with cat meat (*Felix Platter Tagebuch*, 262: 21 January 1557, Montpellier).

with renewed vigour to his now redundant task of delivering the already-eaten pie. Like his other four lazzi, and like lazzo no.9, Albertinus's fifth lazzo features the sin of gluttony. But, using Guarinonius's episode as a starting point, Albertinus radically changes its emphasis.

As in Albertinus's first two lazzi, based on Guarinonius's lazzi nos.22 and 23, the main focus is an episode of bodily incontinence, made more shocking here, to a readership for whom professional actresses were a very recent novelty, by the fact that it concerns a woman. As in lazzo no.9, Zanni's lecherous master gives him the task of delivering a pie to his beloved. But Albertinus's Gusmändl, who intensely dislikes his master's beloved, whom he considers extremely lewd, is not given the pie by his master, but orders it from the pastry cook, and there is no question of the sin of curiosity tempting him into eating it himself, because he includes a powerful purgative among the ingredients with which he provides the cook. This relates to one of Guarinonius's autobiographical episodes. After he spiked a large cheese in his larder with a poisonous purgative to identify the culprit systematically stealing small pieces from it, a 'greedy maid' in his employ broke down on suffering two days of unbearable dysentery, and confessed that she had been using the end of a codpiece lace to fake mouse bites on it.[16] When Gusmändl's pie is ready, he delivers it to his master's beloved, who gluttonously devours the whole pie with great gusto. Around half an hour later, Gusmändl sought an opportunity to bring her back onto the stage, and to promenade up and down in conversation with her. Meanwhile, the purgative took such an effect that she began to complain of stomach pains, and made as if to leave the stage and retire. Whereupon Gusmändl seized her from behind, lifting her skirt, and continuing to restrain her, until at last she began to throw up from above and below, producing a powerful stench for the spectators. Albertinus notes that this prank earned the servant a good hiding from his master, and hearty laughter from his audience.

Albertinus's borrowings demonstrate how, comparably to the development of visual traditions when artists drew on each other's work, literary traditions developed, when writers drew on previous authors instead of, or as well as, their own first-hand theatrical experiences, to augment or replace eyewitness reports with literary borrowings. Valentin has suggested that Albertinus may have used some unidentified German carnival farce to supplement the Guarinonius episode, and the possibility that he is drawing on first-hand experience of the popular stage cannot be ruled out.[17] The question of whether Albertinus augmented this lazzo from his imagination, or from another literary source, or perhaps even by drawing on first-hand experience of the popular stage, is relevant to the interpretation of compositions such as those depicted in Plates 18 or 19. In Plate 18, a coloured drawing based on a print, an unmasked Pantalone with a fur-lined black cloak over his red under-suit, and a Zanni in a dark beige suit, black hat and dark face-

---

[16]   Guarinonius, *Grewel*, 377–8.
[17]   Valentin, *Theatrum Catholicum*, 41.

mask, both white-bearded, molest a scantily-clad woman, and Plate 19 depicts the same theatrical stock roles, engaged in similar horseplay. Such drawings possibly reflect stage lazzi of the type described by Albertinus, who is concerned to reach a readership of women as well as men. Three of his five lazzi feature actresses, and in the fifth, it is a woman who takes centre stage to warn his readers against foolish behaviour, through a graphic demonstration of the dire consequences of the sins of gluttony, and, by implication, lechery.

Foolishness and Folly Literature

Unlike Albertinus, Guarinonius is primarily addressing the Catholic male, and in his 35 lazzi, the sins and follies representing deviations from a healthy and sin-free lifestyle are demonstrated by male actors, with actresses relegated to supporting roles. The context of his lazzi, not a diverting work of fiction (like Albertinus's pirated versions), but a serious medical treatise, prompted considerable criticism. Two years after their publication, Guarinonius addresses this in the fourth and final section of *Pestilentz Guardien*, which provides a carefully considered defence of *Grewel*'s lazzi in the form of question and answer dialogue responses to 13 specific criticisms.[18] The first question in effect censures *Grewel* for trespassing into the territory of spiritual healing, Church-controlled areas of mental healthcare such as Confession, pilgrimage or exorcism. Well aware that Guarinonius's ultimate concern was not the physical, but the spiritual well-being of his readers, this critic nevertheless maintained that 'criticizing sins is the domain of priests, not doctors of medicine'. Making the case that it was perfectly acceptable for physicians to write about the gluttonous sin of alcoholism, Guarinonius responds:

> You say that alcoholism concerns the body, the other [sins] the soul. Isn't irresponsible anger a vice? Is it not one of the seven abominations or deadly sins? Has it never made anyone ill? Who can deny it? Then how should the physician heal his patient, if he can't censure the cause of the illness, namely the anger? [...] Doctors of medicine are responsible for the human soul just as much as the body, and mental illnesses are just as serious as physical ones [...] You should know that I am not merely a simple doctor. In addition to the natural sciences, I studied the moral sciences, namely the ethical, Christian discipline of distinguishing between good and evil, the virtues and the sins.[19]

His fifth response robustly admonishes a reader who challenges his judgment, in including *Grewel*'s 'pathetic' and 'disgusting' comic episodes. In a passage

---

18   Guarinonius, *Pestilentz Guardien*, 164–203*.

19   Guarinonius, *Pestilentz Guardien*, 169–72. On spiritual healing, see Grell and Cunningham, 'Medicine and religion'; Kerwin, *Beyond the body*, 219–24; Lederer, *Madness, religion and the state*, 1–21.

drawing parallels with obscene and scatological behaviour described in didactic biblical passages, Guarinonius rounds on this critical reader for failing to recognize such biblical precedence for his literary strategies: 'Hardly anything could be more pathetic and disgusting than your profound ignorance and folly.' He points out that the Holy Scriptures contain unsavoury passages such as those on the false heathen Pontius Pilate, Sarah's scorn for the word of the Angel, King Saul's physical incontinence, or the sexual incontinence of Lot or King David. He berates his misguided critic for not realizing that, as in the Bible, *Grewel*'s descriptions of sinful behaviour are intended as deterrents, not as examples. In conclusion, he suggests that every time he, Guarinonius, laughs in his book, any reader misguided enough to criticize this literary strategy should weep at his own folly.[20]

Here, Guarinonius encapsulates a major principle of folly literature, in which court or stage fools powerfully exemplify human frailties and temptations. Not least because of their colourful stock costumes, grotesque physical contortions and face masks, stage fools and, above all, the masked servants of the Italian comedy, came to personify folly, and specifically the folly of the sinner in iconographical representations, and to a lesser extent, also in literature. Together with card-sharps and jugglers, who rely largely on manual dexterity, and those, such as professional fencers, sword dancers and tightrope walkers, who specialize in displays involving physical risk, Guarinonius defines travelling players as a sub-group of professional fools and acrobats. He amply demonstrates his awareness of their lowly social status, and of the moral threat of secular drama, especially that staged by the itinerant Italian charlatans.[21] His own Italian background, emphasized by his liberal use of Italian words and phrases in the reported speech of the servant–master pair, adds a further layer to the allegorical function of the commedia dell'arte episodes in his treatise.

The relationship between early modern folly, or foolishness, and the modern concepts of intellectual disability and mental illness is far from straightforward.[22] Modern medical interpretations of early modern folly are powerfully distorted by its cultural reflections in images and literary texts.[23] Unlike the modern concept of mental disability as a physical illness, folly suggests a strong element of sinful character weakness, introducing the potential for growth and redemption through the acceptance of personal responsibility. Or, as Bodin puts it, 'folly not originating from illness is one of the signs indicating that a person is possessed by an evil spirit'.[24] It foregrounds irrational moral disorder, an inability to comprehend religion not present in the strictly pathological later psychiatric concepts of madness, and is closely linked to the concept of sin, particularly

---

[20]   Guarinonius, *Pestilentz Guardien*, 182–3.

[21]   Guarinonius, *Grewel*, 66, 214, 1256.

[22]   Plat[t]er, Cole and Culpeper, *A golden practice*, 26–7; Schupbach, 'The cure of folly', 279; Goodey, 'Foolishness', 289–90; Lederer, *Madness, religion and the state*, 9–10.

[23]   Midelfort, *A history of madness*, 228–76.

[24]   Bodin, *Demonomanie*, sig.155ᵛ.

in the God-denying fool of the Old Testament psalms, repeatedly evoked by Guarinonius as the greatest of all fools.[25] Guarinonius, for whom the concepts of folly ('Narrheit') and madness ('Thorheit') were virtually interchangeable, saw fools everywhere.[26] Folly and fools – most especially Italian stage fools – are a major literary *leitmotiv* of his essentially serious medical treatise. Its copious deployment of folly-related vocabulary and rhetorical devices is motivated by counter-Reformational concerns.[27] In direct addresses, they often serve to distance the reader socially and intellectually from Guarinonius.[28] Sometimes, they are used to highlight readers' failings, as when listing sins ('one fool likes his money, another his cap, the third likes women, the fourth variegated colours, the fifth his folly stick'), or denouncing barber-surgeons' use of almanacs ('certainly a plump and well-fattened madness, richly deserving and worthy of the folly stick, cap and bells'), card-playing or the time-honoured custom of drinking alcoholic toasts to the 'health' of friends and lovers:

> Oh, unconsidered madness above all madnesses! Oh, worthy folly that should be crowned and honoured a hundredfold with foolscaps and asses' bells. [...] How can your toast help this or that person? Explain what type of bizarre method for promoting health this is, that endangers your own?[29]

A whole chapter of *Grewel* turns on the laboured metaphor of comparing human diet to the patched garments of professional fools.[30] Guarinonius repeatedly identifies genuine happiness as a virtue in its own right, and the key to longevity and health: 'Nothing better, more certain, more magnificent and splendid than

---

[25]   As in two couplets from chapters on astrologers, witches and fortune-tellers, and on deniers of God, in the unpublished second volume of *Grewel* (Innsbruck UL, Cod.110, IV, ff.452^v–453^r; see also Guarinonius, *Grewel*, 69, 154–5), drawing directly on the opening verse of Psalms 14 and 53: 'The fool hath said in his heart, *There is* no God' (*King James Bible*: Psalms 14 and 53, v.1; see also Psalm 36, v.1: 'The transgression of the wicked saith within my heart, *that there is* no fear of God before his eyes').

[26]   'Stultorum plena sunt omnia' (Guarinonius, *Grewel*, 1043).

[27]   Brandauer, 'Die poetischen Teile', 16; Gebhardt, 'Der "Gegenreformator" Hippolyt Guarinoni', 98–9.

[28]   As in: 'Oh you Fool', 'Dear Fool', 'Who could be foolish enough to deny this?', 'Shame on you fool', 'Welcome, Mr. Gut-and-Guzzle Fool', 'Oh, you coarse guzzle-fool', 'You guzzle-fool of all guzzle-fools', 'You more than thousandfold fool above all fools' (Guarinonius, *Grewel*, 77, 90–1, 165, 178, 647–8, 1073). One critic of *Grewel* is addressed as 'you most vulgar of all fools', others are rhetorically asked: 'Why have you become a fool?', 'Do you see your folly?' or 'Do you not understand that you are turning yourself into a public fool?' (Guarinonius, *Pestilentz Guardien*, 176–8, 196). See also Siller, 'Die Sprache des Hippolytus Guarinonius', 40–1.

[29]   Guarinonius, *Grewel*, 68, 709, 998, 1259.

[30]   Guarinonius, *Grewel*, 523–5 (Book 4, Chapter 2: 'Simple example whereby most characteristics of human diet can be explained').

spiritual and mental happiness, can be devised or invented for a long healthy life'.[31] *Grewel* explicitly refers to those favoured imaginary sites of folly literature, the gluttonous Land of Cockaigne and the anarchic Ship of Fools, and particularly emphasizes the health-threatening dangers of foolish behaviour in eight central chapters identifying wine and beer taverns as major social hothouses for key health-threatening human sins and follies.[32] In a passage following on directly from a criticism of the unseemly jollity often generated by fools and jesters hired to entertain at feasts and weddings, Guarinonius warns that happiness is founded in reason, not 'bestial' sin. Quoting the motto 'Stultitia gaudium Stulto' (fools rejoice in folly), he notes that 'virtue is not to be sought amongst fools', because the happiness they offer is not genuine but harmful. That there are, despite this, many in this world who seek fire in water, fish in the ground, and virtue in fools, he continues, is due to their own folly, which leads them to greatly prefer to listen to and follow a fool than a virtuous, educated man, and to forget that 'no-one escapes unfooled from the fools'.[33]

Guarinonius's moralizing literary use of the Italian comedy's stage fools to counterpoint the serious content of his treatise, may be compared to the iconographic inclusion of commedia dell'arte fools in the grotesque scenes used in certain late sixteenth-century visual programmes. One such is the frieze of 16 grotesque Italian comedy scenes of 1576, destroyed by fire in 1961, with which Christoph Schwarz[34] framed an illustration of princely virtues in the Bavarian Castle Trausnitz cycle.[35] Here, stock commedia dell'arte characters personify sinful folly. They elicit complex critical responses reinforcing perceived links between the demonic, the monstrous and the grotesque: between diabolical stage devils and transgressive carnival, stage or court fools; evil sin and ridiculous folly; fear and laughter. Spectators are simultaneously warned of the humiliating consequences of various types of sinful and foolish behaviour, and offered the healing redemption of therapeutic laughter. Guarinonius's treatise in a sense transmutes quack theatrical episodes into the literary equivalent of such visual grotesques.

Dramatically, the function of Grewel's theatrical scenes has parallels with stage devils and the figure of Vice in late sixteenth-century popular drama, and even more with the stage quacks central to the so-called merchant scene of late medieval religious plays. This significant theatrical forerunner of the folly literature tradition increasingly dominated some medieval mystery plays. Notwithstanding their extremely tenuous New Testament credentials, speaking

---

[31]   Guarinonius, *Grewel*, 169.

[32]   Guarinonius, *Grewel*, 344, 777, 789–90, 809, 819–63 (Innsbruck UL, Cod.110, IV, ff.63–71).

[33]   Guarinonius, *Grewel*, 237–8.

[34]   One of whose religious paintings is praised by Guarinonius, a keen amateur painter (*Grewel*, 231).

[35]   Katritzky, *The art of commedia*, 50–3 and plates 22–3.

quacks had already established themselves in Easter mystery plays by the eleventh century. From the twelfth century onwards, they make an increasing impact on religious drama, providing a profane secular counterpart to the healing Christ of the Gospel miracles.[36] In the merchant scene, an itinerant quack sometimes sells the three Marys[37] herbs and spices at the tomb of Christ. Its most fully developed versions replace the lone quack with a small troupe, led by a married quack couple, who pad out his essentially brief selling routine with bawdy comic interchanges of total biblical irrelevance. They typically prepare and market their medicines and cosmetics, puff their skills, barter and banter with the Holy women, and crack surprisingly robust jokes, often of a medical nature. The merchant scene's dramatic function was to heighten the intensity of the contrast between profane and spiritual concerns in religious plays, by ridiculing earthly pleasures.[38] The concrete examples through which religious stage quacks exemplify human folly have two complementary intentions: to cure spectators' souls through didactic counter-example, and their minds and bodies by entertaining them sufficiently to actively promote healing through the liberating, visceral laughter then regarded as the most effective therapy for melancholy.

Folly literature is informed by these dual healing aims. Promoted by Brant's *Ship of fools* (1494) and Erasmus's *Praise of folly* (1511), they were comprehensively explored by François Rabelais, who studied medicine at Montpellier with several of Felix Platter's most influential teachers. In the preface to his 1575 German adaptation of the 1534 first volume of Rabelais's four-volume *Gargantua et Pantagruel*, Johann Fischart notes that, as a physician, Rabelais's graphic descriptions of gluttonous and scatological behaviour have the didactic aim of shocking readers out of the path of sin and guiding them back to shame and propriety, and the therapeutic aim of using laughter to expel melancholy.[39] Thomas Murner's sardonically brutal advocacy of quasi-surgical 'exorcism' as a cure for folly, in *Narrenbeschwörung* (1512), inspired enthusiastic iconographic representations, and influenced literary works such as the Shrovetide play of Hans Sachs noted in the previous chapter. Rabelaisian 'textual therapy'[40] had a wider impact, informing the seventeenth-century popular publications of numerous English authors, including qualified medical practitioners.[41] Thomas Heywood's

---

[36]   Linke, 'Vom Sakrament bis zum Exkrement', 135–6; Veltruský, 'The old Czech apothecary', 273; Katritzky, *Women, medicine and theatre*, 33–43.

[37]   Thomas Platter notes that their relics, in a church near Arles, can only be viewed on high feast days, by cooperation of key holders in three different locations (*Thomas Platter d. J*, 174: 10 February 1597, Saintes-Maries).

[38]   Linke, 'Zwischen Jammertal und Schlaraffenland', 352, 361–2, 370.

[39]   Fischart, *Geschichtklitterung*, 14–15; Könneker, *Satire*, 229–30.

[40]   Alison Williams's expression ('Rabelais's jokes', 678).

[41]   Gowland, 'Melancholy', 84–5; for further European examples, see Katritzky, *Women, medicine and theatre*, 159.

1624 defence of his use of this literary strategy refers directly to the commedia dell'arte most enduring stage fool, Zanni:

> It may be likewise obiected, Why amongst sad and graue Histories, I haue here and there inserted fabulous Jeasts and Tales, sauouring of Lightnesse? I answer, I haue therein imitated our Historicall and Comicall Poets, that write to the Stage; who least the Auditorie should be dulled with serious courses (which are meerely weightie and materiall) in euerie Act present some Zanie with his Mimick action, to breed in the lesse capable, mirth and laughter.[42]

Some critics have sought to demonstrate that Guarinonius was oblivious to the theoretical fundamentals of literature.[43] While he never commented on literary style or form, and projects a far less sympathetic author-physician persona than Rabelais, he too uses the medium of print to extend his circle of patients, and it is clear that the dual healing aims of folly literature underpin his use of lazzi in *Grewel*. Their inclusion reflects his perception of sins as representing specific pathways to both spiritual ill-health and unhealthy lifestyle choices, against whose physical and mental symptoms his readers must be warned in the strongest terms. *Grewel*'s lazzi also exploit the inherent comicality of foolish sins and sinful folly to promote therapeutic laughter. They share the religiously-motivated didactic agenda of mystery play quacks: deployed to lure spectators in as quasi-extras with their sales-pitch, inspire them to recognize and laugh at their own human folly, and to reject it in favour of spiritual redemption. The framing of *Grewel*'s lazzi within its moralizing context demonstrates the multiple intentions of the folly literature tradition with exceptional clarity, providing dramatic *exempla* whose laughter-inducing warnings against specific sins and vices offer Guarinonius's readers a literal cure for folly.

In Summary

In many ways, Guarinonius was a forward-thinking physician. *Grewel* is widely identified as a breakthrough in medical approaches to the municipal management of hygiene, and certain aspects of its scientific content anticipate future medical developments. But to an even greater extent than most other physicians of his own time, or even many earlier physicians, not least Felix Platter, Guarinonius's medical publications are suffused with the assumptions of his faith and the events of his life. He neither compartmentalized his approach to scientific objectivity from his religious agenda, nor drew clear lines between his scientific, theological and life writings. *Grewel*'s ecclectic literary presentation drew on outmoded and old-fashioned approaches. This applies particularly to its theatrical inclusions, whose

---

42   Heywood, 'To the reader', in *Gynaikeion*, sig.A4ᵛ.
43   Gemert, 'Medizinisches Naturverständnis', 1136.

choice and positioning express a carefully planned literary programme, drawing heavily on late medieval conventions of folly literature, which themselves closely follow classical literary and medical approaches to the treatment of melancholy. Essentially, even for its date of publication in 1610, the treatise looks back to earlier ways of presenting literature and medicine. Sidelined by the relentless progression towards enlightenment and specialization that continues to shape the modern medical and theatrical professions, this holistic literary approach is now gaining renewed relevance with the rise of medical blogs. Although, as amply indicated by its embedded dates, *Grewel* was continuously written from start to finish in comparable manner to the modern blog, it is no exemplary forerunner of the genre. While it undeniably contains both good literature and good medicine, they rarely coincide. *Grewel*'s ambitious literary, medical and moral aims are tainted by the uncompromising prejudices of its author.

Guarinonius sought to widen *Grewel*'s popular appeal both by sporadic deployment of rhetorical structures, expressions and sayings influenced by quack monologues, and by including descriptions of actual quack routines. Notably, *Grewel* features quack commedia dell'arte entertainment in the form of numerous lazzi descriptions, to attract, hold the attention of, and influence readers, to promote healing laughter, and to encourage its sale and the acceptance – and effectiveness – of its contents, in private, civic and court spheres.[44] In *Grewel*, Guarinonius addresses his own contemporaries, and more precisely, pious German-speaking Catholic men. Many of his reasons for choosing to include theatrical passages in this medical treatise are profoundly unappealing to multicultural sensibilities. However, through his structured inclusion of episodes involving the Italian stage 'fools', and through the influence of these theatrical passages on later writers, *Grewel* deserves recognition as a significant contribution to the tradition of German folly literature.[45] All performance is ephemeral, and unlike scripted drama, early improvised commedia dell'arte and itinerant quack performances from the start lacked even fully written out playtexts. If Guarinonius's polemical and literary agenda had not motivated this complex, opinionated physician and man of letters to recall and describe them in such detail in his medical treatise, some of the most significant early modern commedia dell'arte lazzi would be lost to modern scholarship. By virtue of its commedia dell'arte interpolations, *Grewel* represents a substantial and enduring cultural monument to the early modern period's quest to interweave medicine and theatre.

Early modern negotiations between science and showmanship contributed towards stabilizing and entrenching the contested boundaries between medicine and theatre. The present book has sought to investigate interchanges and interdependencies between health and performance with reference to specific

---

[44]   Neuber ('Vom Grewel deß Trawrens', 78), without drawing the parallel with the way in which mountebanks promoted their medicinal wares, compares the treatise to satires which, like Burton's *Anatomy*, in themselves offer a remedy for melancholy.

[45]   Neuber, 'Vom Grewel deß Trawrens', 78–9.

passages in the writings of Guarinonius and the Swiss physicians Felix and Thomas Platter. Many are slight in themselves. At their most potent, as evidenced by the ceremony of the Royal Touch, they contribute materially to early modern political power systems. Taken as a whole, they substantially inform our understanding of the theatrical and medical culture of their time. The three physicians' accounts of fairs, carnivals and other festivals offer rich perspectives on a vibrant Christian festive year whose influence had already greatly waned in Protestant England. To varying degrees, according to regional confessional allegiances, this informed every aspect of mainland European theatre culture and, through annual markets, the activities of itinerant medical traders. The physicians also provide insights into the ceremony and traditions of the most influential coherent group of non-participants to the economic and cultural support systems of the Christian festive year, the Jews. Their accounts offer numerous instances of medical professionals' routine privileged access to diverse spheres of the ceremony, spectacle and routines of early modern festivals. In particular, their union of religious ceremony, cultural performance and martial arts made physicians indispensable to court festivals. The three physicians' writings on magic and superstition illuminate aspects of their relevance to medical and stage practice. An inquiry into the significance of magical impotence for the Jacobean stage, in the light of Thomas Platter's account of the occult ritual of ligature in Languedoc, demonstrates the theatricality and transregional nature of one particular supernatural medical practice, and confirms that travel journals can represent an invaluable documentary source for the theatre historian, even when, as with Platter's account of this ritual, their connection to the stage is indirect and previously unrecognized. The three physicians also provide insights into the key role of theatricality in the understanding of early modern human monstrosity, and the varied exhibition sites of monsters, as locations of intense negotiation between medicine and theatre. Above all, their quack-related descriptions of itinerant trading and stagecraft provide uniquely informative evidence on the profound interdependency of the itinerant theatrical and medical marketplaces. They confirm that some quacks used performance itself as their most effective medicine, by harnessing the therapeutic power of music and laughter, to stage healing as performance. They also offer new information concerning the mechanics of how quacks did this, and their strategies for making it pay. The identification of the quack troupe leader Zan Bragetta as the renowned professional actor Giovanni Paulo Alfieri, made possible by close interrogation of Thomas Platter's account of Bragetta's 1598 Avignon season (one of the key passages translated into English in this book's concluding section) in the light of newly-discovered archival documents, confirms the fluid boundaries between early modern performing and healing.

The interest of all three physicians in participating in and recording theatrical events closely relates to their medical practice. Felix Platter took pride in his secular lute-playing and dancing skills, and used them for professional advancement as a physician. Thomas Platter underplayed his own abilities as a performer while coolly judging those of his itinerant medical rivals. Hippolytus Guarinonius energetically promoted sacred music and spectacle in the Tirolean town of Hall, while adopting and reformulating to his own literary agenda the secular commedia dell'arte stage business quacks used as a medical marketing strategy. In their writings, all three physicians illuminate, in fresh and immediate ways rarely offered by traditional historical documents, mutual interchanges and influences between early modern healthcare, theatre and spectacle, in the decades that shaped the emergence and character of Europe's modern acting profession.

PART V
Source Texts

Translations by M.A. Katritzky and Verena Theile

PART V

Felix Platter: The 1598 Wedding of Johann Georg, Count of Hohenzollern and Franziska, Countess of Salm[2]

His gracious highness[3] set off from Hachberg on Thursday 28 September, at eight o'clock in the morning, in the following formation: in front ride ten of his gracious highness's personal mounted escorts and guards, one of whom leads a riderless horse, one of his gracious highness's own. They are followed by a trumpeter on horseback. Behind them ride 26 aristocrats, always three to a row, namely Martin von Remchingen, provincial governor of Hachberg; Heinrich vom Starschedel, equerry; [Hans] Caspar vom Stein, chief magistrate of Badenweiler; Rûtprecht Castner, chamberlain; Jacob [II] von Rotburg, forest warden; stablemaster, Hans Jakob Nagel; Albrecht and Melchior Besolden; Wolf Wilhelm von Eptingen; Adam Hektor von Rosenbach; Hans Melchior Schenk von Winterstetten; Ludwig von Bütikum; Hans Diebold [d.J.] von Reinach; Melchior and Lüpold von Baerenfels; Caspar von Hohenfürst; Hans Ludwig von Andlau; Hans Melchior von Landsberg; Hans Georg Volmar; Christoph and Hans Caspar von Rockenbach; Wernhardt von Offenburg; Ludwig Efinger; Ludwig Reutner; [Johann] Albrecht Gebwiler [d.J.].[4] Then the following three on horseback in one row: Dr Hans Georg Kienlin, the lawyer, and Dr Felix Platter, the doctor of medicine, who sometimes also ride in the carriages, and Joseph Arhardt, the

[1]   Chapters 16–18 were made possible through the generous support of the British Academy, Arts and Humanities Research Council, and Herzog August Library (Wolfenbüttel), and the invaluable expertise of co-translator Verena Theile (who expresses her gratitude to David Collins, Mike Herzog, Bruce Maylath, and Resi Kremer for their help with these translations, and a warm thanks, too, to Gillian Bepler and the Freunde der Gesellschaft der Herzog August Bibliothek).

[2]   Basle UL, Codex A λ III.3, 6–9, ff.1–10 (Platter, *Felix Platter Tagebuch*, 484–513). This section of Felix Platter's journal was first published by Geßler (*Felix Platters Schilderung*: 'modernized' edition). The present translation standardizes the spelling of proper and place names. Information taken from the extensive editorial annotations of Valentin Lötscher (*Felix Platter Tagebuch*) and Casimir Bumiller (Frischlin, *Hohenzollerische Hochzeyt*) is not always further acknowledged here.

[3]   Felix Platter's noble patron, Georg Friedrich, Margrave of Baden-Sausenberg and Hachberg (1573–1638). See also Diagram 2b, this volume.

[4]   A nephew of Felix Platter's former lute student, Karl Gebwiler (on whom see Chapter 11, this volume).

steward of Hachberg Castle. Behind them ride three trumpeters in front of his highness and behind them the margrave himself, and next to his gracious highness eight footmen with halberds march dressed in red and yellow, and three lackeys run wearing black velvet.

Behind them rides the ladies' steward, Franz Conrad Höcklin, followed by the margravine in her two-horse sedan, with two guards on foot steadying the sedan. Thereafter follows a precious carriage with velvet and gilt fittings, in which ride the bride and three other unmarried ladies, and two further similar carriages, in which sit the ladies' housekeeper and seven unmarried noblewomen; and each carriage is drawn by six horses and accompanied by nine coachmen and guards. Behind these, eight noble margravial pages ride in formation as described above, the first three carrying the ceremonial helmets, and one rider sits on the third sedan horse, which serves for the use of the tired. They are followed by 36 mounted guards of the above-noted landed gentry and noblemen, as each is accompanied by one servant, many by two or more.

Behind this formation follows the maidservants' carriage, in which there are six maids, with six horses and two footmen. Next is the coach of the provincial governor of Rötteln, Hans von Ulm, with three people, drawn by three carriage horses. Then follows the carriage of Dr Joseph Hettler, the regional record keeper, in which he, his scribe and servant sit, together with the coachman. Then come the chancellery carriage and the musicians' wagon, an instrument and silver wagon laden with silverware and money which transports 22 people: the court preacher [Michael] Baldtauf, the secretary Thomas Stotz, personal secretary, barber, silver servant, two personal cooks, the knights' cook, stable boy, unmarried noblewomen's guard, three tailors, seven musicians, one painter, an armourer or blacksmith, and each carriage has six horses, and nine coachmen and guards. Likewise, another four, two quartermasters, one chef, and a carriage master, always ride in front, with three hunters and three kitchen apprentices on foot. Additionally, six margravial riders lead six fully saddled, unmounted racehorses by hand, and several servants of the landed gentry lead carriage horses, and other lackeys walk with them. Eight transport wagons and one cart are always sent on a day ahead, loaded with all kinds of necessities and things, requiring 25 coachmen and guards and 50 carriage horses.

In this formation, and with the number of people and horses described above, approximately matching those in the quartermaster's lists, totalling 218 people and over 200 horses, we left Hachberg. We climbed up towards Bildstein, where there is a lovely hunting lodge owned by the margrave, onto the plateau, across to the other mountain, down towards Haslach in the Kinzig valley, in the territory of Albrecht, Count of Fürstenberg. His gracious highness stayed at the castle in the village, and the rest found quarters here and there. That same evening [Jacob] von Geroldseck arrived there with his entourage, to join his gracious highness. On Michaelmas, Friday 29 September, it rained heavily. We rode repeatedly through the River Kinzig, and with only one short stop travelled through Hausach and Wolfach towards Schiltach, outside which we were received by the representatives of [the Duke of] Württemberg, to whom it belongs. On the morning of Saturday 30 September, we travelled up a steep slope, and then for a long while across a plateau, until we saw Sulz Castle. Then we descended the slope in rain down to the little town of Sulz [am Neckar], where our night quarters were, and both nights' quarters on Württembergian soil were paid for by [Friedrich,] Duke of Württemberg.

On Sunday 1 October, travelling up the slopes, we soon reached the realm of Hohenzollern, passing by the castle near Wehrstein, from which salutes were fired. Then we reached Haigerloch, a town located low down by the water, with the castle up on the mountain; from there, passing by an old castle named Stein, into a village, Rangendingen. There his gracious highness's unmarried sister Elisabeth [Margravine of Baden], met us herself, riding in her own carriage from Durlach, drawn by six coach horses. The noblemen who rode with her were [Georg] Christoph von Venningen, Carl von Schornstetten, Erasmus von Erlach, Georg Friedrich von Rixleben and Melchior Sigelmann, together with their mounted guards with thirteen horses. Three of the Rheingraf counts also joined us there, including the father of the bride, and with them many servants and aristocrats from Lorraine; also the nobleman [Eberhard von] Rappoltstein, and [Friedrich] Count of Hohenlohe. Here we prepared for the formal entry. The margrave, luxuriously clothed, was mounted on a well-ornamented horse decorated with feathers; and with his gracious highness rode three noble young lancers wearing ceremonial helmets covered in velvet and leading lambs; and we proceeded together in this way until we reached a broad meadow not far from Hechingen.

There we were met by the father, Eitel Friedrich [IV], Count of Hohenzollern together with his son, the bridegroom, Johann Georg, Count of Hohenzollern. Together with many counts, gentry, and noblemen, elegantly and beautifully turned out, with 120 horses, many fanfares and six trumpeters, including some borrowed from the Bavarian court, they rode with the groom's carriage. The counts and gentry riding in front of the margrave rearranged themselves, as did our noblemen and mounted guards, and so we proceeded together to the little town of Hechingen. Then salutes were fired from large cannons at Hohenzollern[-Hechingen] Castle, and the several hundred-strong entry took place at five o'clock, in the following formation: at its centre was the bride, next to the margravine,[5] presenting herself in the middle of an expensively decorated open carriage. They were followed by many carriages and wagons, including one decorated all over with gilt fittings, empty, drawn by six beautiful horses, which the father of the bride, according to custom, was giving her in addition to her dowry, clothing and jewels, so that she was endowed with all the necessities. They proceeded in this way, down through the town, passing the troops of soldiers standing to attention on both sides, and into the glorious castle of Hechingen. After many greeting were exchanged in the

---

[5]   The bride Franziska von Salm, and her sister Juliane Ursula von Baden (née von Salm), daughters of the late Franziska von Salm, second wife of Wild- und Rheingraf Friedrich I, Count of Salm-Neufville.

courtyard, the high nobility were accommodated at court, the rest were lodged in the town, so that few remained who found no quarters.

According to the quartermaster's records, the number of people who attended this wedding, including princes (in person or by delegation), counts, gentry, nobility and officials, mounted guards, servants, and also the number of horses, was as follows:

> Georg Friedrich, Margrave of Baden, with Margravine Juliane Ursula, his gracious highness's wife and her three unmarried sisters: Franziska [von Salm], the bride; Elisabeth [von Salm], nun of Remiremont, and Anna [von Salm], all four née Wild- und Rheingraf countesses; and an unmarried Rheingraf countess, Otten. People 218, horses 201.

> [Joachim Friedrich,] Elector of Brandenburg's delegate, Hans Jakob Wurmser of Strasbourg. People 8, horses 7.

> [Maximilian,] Duke of Bavaria's delegate, Frobenius Truchseß von Waldburg. People 22, horses 22.

> [Friedrich,] Duke of Württemberg's delegate, Sebastian Welling of Fehingen, with Acharius of Gůtenberg, the Württembergian guard. People 14, horses 14.

> Franciscus, Duke of Vaudémont's delegate, the noble Eberhard von Rappoltstein,[6] with his wife Anna, née Wild- und Rheingraf countess. People 32, horses 31.

> [Georg Friedrich,] Margrave of Brandenburg-Ansbach's delegate, the nobleman Thomas von Kriechingen. People 12, horses 10.

> Ernst Friedrich, Margrave of Baden-Durlach's delegate, Carl von Schornstetten. People 6, horses 5.

> Wild- und Rheingraf Friedrich [I, Count of Salm-Neufville], noble father of the bride, with his grace's sons, Rheingraf Philipp [Otto, Count of Salm] and Rheingraf Johann [Count of Salm], of whom Rheingraf Johann was also a delegate of Johann, Count of Salm and the Abbess of Remiremont [sic], Claudia, née von Salm.

> Next, there were Rheingraf Friedrich's wife, Sibilla Juliana,[7] and two unmarried noblewomen, Agnes and Irmgard, all three sisters née Countesses of Isenburg.

---

[6]   1570–1637. He and his father Egenolf von Rappoltstein were personal friends of Felix Platter.

[7]   Stepmother of the bride.

Item, [Baron Johann] Ludwig of Hohensax, a young nobleman, with them. People 45, horses 44.

Wild- und Rheingraf Adolf [Heinrich, Count of Salm] and his wife Juliana, née Countess of Nassau, and the unmarried Anna Maria, Countess of Zeiningen. People 25, horses 22.

Wild- und Rheingraf Otto [Count of Salm-Kirburg] and his grace's wife, and with them the noble Ernst Peter von Kriechingen. People 13, horses 12.

Eitel Friedrich [IV], Count of Hohenzollern, father of the bridegroom; his wife Sybille, née Countess of Zimmern;[8] their son, the bridegroom, Count Johann Georg; two unmarried noblewomen Juliana and Eleonora; also the widow of [Baron Karl] Truchseß [of Waldburg], née von Hohenzollern; counting only nobility and official staff. People 93, horses 93.

Karl, Count of Hohenzollern; his grace's wife Elisabeth, Countess of Cuilenberg;[9] two unmarried noblewomen, Maximiliana and Johanna. People 49, horses 36.

Friedrich, Count of Fürstenberg; his grace's wife Elisabeth, née Countess of Sulz. People 36, horses 25.

Friedrich, Count of Hohenlohe. People 20, horses 15.

Two counts of Helfenstein, Georg and Frobenius, both presidents in the supreme court. People 20, horses 18.

Emich, Count of Leiningen. People 12, horses 10.

Delegate of Joachim, Count of Fürstenberg.[10] People 3, horses 3.

---

[8]   Of the siblings of the groom's mother, Sybille (1558–99), death or illness prevented Katharina (born and died 1553), the childless Wilhelm (1549–94), Barbara (1559–c.95) and Maria (1555–25 October 1598) from attending. Apollonia, Johanna, Kunigunde, Ursula and Eleonora attended with their families, and Anna's husband sent a delegate.

[9]   1567–1620. First married to Jakob III, Margrave of Baden (1562–90), a brother of Georg Friedrich, Margrave of Baden. Her second husband, Karl II von Hohenzollern (1547–1606), abducted her from the Netherlands to Sigmaringen in 1591 with the aid of 60 armed cavalrymen. Her third marriage, in 1608, was to Johann Ludwig von Hohensax (died 1625).

[10]   His wife Anna (1544–1602) was a sister of Sybille von Zimmern.

Johann Georg, Count of Hohenzollern.[11] People 5, horses 5.

Delegate of Wilhelm, Count of Oetingen, People 4, horses 4.

Baron Berchtold of Königseck; his grace's wife Kunigunde, née Countess of Zimmern.[12] People 16, horses 14.

Baron Heinrich Truchseß [of Waldburg]; his grace's wife Anna Maria, née Mechselrein. People 22, horses 22.

Baron Joachim of Mörsperg. People 6, horses 6.

The noble Schenk Johannes von Limpurg[-Gaildorf]; his grace's wife Eleonora, née Countess of Zimmern;[13] and the noble Schenk Heinrich von Limpurg[-Sontheim]. People 32, horses 29.

Jacob von Geroldseck, together with his grace's wife Barbara, née von Rappoltstein.[14] People 30, horses 23.

The noble commissary S. Johans, delegate of Baron Augustin of Mörsperg. People 2, horses 2.

The unmarried Elisabeth, Margravine of Baden. People 17, horses 19.

Apollonia, Countess of Helfenstein, widow, née of Zimmern.[15] People 6, horses 12.

Katharina, Countess of Hohenzollern[-Haigerloch], widow, with two young noblemen, the counts of Hohenzollern[-Haigerloch], Christoph and Karl. People 10, horses 7.

Baroness Kunigunde of Königseck, née Baroness of Waldburg.[16] People 16, horses 14.

---

[11]   1580–1622. In giving the age of the bridegroom (Johann Georg, Count of Hohenzollern, 1577–1623) as 17, Platter is possibly mistakenly referring to this same-named cousin, son of his father's younger brother Joachim von Hohenzollern (1554–87), although Bumiller supports a recent revision of the groom's birth date to 1582 (Frischlin, *Hohenzollerische Hochzeyt*, 259n4).

[12]   1552–1602. A sister of Sybille von Zimmern.

[13]   1554–1606. A sister of Sybille von Zimmern, also recorded as Elisabeth.

[14]   Sister of Eberhard von Rappoltstein.

[15]   1547–1604. A sister of Sybille von Zimmern.

[16]   Sister-in-law of Kunigunde von Königseck née von Zimmern.

Ursula, Countess of Ortenburg, née Countess of Zimmern;[17] and an unmarried noblewoman, Polixena. People 8, horses 7.

The noble Johanna Truchseß [von Waldburg], née von Zimmern;[18] and two unmarried noblewomen, Sabina[19] and Johanna. People 14, horses 14.

The grand total of people and horses, as far as can be ascertained from the quartermaster's personal records, amounts to 819 people and 746 horses. However, further delegates, from the city of Reutlingen, and the domain of Hohenzollern and other places, not included here, are listed in the Hechingen quartermaster's public records. So those who attended the wedding and were lodged, fed, and entertained totalled 984 people, of whom 68 were aristocracy, and 148 were noblemen and women; and 865 diverse riding and carriage horses were stabled.

When these people had arrived and assembled together, they prepared for the wedding, which took place before the evening meal, but not until late, at eight o'clock. At this hour the bridegroom, the young 17-year-old[20] count, entered. At his side walked Margrave Georg Friedrich, and their arrival was heralded by 11 trumpeters, one of whom played especially purely and well. The high nobility walked in front, followed by the counts and gentry, accompanied by many torches before and behind them. They marched into a great hall, about 25 feet long and wide, and very high, with a beautiful ceiling and richly tapestried all over. They were soon followed by the bride, the noble Franziska, led by two princely delegates, with her hair put up and dressed, in a very precious tiara, jewels, necklace and clothes. In front of her grace walked two stewards, many shawm, cornet, and trombone players, and then followed the unmarried and married aristocratic women, and finally also the minor noblewomen, in a long procession, each one dressed and decorated more exquisitely and specially than the one before. The wedding couple was placed side by side, and a priest[21] joined them in matrimony with many ceremonies, and German and Latin speeches. There was magnificent singing and instrumental music in the hall, into which in the meantime many torches and small and large candles, all of wax, had been brought and lit.

At around nine o'clock, when this had finished, the wedding couple was led in a similar procession to a great hall nearby, which was 54 feet long and 25 wide, and very high, with an elaborately decorated ceiling of varnished joinery, and every wall plastered and artistically decorated in low-relief. In one place, great quantities of silverware were set up next to each other on several display

---

[17]   Born 1564. A sister of Sybille von Zimmern.

[18]   1548–1613. A sister of Sybille von Zimmern. Mother of Heinrich and Frobenius Truchseß von Waldburg.

[19]   In 1599, she married Joachim von Mörsperg.

[20]   Platter may be right (see note 11, above).

[21]   Dr Johann Jakob Mirgel, Bishop of Konstanz.

sideboards. There were also two beautiful carved stone fireplaces, one at the front and one at the back, in which great fires continuously burned, and also many big candles standing at all the windows, and two chandeliers hanging in there, in each of which burned 15 candles, arranged to look like two pope's crowns burning inside them. The aristocracy gathered along the length of this great hall, the noblemen to the right, and the unmarried and married noblewomen to the left, and then two stewards entered carrying silver-gilt maces. In front of them walked two pageboys dressed in yellow and black velvet, the colours of the house of Hohenzollern, carrying burning torches. They were followed by others carrying large gilt platters, water jugs and exquisite hand towels. With much ceremony, they poured water for all the aristocracy, who then sat down at two long banqueting tables, half the length of the hall and placed next to each other, in such a manner that the groom, and next to him the bride, sat at the head of the table. To his right sat the margrave, and to the left of the bride sat the margravine. They were followed by the princely delegates, counts and nobility, but always with the most high-ranking of the noblewomen between them, until the banqueting table was completely occupied. Then the remaining married and unmarried noblewomen were all seated at the other table, so that both long tables were occupied by 68 aristocrats. After the remaining noblewomen, together with the landed gentry, gentry and most distinguished officials, had waited for a while around the long tables, they were seated at four round tables also set up in this same hall. Then the rest were seated in a large room downstairs in the castle, in which many tables had been set up, including one for the clergymen. They were all so full that no seat remained unoccupied, and the maidservants, of whom there were also many, were given a special place. The remaining male commoners, including the coachmen and guards, boys and lackeys, of whom few were admitted to court, were all fed in town in their lodgings, at 120 or more tables.

Regarding the food and tableware for this meal and those of the next eight days, their preparation and presentation were exceptionally costly and varied in the aristocrats' hall, especially at the long tables. All the cutlery, platters, plates, candelabra and whatever dishes were used were silver, mostly even silver-gilt. The drinking vessels were unusually large and so were the bowls used for serving the confectionery. They were wide and tall, with pedestals. Set up in the middle of each one there was a tall artistic sugar sculpture, featuring buildings, plants and all types of animals, beautifully and skilfully made at great expense, and changed for each meal. The serviettes or napkins were always placed on the plates formed and folded into different shapes. All kinds of delicious food, pastry, tarts, confectionery, numerous and beyond description, were served by several noblemen assigned to seneschal duties. And throughout this banquet, some 30 musicians sang and played wind instruments and all sorts of others, including violas, harps and spinets, modestly and not too loudly making beautiful music the like of which I had never heard, in their special place in the hall. Half of them were the regularly employed musicians and instrumentalists of the count, whose director of music is Narcissus Zängel and whose organist is [Jakob] Hassler. The rest, all well rewarded for their services, were sent from afar, from the imperial court of Prague, from Munich (including, among others, Ferdinand di Lasso, son of Orlando), and from Sigmaringen, who sent their director of music, Melchior Schramm.[22] The other meals, for those not seated in the aristocrats' hall, were also considerable. Second helpings of many dishes were offered, and dessert was provided. In this way a great deal was consumed in the town by the servants in their lodgings. In particular, they drank many measures of wine, even with the morning meals, carried up to the rooms, or otherwise given out on request; a lot was consumed. In this way, the nobility sat at the banqueting tables for three hours, the others at court for two hours, except when they had to serve again, and everyone was permitted to circulate and look around the banqueting tables, and to listen in on conversations.

During this time, professional entertainers also performed their vocal and instrumental acts. One among them, called Pauli, spoke and sang fast rhymes with which he could wittily mock the aristocrats and minor nobility. By revealing how they had behaved badly in divertingly delivered rhymes, he created much entertainment and laughter, and earned a reward of over 100 crowns.[23] After completion of this evening meal, which lasted until midnight, and after much time had been taken up bringing water to table for hand washing, getting up and other ceremonies, and also after retiring for a while so that the tables could be cleared and put away, the trumpeters softly began to call everyone to the dance. The dances were led by several counts and gentry, preceded by their stewards. The first to dance to the sound of the trumpets were the groom and his bride; thereafter the margrave; then the princely delegates as well as several counts and gentry. Always just one danced with the bride, the margravine, or another highborn lady; with torches carried before them by two pageboys dressed in velvet as described above, and behind them by the next two noblemen to dance. And the dance lasted until two in the morning, when the wedding couple was finally conveyed away to bed, in the same manner in which they had been led here.

On Monday 2 October we prepared for church, and everyone put on costly clothes and groomed and ornamented themselves according to or beyond their means and status. After we had gathered in front of the chamber of the groom and bride, who were together, they were led into the castle chapel with the same

---

[22] Shortly after his voice broke in 1569, from 1570 to 1571, Schramm held the post of organist at the imperial convent in Hall, established in 1566, where Guarinonius later served as court physician (Senn, *Aus dem Kulturleben*, 175; Schmid, *Musik*, 32).

[23] On Pauli of Zell, see also Chapter 6, this volume. Coinage is here translated as follows: florins ('gulden' or 'fl.', the common currency of the southern German-speaking regions, of which, c.1600, one was worth exactly 15 Batzen, each of which were in turn worth 4 Kreuzer), groats ('batzen') , thalers ('taler', the common currency of the northern German-speaking regions, of which, c.1600, one was worth approximately two German florins, or one-and-a-half French crowns or three Spanish pistoles), crowns ('kronen'), pistoles ('pistolen').

procession and celebration as that which took place on the previous evening. The bridegroom was led by two princely delegates, the bride by the margrave with a large entourage. The noblemen and representatives of the margrave's group remained standing outside by orders of the ruler, and soon the ruler himself also came back out of the church again, as did the Rheingraf counts and other Protestant gentry, and also the margravine and other women who had converted to this religion.[24] In the chapel, which was beautifully decorated, Mass was held, accompanied by the musicians. The organ and other wind instruments were played together with the other instruments, making an extremely strong, well-tuned and harmonious sound. The couple was joined in marriage with all the customary ceremony, conducted entirely in Latin. After which the previously excluded male and married and unmarried female gentry returned, and again with the same formation and celebration escorted the newlyweds back to their chamber, and soon after to the midday meal. This was of the same type as described above, except that this time it was arranged and took place in the most costly manner, with sugar sculptures, and many various and unusual courses. Also with lovely music, and followed by a dance at which more people danced than the night before, and there were no longer trumpets. Instead, because they are quieter instruments, violas, fifes and spinets were played, as again in the same manner during and after the evening meal, and the same order and custom was followed on the following two days. So that one seldom sat down to the midday meal before one o'clock or left it before four o'clock; or, after the dance and a short break, started the evening meal before ten o'clock, or left it before one o'clock, or went to bed before three or even four o'clock after the customary dance.

On Tuesday 3 October, at around four o'clock in the afternoon, after the usual dance, we began to present the newlyweds with gifts, because each aristocrat, whether personally or through delegates or officials, presented his gift and placed it on a table while making an elegant speech, and this was always acknowledged with a speech of thanks by Dr [Johann] Pfeffer, the Count of Hohenzollern's chancellor. This took a good while, as many valuable gifts were presented. The margrave presented the largest cup, the other counts and gentry, and the cities of Reutlingen and Rottweil, gave all kinds of silverware and jewels. A valuable necklace was given by the Count of Hohenzollern, the bride's father-in-law, and another by [Elisabeth von Salm] Abbess of Remiremont; the domain of Hohenzollern gave twelve large cups. Afterwards, everything was inventoried, and its worth estimated at more than ten thousand florins. After the evening meal and dance, close to midnight, a herald arrived, wearing silk livery in the Hohenzollern colours, carrying in his right hand a gilt sceptre and in his left a great round painted and inscribed plaque called a 'cartel'. After he had marched around three times, preceded by trumpeters, he stood in the middle and read out the 'cartel': that two

---

[24] The bride's family was Protestant, that of the groom was Catholic. Margrave Georg Friedrich was a Lutheran, his brothers Ernst Friedrich and Jakob III were respectively Calvinist and Catholic.

knights were present who would bring the child Cupid – or Love bound – and if any knights present wished to rescue him through chivalrous contest, they should present themselves tomorrow at midday at the tournament field, in order to volunteer as 'avanturier' or daring challenger, against the 'maintenir' or defender. He also read the regulations according to which everything would be conducted, and the three trophies awarded. After this, the herald marched around again, then left, and hung up the 'cartel' in the courtyard, so that it would be read by everyone.

On Wednesday morning, however, the parade was postponed due to the rain and the day was well spent in other celebrations and diversions. In the afternoon, several of the gentry practiced running to the ring with their horses, of which a considerable number were of Turkish, Neapolitan and other such stock, including many bought at a very high price and highly valued, especially a black mare belonging to the margrave, valued at 500 florins. The Count of Holach rode a dappled horse, which he put through its paces. First he whistled for it to dance, and for a long time the horse danced around impressively; then the count dismounted and talked to it, and it lay down completely on its side, with its head on the ground, and he sat on it for a good while before it rose again at his command. He also jumped a high fence with it, and when he tried this a second time, the horse stumbled and fell back with him, but he was not injured.

On Thursday 5 October, seven companies secretly made their preparations here and there to take part in the disguised and masked parade for the running at the ring. At around noon, one by one, each company, preceded by its pipers and instrumentalists, proceeded to the tournament field, where four trumpeters immediately rode up in front of them, and two mounted marshals, Martin von Remchingen and Georg Christoph von Venningen, received them. They accompanied them until they had paraded round three times, and thereafter arrived at the place where they all lined up with their horses. Firstly, parading as hunters, were the two knights or cavaliers who were to be the challengers, namely Brid'amour (that was the margrave) and Scipio ([Eberhard] von Rappoltstein), in green velvet coats with flowing sleeves and hats, all richly trimmed with real gold embellishments, as were the horses' saddles and tack. Their boots were white, turned down at the top and trimmed with gold. Their weapons, spurs, reins, buckles and bits were all gilt, and they carried long, gilded arrows in their hands. The margrave had a white, and von Rappoltstein a red, silk garter tied around their right arm. They were preceded by four noblemen, Nagel, von Rosenbach, von Rixleben, and Sigelmann, all clad entirely in green silk, and their horses' tack decorated in the same fashion, likewise edged with gold embellishments. On their heads they wore green wreaths like ivy, and bunches of the same foliage, all made of silk, decorated the horses. Around their necks were gilt hunting horns, which they occasionally blew. Between them and the defenders, one who was costumed to look nude, called Horatio, led Cupid, a little boy also costumed to look completely nude, with little golden wings, bound to cords, symbolizing that 'Ratio' (or Reason) should hold Cupid (or Love) captive. Behind them three hunters followed on foot, likewise all dressed in green silk, with green felt hats, like those typically worn by hunters; each leading four white hounds on green leashes. Lastly, six mounted escorts led on six race horses by hand after them, saddled and bridled in the same costly manner as the knights' horses. These two defenders met their challengers one after another.

Then followed the second company of challengers: ten knights riding in pairs, costumed like Zannis,[25] especially the last two, who wore ugly masks or makeup. They were Karl, Count of Hohenzollern, the Count of Holach, [Wild und-] Rheingraf Otto [Count of Salm], the Count of Zeiningen, Schenk Heinrich von Limpurg, Frobenius Truchseß [von Waldburg], von Schornstetten, Wolf Fuchs, Christoph Fuchs, and the revenue master. They wore blue or in several cases brown nightcaps, with white caps underneath, with attached cowls and aprons down to their boots, short cloaks like collars, blue, brown or yellow in colour. The first called himself Joan Badello, and placed a ten florin wager with the judges in order to take part in the tournament. The second, Joan Frimocollo, ten florins, the third Scherisepho eight florins, the fourth Peterlino eight florins, the fifth Jhan Fourmage five florins and five groats, the sixth Joan Fritada four crowns, the seventh Francotrippo nine florins, the eighth Pergomasco five florins, the ninth Zani four florins seven groats, the tenth Zani, five florins and seven groats. The defenders won nine contests and Frimocollo one. Their seconds, who ran after them and gathered up their spears, were the Counts of Fürstenberg and Helfenstein. The third company featured two knights completely covered, including the boots, hands, hips, and neck, with black armour with costly silver decorations in traditional fashion, as if they were nude. On their heads they wore tall morions of the same type, topped with tall black and white feather plumes. The horses had cloths decorated with the same black and silver colours. In their hands they carried silver regimental maces, and the one on the right, who was called King Philip and was the old count, Eitel Friedrich of Hohenzollern, had a silver crown on his helmet, and the second, called Attalus, was [Baron Berchtold of] Königseck. In front of them rode two lancers and ran two lackeys, costumed in the same manner, as were the horses. Philip wagered 20 florins with the judges and won; Attalus wagered 15 florins, which he lost.

The fourth company featured two more cavaliers, equipped exactly like those of the third, including their horses and those who accompanied them on horseback or on foot, except that while the armour of the previous was silver on black, these had gold on red, and even the crown of the one who rode on the right was gold. He called himself Alexander the Great[26] and was the young Count of Hohenzollern, the groom, and wagered ten crowns and lost it. The other, called Antipater, who

---

[25]   On the characters of the second company see Chapter 7, this volume.

[26]   The third, fourth and sixth companies draw on historical figures from fourth century (BC) Macedonia: King Philip II and his generals Attalus and Antipater (who also served under Alexander), and Alexander and his ambassador Eurylochus and commander Philotas (this latter the central figure of plays of 1604 by Samuel Daniel and 1759 by Gotthold Ephraim Lessing).

was a Count of Helfenstein, wagered twelve florins and won. The fifth company featured a knight dressed in women's clothes, wearing a long, green coat and a black velvet bonnet decorated with black and white swallows' feathers. Long black and white silk ribbons, which fluttered elegantly during the tournament, were tied around the bonnet, also around himself and his arms, also to his horse. In front of him rode two maids costumed like women of dubious virtue, with broad, Swabian, fringed hats, brown pleated skirts, and white boots, each carrying a large gilt double-handled cup in her hands. In front of them rode one with a lance from which hung a white and black banner, and four beautiful unmounted horses were led in after them. The cavalier called himself the Whore of Speckeberstadt,[27] wagered ten thalers and lost them; this was the old Rheingraf, Friedrich [Count of Salm].

The sixth company consisted of two knights, 'avanturier' or daring challengers, clad in silver-plated armour and ceremonial helmets in traditional fashion, with beautiful gilt studs shaped like lion-heads at their shoulders and knees; their necks, arms, and hips as if they were nude; and their horses' armour likewise after the classical manner. They presented a rhymed script whose content was: that often, while voyaging to explore the world, they had been betrayed by the sweet song of a siren or sea wonder and come to great harm. Finally they had captured her with the help of a Moor who was a wizard, and brought her with them to show her to this glorious gathering, and in order to practice chivalric pursuits with her here. The siren they led was half like a beautiful woman, nude down to the navel, with breasts and long blonde hair; from the navel down she was like the lower half of a fish, blue and silvery, big and curved in on herself, just like sea wonders are painted. Thus she sat and occasionally moved back and forth on a deep sea made of cloth painted like the ocean, with ships and fish painted on it, rather big, wide and enclosed, which moved around the tournament square by itself with the siren. From within, as if the siren were singing the song 'Venus, you and your child [are blind]', one could hear beautiful singing and the sound of violins.[28] A Moor followed the siren on foot, led by her bound to long cords, and thereafter Fortuna, costumed as if she were nude, carrying a marine anchor in her hands. Two lancers dressed in yellow also rode in front. One, calling himself Philotas, who was Joachim, Count of Hohenzollern,[29] wagered four crowns and won. The second, Eurylochus, who was a rich nobleman from Munich, wagered six florins

---

[27] Literally: 'Fat-wild-pig-town': satirical reference to the nearby town of Eberstadt. The intention of this company was to symbolize the sins of gluttony and lechery.

[28] Schmid identifies this as the villanelle published by Jakob Regnart in 1576 (*Musik*, 606).

[29] According to Lötscher, Platter here mistakenly names the father of Johann Georg, Count of Hohenzollern, who died in 1587, in place of his son. In fact, Platter must here be referring to a young relative of the same name, the Joachim, Count of Hohenzollern who directly after the wedding accompanied Margrave Georg Friedrich to serve at his court in Hachberg.

and lost. Of the other knights, challengers who had brought the stage props and musicians from Pforzheim, one called himself Lysander and was Cůnrath Kechler of Schwandorf. He wagered nine florins, lost. The other, called Flores, was Adam von Auw, who wagered fifteen florins and won.

The seventh company, which paraded last, consisted of four knights in full armour, completely gilded, with beautiful red and yellow feather plumes on their helmets and braided horse tails. Their horses were covered in red horse blankets with gilt suns, moons, and stars all over them, and everything shone attractively on them. One, called Perion of Gaul,[30] who was Rheingraf Adolf [Count of Salm], wagered twelve florins. The second, Angriote, was von Geroldseck; he wagered twelve pistoles. The third, Quedragant, was the equerry [vom Starschedel]; he wagered six florins six groats. The fourth, Madanil, was von Rotburg; he wagered five florins three groats. They all lost. Their three seconds, who rode in front of them dressed in black velvet, carrying gilt maces, were von Erlach, Volmar and von Canneck. Behind them rode three lancers with banners, dressed in red, with long coats, and caps, all embroidered with gold trimmings; these were von Andlau, von Bütikum, and Schenk. Calling themselves Frandalon, Vaillades, Galvanes, they each wagered five florins three groats. They all lost as well. Finally, two of the margrave's first company also competed. Von Rixleben wagered five florins and lost, and Sigelmann wagered six florins and won. Because it was getting dark, the remaining two, Nagel and von Rosenbach, did not participate. And then all of the companies paraded together around the tournament square three times, in their correct order, to the sound of fanfares and instruments, and then back toward the town, everybody returning to their quarters. After dining at court, at around midnight trumpets were sounded, and the judges stepped forward to hand out the awards. These were precious pearl wreaths, each decorated with a jewel. With much reverence, they approached the bride, who presented them. The first award was for the margrave, for capturing the ring the most times in the tournament's first three rounds. The second, called the Elegance Prize, she gave to the bridegroom as the one who had conducted himself most elegantly. The third, called the Spear Prize, was presented to the Count of Leiningen, as the one who had deployed his spears most entertainingly. In addition to these three, they also handed out a fourth to the old Count Eitel Friedrich, who despite his age, had conducted himself well in honour of the ladies. Then, as customary, after receiving their prizes, each of them danced with the bride, led by torches and to the sound of trumpets.

On Friday 6 October it rained, so not much could be undertaken. The margrave set out to [Friedrich,] Duke of Württemberg in Tübingen. He ate the midday meal with his gracious highness in Tübingen Castle and returned to Hechingen in the evening. On the afternoon of Saturday 7 October, the Count of Hohenzollern arranged a hunt in the game park. It stretches around the mountain on which

---

[30]   King Perion of Gaul was the father of Amadis de Gaul, hero of the fifteenth-century fictional prose romance from which the characters of the seventh company are taken.

Hohenzollern Castle is situated. It takes up a great expanse, and is surrounded and completely enclosed with oak fencing that would take eight hours to ride round. 900 head of red deer were commonly kept and grazed within it. It also supports many domesticated animals, including many cattle which had been castrated, and thus were called 'nuns',[31] which we also ate at court; no foxes, but rabbits, of which likewise many lived within it. In this park, up by the forest on the mountain, a considerable area had been enclosed with stretched sheets of cloth, into which numerous deer had already been chased by the hunters. By the place at which the game was to be chased out by the dogs and exit from the sheeted area, three hunting lodges, or little huts constructed of leafy branches, were set up, from which to shoot the game as it ran past. With their guns, the margrave waited in the highest one, von Rappoltstein and the forest warden von Rotburg in the middle one, the Rheingraf count and the Count of Holach in the lowest one. Behind them, the women sheltered in a long hunting lodge. And thus, game was chased out with the dogs, and sometimes two came, occasionally more, even eighteen at a time; running out alone or one after another, several together. First the margrave shot at them. His second shot hit a stag in the chest, which immediately plunged down the cliff and remained there, caught or dead. Numerous stags were allowed to get away because since the season for hunting them was over, they did not like shooting stags, and waited for deer. The Rheingraf count shot down a young stag and von Rotburg dispatched it with his rapier, driving away the dogs. The dogs brought down a deer and a stag right behind us in the forest. It was getting late and night fell, so we returned to Hechingen, where we arrived in total darkness.

On Sunday 8 October, the margrave rode with Count Eitel Friedrich, the Rheingraf count and a few others to Hohenzollern, in the meantime we walked around to explore the sights. First, we walked in the pleasure gardens, located just outside the town by the tournament square, and saw how the beds and archways were all beautifully separated and edged with plants and neatly trimmed. The fig house, within which many small fig trees grew planted into the ground, was covered in winter with a complete and fully erected house. Before the winter, this could be pulled over it via two tracks permanently installed at the base of the fig house, which had grooves with little wheels in them. It was already pulled over in preparation, and in spring it would be completely taken away and pulled to another place. We also inspected the summer house, in the middle of the garden on a small lake, constructed faced with wooden boards, standing on posts and vaulted underneath, and finished with rather pretty decorations on the outside, including beautiful little simulated towers visible in four places. Inside is a beautiful spacious decorated hall, with all kinds of paintings and plasterwork. We also walked over to the aviary, also in the garden. It is very large, with many trees in it and every type of breeding nest, also little fields which are tilled and planted, and in the middle there is a house. It was so tightly enclosed all around with woven latticework

---

[31] One early modern German expression for farm-animal castrators was 'Nunnen-macher' (nun-makers).

that even a small bird could not get out. On top, it was covered all over with wire mesh, in frames resting on posts. Inside are all kind of small and large birds, apart from birds of prey, including many partridges and hazel grouse, and numerous pheasants, even though many had already had their necks twisted for the wedding. Among them I saw one with white spots, said to have been bred from a common hen. All of them breed and hatch their young. In the summer, they are fed with whatever is being sown, and in the winter they are given all kinds of food in the house, where they are placed and kept in a warm room. The count also has a small lake not far from the garden, completely enclosed by woodland, known as the wooded lake, and occupied by all kinds of fish.

In the afternoon, to view the rooms and buildings, we also looked around the castle, which covers a large area built in the shape of a square, but longer than wide. Inside the front part of the castle, entered through two gates, are many rooms including the chancery. The stables are round a long, wide courtyard. Behind that, the walls of one half of the castle enclose a capaciously constructed courtyard in which some 300 horses could be kept, and then the other half of the castle surrounds a constructed formal garden. Throughout, the castle is three stories high, with many beautiful, high rooms in it, so that besides the regular occupants, 68 aristocrats[32] were then being accommodated there, and they still had plenty of space. Most rooms were hung and decorated with tapestries, skilfully worked with gold, silver, silk and other threads. Downstairs, there were big vaulted kitchens; a chapel with many plasterwork reliefs and other decorations, an organ and paintings. There was a spiral staircase at each corner, including one constructed in such a way that one could ride up it. These led to wide hallways passing in front of every room, through which one could walk round. These passages were beautifully vaulted and the tops of the vaults were doubly pierced and wonderfully skilfully carved, and all the door and window frames in the whole castle were carved with many sculptures and pillars. The spout and surrounds of a well in the courtyard in front of the kitchen have also been beautifully decoratively. And in the middle of the garden, transformed and separated into unusually-shaped beds, there also is a beautiful fountain, and the plastered vaulted cloisters along all four sides of the garden are likewise beautifully carved. Their walls have been painted with hunting scenes all the way round, depicting and showing lifesize hunters and people, as well as wild animals and deer.

On Monday 9 October, most of the remaining male and female gentry departed, and the margrave, too, prepared for his departure. He made his formal farewells at court, and here and there where the margravial entourage had been lodged, and after partaking of the morning meal, they departed from court with many fanfares, in the customary formation. And accompanying his gracious highness as far as Hachberg were Rheingraf Friedrich [Count of Salm] with his two sons, Rheingraf

---

[32]   The 68 highest-ranked wedding guests. The castle then had 127 rooms (including an extensive library of over 1000 volumes and a curiosity cabinet), and Count Eitel Friedrich and his family were attended there by a regular staff of 102 courtiers.

Adolf [Count of Salm], the noble Schenk von Limpurg, von Rappoltstein and von Geroldseck, and a young count, Joachim von Hohenzollern, who was being dispatched to his gracious highness's court. Furthermore, the old Count Eitel Friedrich, together with his son the bridegroom, and the wives and ladies of both, accompanied his gracious highness for a quarter of a mile. After many pleasantries and farewells they parted from one another, and that night we made our night quarters again near Sulz. There we viewed the salt pans in a building outside the town, in which salt is refined. Saltwater is constantly conveyed into them through channels consisting of eight long boxes like sifting pans, covered with lids and elevated, each standing there on its own like a long passage. Into which boxes the saltwater from the salt spring in the town flows, also through channels, and is collected. Before that, it is repeatedly forced against many suspended straw boxes, so that it evaporates, that is, so that the watery moistness sticks to the straw and dries out, eliminating a large part, so that what remains is more concentrated and richer in salt, and can be refined more quickly. We also visited the salt spring in the town, which is very deep down, from which saltwater is constantly scooped up by numerous pumps with wheels. The wheels are driven by running water driven by another wheel, with someone walking inside it, drawing up buckets. Likewise, in the winter, when the water wheels are frozen still, it is drawn up by hand and poured into the channels that convey it away.

On Tuesday 10 October we travelled to Schiltach, where Eberhard, Count of Tübingen, chief governor of Hornberg, met us, and later travelled on with us towards Hachberg. We were fed well in Schiltach, as also in Sulz, and again, as before, both nights' lodgings were paid for by the Duke of Württemberg, which, as I was told, amounted to a considerable sum of money. The following day, Wednesday 11 October, we rode to Haslach. As the Count of Tübingen rode through the River Kinzig, which was swollen with rain, with a strong current, his horse stepped onto a big stone, fell headfirst into the water, picked itself up again and fell again into the water, so that the count would have been thrown from his horse if he hadn't grabbed hold of the horse of the stablemaster, riding next to him. During this accident, the stablemaster's hat, which had a pearl cord, floated downstream, but was retrieved again. On Thursday 12 October, it rained so much that we reached Hachberg very wet. The ruler had arrived earlier with several noblemen and they were already playing a ball game in teams. A great crowd was together there, all lodged in the castle, with many horses stabled at the farm and in Emmendingen. On Friday, everything was arranged and organized splendidly at the banquet, music and dances. Afterwards, after midnight, a herald carrying a gilt sceptre entered, dressed in the margravial colours in a red silk robe with yellow sleeves. Led by trumpeters, he marched three times around the great hall in which we had danced, and then read out a 'cartel' which he was carrying: how a knight of rather advanced age named Cheerful Fred[33] had arrived, who wanted to hold and be the challenger of a tournament on the following Sunday, on horseback and

---

[33]   Fritz Wohlgemut.

with swords. If several of the noblemen present were willing to engage with him in full armour as 'cavaliers' at this, he would try to hold his own against them. He also read out the rules according to which this should take place, and under what conditions, and which three should earn the prize, and with that he left.

On Saturday, a wild boar[34] hunt was arranged, in the forest not far from Hachberg, of which a part was enclosed by stretched sheets of cloth. They went there at eight o'clock and began the hunt, and the hunters and peasants chased the red deer and wild boar out of the woods with dogs, to a place close by, sloping and likewise enclosed with cloth sheets, where his gracious highness and several other gentry and noblemen were ready with boar-spikes and guns, and the womenfolk and others watched from inside the hunting lodge. In addition, trumpeters sat in the trees in the forest, and signalled when they saw game move toward the place where they were to be caught. And once the first deer was caught, having run into the cloth, and been restrained there by the dogs, von Rotburg dispatched it. Then the dogs brought down a second one in the woods, which was also captured. The third deer was chased out of the woods by the dogs. They would have preferred to let it go, as the hunt had been arranged for wild boar. So the cloths were lifted to allow it to run out of the enclosure. But the dogs likewise forcefully broke free, and chased it into some water down in the valley, into which it ran, bringing it down, so that the peasants following them had to kill it as well. It took a lot of trouble to bring the dogs back into the hunting enclosure. Here they later chased five young wild pigs, year-old boars, out of the woods and brought them down with loud barking, and groaning of the boars. Of which three were killed, and the peasants freed two from the dogs alive and tied them up. On his gracious highness's order, they threw one into the women's carriage, out of which they fled, and when it escaped, the young dogs throttled it. They also caught a wild pig right in front of his gracious highness, a two-year-old, and when the large dogs secured on chains were unleashed, they caught a three-year-old wild boar. The peasants pushed a cudgel down its throat and tore it away from the dogs, which they drove off, then tied its feet, and laid it live onto a cart. But it was so exhausted and panted so strongly, that it arrived dead at Hachberg. There the seven boar and three deer were gutted and laid out in a row in the yard, according to custom, and their offal was gathered together in a barrel to share between the dogs. Then the game was taken to the slaughterhouse.

On Sunday, the sermon was held, and music accompanied the hymns; and because it rained a lot, the tournament was postponed until the weather let up. But a great deal of practicing took place, and while they were testing their skills prior to the main tournament on the tournament square, the stablemaster's arm was slightly wounded. The sword tournament on horseback was postponed until Tuesday 17 October because of persistent rain, which continued even on that day,

---

[34]   Generically male in English, but female in German. Platter also refers to them as wild pigs or 'black game' (as opposed to red game, or deer), and uses the terms for one-year-old ('Frischling') and two-year-old ('Bache') boar.

so that the tournament did not take place on the tournament square, which was under deep water, but on gravelled land in Emmendingen so surrounded by water that it looked like an island. And so that the horses didn't fall into the water, this area was surrounded and enclosed by stretched sheets of cloth all round, as with the hunt. The parade took place here in the afternoon, led by fifteen mounted cuirassiers with closed helmets, with trumpeters, preceded by riders carrying regimental maces and banners. They paraded in the traditional manner, bowing before the judges and womenfolk gathered there, before lining up in formation. First, the old Rheingraf Friedrich [Count of Salm] came forward to challenge or defeat one after another. His grace's son-in-law, Georg Friedrich, Margrave [of Baden], came forward against him. They engaged in five rounds in a row, each time hitting each other's ceremonial helmets so powerfully with their drawn swords that a particularly severe blow dented the Rheingraf count's morion. The margrave was slightly injured under his arm, in his armpit, without, however, incapacitating his gracious highness. Then von Rappoltstein met with the Rheingraf count in battle, who however, was hit in the second exchange, and, losing his balance in his heavy armour, fell off his horse, but was soon righted again without injury. In the third meeting, between the Rheingraf count and von Geroldseck, all three rounds were fought honourably. As also in the fourth meeting, between the Rheingraf count and von Limpurg. In the fifth, however, Rheingraf Friedrich [Count of Salm] was so badly wounded on his hand by his son Johann during the first round, that he no longer wished to challenge or participate in the tournament.

So the sixth meeting was between Johann Georg, Count of Hohenzollern and Wolf Wilhelm von Eptingen. The count's weapon dropped out of his grasp, so that he had to dismount and, hampered by his armour, which made everything difficult, mount again and complete the round. The seventh exchange was between the forest warden von Rotburg and von Reinach, and during the third round von Rotburg's right hand was severely injured at the wrist, so that he could not compete in the remaining rounds. The remaining meetings involved von Baerenfels, Schenk, von Steinkallenfels, von Landsberg and von Bütikum, always two paired up. Once they were over, the 'Foille' or concluding fight followed, during which everyone picked an opponent; the margrave competed with von Geroldseck. This resulted in a tough fight which lasted a good while, and went well except that von Steinkallenfels pursued von Landsberg so hard that he went through the cloths to the edge of the island, and fell backwards on his horse, in full armour into the water. But he was soon helped out again. And when this tournament was finished, everyone returned to Hachberg. After the evening banquet and dance where completed, the trophies were distributed with the customary ceremonies. The first was presented to von Geroldseck, the second to von Steinkallenfels, and the third to the Rheingraf count, as those who had conducted themselves most chivalrously. On the morning of Wednesday 18 October, everyone made their farewells and joyfully set off for home, and this is the farewell saying that I left on the wall: 'Eventually, you can have enough of court life, even though it's a good life for those who enjoy it.'

On Wednesday 8 November, Georg Friedrich, Margrave of Baden sent for me at Kandern.[35] And at a hunt on that day, his gracious highness killed 23 wild boar, two deer, and a rabbit, and before that, his gracious highness also killed many wild boar, including six whelps, at a hunt around Sulzberg. After the evening meal, his gracious highness disciplined two young women from the women's group, and then the chief forest warden performed the traditional ceremony of the hunting knife with several noblemen and others. In this, the accused, those who had trespassed hunt regulations by word or deed, had to kneel on a captured boar, where they were struck twice on their backside with the flat side of the blade, then for a third time on the shoulder, and each blow was accompanied by an announcement that this was done in the name of his gracious highness and of those gathered there. He was then asked whether he deserved this, if he said yes, he was free; if he said no, he was struck again.

---

[35]   This seat of the margrave's hunting palace lies 20km north of Basle.

Chapter 17

Thomas Platter in Avignon: Jewish Life and a Performing Quack Troupe in 1598[1]

On 13 October I took a printed health certificate reading as follows:

> Today, 13 October 1598, having lived here for a year, Thomas Platter, Doctor of Medicine and his page left Montpellier, God be praised in good health, in order to travel to Sommières and Uzès.

> Fesguet.[2]

Then I left Montpellier again. My fellow countrymen accompanied me as far as Castlenau. There we had a drink, and I rode on alone with my lackey through Faumanie, back toward Sommières. On 14 October, I rode through Saint-Mamert-du-Gard etc., taking the main road to the village of La Calmette, where I had the midday meal, and afterwards, by the route repeatedly described above, arrived again in Uzès that night. [...] On 17 October, I sent my lackey to Avignon to find out if the noble Lasser von Lassereggs were still there. When I found out that they were, I began to prepare for the journey. On 19 October and the following days to the time of my departure, I collected final payments from my patients and made my good-byes. I also purchased much fruit and other unusual things. Together with my books, notes and clothing, I packed them in

---

[1] Basle UL, MS.A l V.7–8: ff.237ᵛ, 238ʳ, 239ʳ, 239ᵛ, 241ᵛ–266ʳ; *Thomas Platter d.J*, 285–308 (13 October – 24 December 1598, Avignon). As noted above (Chapter 5), Platter's account of Avignon's Jews draws heavily on a 561-page German language publication written by an academic colleague of Felix Platter (Buxtorf, *Synagoga Ivdaica*, Basle 1603). The bold passages in the present translation indicate equivalent or near-equivalent passages here quoted verbatim, as substitutes for literal modern English translations of Platter's wording, from the 334-page English edition of this work (Buxtorf, *The Jewish Synagogue*, London 1663). The sequence of the quoted passages follows Platter, not Buxtorf, and the indicated omissions are not to Platter's accounts of Jews and actors in Avignon in 1598, of which each included section is here represented in its entirety, but to the 1663 English edition of Buxtorf's monograph. Titles of the omitted sections of Platter's account of Avignon's Jews, which also follow Buxtorf, are here footnoted, the first being 'On several Jewish laws and practices'.

[2] Thomas Platter provides a German translation for the original French wording of the certificate, authenticated with Montpellier's civic seal and signed by the city's First Consul, M Fesquet.

a hamper, whose final weight was recorded at 200 pounds. This I had sent from Uzès to Lyon and from there to Basle. [...]

Journey to Avignon

On the morning of 26 October, I visited several of my closest friends, giving them gifts according to the custom. For whom my farewells and their reciprocations were very difficult, since I had now lived amongst them for a good while. But eventually the time to part arrives. [...] On 27 October [...] after taking the midday meal in Villeneuve I crossed the bridge into the city of Avignon, where I lodged at the Petit Paris with the highborn Lasser von Lassereggs. I stayed in Avignon with these two brothers until 24 December. I learnt the Spanish language from them and practiced many unusual skills with them, on which they spared no expense, all of which I wrote up as diligently as I could. I also witnessed the following things, which are not described above. [...] At that time there was also a (*synagoga judaica*) Jewish synagogue in Avignon, and always around 500 Jews living in one particular street, as indicated in fol.80 above. I often observed them practicing all kinds of unusual customs both in and outside their temple, and I frequently spoke (*conferiert*) with them, given that almost every day several came to our lodgings bringing goods for sale. For this reason, I now want to describe them in a little more detail than previously.[3]

On the Circumcision of the Jews[4]

During the two months I stayed in Avignon, I saw two little boys being circumcised in their temple. Partly from what I saw, and partly from what I heard from them or read, this took place as follows: **he that circumciseth [...] ought to be a Jew, a man, not a woman. One well exercised in cutting.** The first circumcision that I saw was performed by the child's father. On both thumbs, he had **long nails, pointed at the top**. The knife was of sharpened iron or steel, with a yellow tin handle, **much like to Barbers Rasours**, but less broad. The child was bathed before the circumcision, washed clean and swaddled, that it **may be cleanly in the time of Circumcision; for otherwise it is not lawfull to say any prayer for it. Hence if the child [...] beray himself, he who circumciseth will not [...] pray for him, untill he be washed and swadled up in other linnen. The ordinary time appointed [...] is the eight day following the Nativity [...] while it is yet morning, and while the child is fasting, because such plenty of**

---

[3]   Here follows Platter's here omitted first sub-section ('On several Jewish laws and practices'), which is in turn directly followed by 'On the Circumcision of the Jews'.

[4]   Source of bold translations: Buxtorf 1663, 45–55 (Platter's original German language source: Buxtorf 1603, 106–27).

blood will not issue from the child then. And everything had been prepared very early that same morning. **First of all** there were **two chairs [...] adorned with** beautiful **Tapestry, and silken and velvet furniture [...] near unto the Ark, anciently styled the Ark of the Covenant, in which the book of the Law is kept; for such a place is holy in esteem.** Then the Godfather [...] drew **near,** and stood by **the foresaid chair, [...] he that is to circumcise the child being place near unto him. After them follow other of the Jews, one of which with a loud voice gives warning that they should [...] bring the things requisite for the Circumcision. [...] some certain youths hasten to the place, one of them carrying a great Candlesticks in which are twelve wax lights burning, to represent the twelve Tribes [...] two [...] carrying two Goblets full of Claret wine, another brings the knife wherewith the child is to be circumcised, another one Bason full of sand, and a third another filled with the oyl of Balsome, in which are steeped some** clean soft, fine **rags,** to be laid afterwards to the sore of the [...] **infant. These drawing near [...] cast themselves into a certain ring or circle** round the circumciser, **that they may better see and learn [...]** because **These places the youths purchase with mony,** bidding for them publicly in the temple, as for other religious offices. **Some others also there be, that flock thither with odours and sweeet meats [...]**[5] **that they may comfort and refresh the Father or Godfather [...] so be it that any of them should fall into a swound by some conceived grief for the cutting off the foreskin [...] The Godfather [...] placeth himself in one of the aforementioned chairs [...] opposite to him** stood the circumciser and sung **that Song registred in the second book of** *Moses,* **which the Israelites sung, when they had passed through the Red sea, with many more of the same sort, then the women bring the infant to the gate, when the whole Congregation rising up, the Godfather** goes to the door and takes **the child from them, sitting down with him in his seat again.** And everyone cried (in Hebrew: ***Baruch habba,*** because in the temple they only speak Hebrew): ***'Blessed is he that cometh.'*** Because they **are of the opinion that** the angel of the covenant, that is the prophet *Elias* **comes with the Child, & seats himself in the empty chair** next to the godfather, **to see** that **they rightly observe and keep the covenant of Circumcision. [...]** So soon as *Elias* **his chaire is brought [...], then are they bound to say in expresse terms, This seat is provided for** *Elias,* **the Prophet.** Otherwise **he comes not to the circumcision. [...] Moreover, that Elias may tarry till the circumcision be totally finished they leave the chair in the same place, for the space of three whole dayes. [...] When therefore the Godfather hath the child** on his lap, the circumciser **looseth his swaddling, takes hold of his yard, laying hands apon the former part thereof by the foreskin, thrusts down the gland thereof, which done, he rubs the foreskin, that by mortifying of it the child may be lesse sensible of the cutting: then taking the knife prepared for circumcision**

---

5   Buxtorf adds: 'made by the Art of the Apothecary, with strong and delicious wine, Carrawaies, Cinnamon and such like' (1663, 47).

out of the boyes hand that carried it, he says loudly: *Blessed be thou, O God our Lord, King of the World, who hast sanctified us by thy Commandements, and given to us the Covenant of circumcision.* […] whiles he is thus speaking, he cuts away so much of the fore-skin that the top of the yard may be seen bare and naked, which he throws in haste into the Bason filled with sand, restoring the knife to him from whom he took it, and takes one of the Cups full of red Wine, out of which he sucks a mouthful, which he presently spues out again upon the Infant's face if he perceive him to faint: instantly upon this he takes the childs yard in his mouth, and sucks as much bloud out of it as he can possible, to the end that it may sooner leave bleeding, which bloud he casts out again, either into one of the bowls of red Wine, or into the bason of Sand. This he doth three times at the least. […] After that the flux of bloud be somewhat appeased, then the circumciser grasps the cut skin on the child's penis with the pointed, sharpened nails of both thumbs, tears it apart, tucks it in, that the head of the yard may wholly appear (which they call exposure, and is far more painful for the child than the circumcision itself), then takes the linen rags […] steeped in […] Oyl, applies them to the childes yard, and binds them about three or four times, then taking the Infant, folds him up in his swaddling cloaths. Then the Father of the child, who in this case was the circumciser, saith: '*Blessed be thou, O God, our Lord, King of the world, who hast sanctified us by thy Commandements, and hast commanded us to fulfill the Covenant made with Abraham our Father*'. Whereupon the whole Congregation answered, saying: 'As happy an entrance shall this little Infant have into the possession of *Moses* his Law, into Marriage and the practice of good works, as he hath had into the covenant of *Abraham* our Father'. Then the circumciser washes his mouth and hands completely clean, the Godfather of the child rises up with him, placeth himself directly opposite the circumciser, who takes one of the bowls full of red wine, and saith a certain Prayer over it: then he prayes also over the Infant and sayes: *O God which art our God, the God of our Fathers, strengthen and keep this Infant, to the comfort of his Parents; and make that* among the people of Israel *his name may be called* (for at this instance he names the child […]) *Isaac, which was the Son of Abraham: let his Father rejoyce because he came out of his loyns: let his Mother rejoyce in the fruit of her womb,* as it is written in Proverbs 23 v.2: *Thy Father and thy Mother shall be glad, and she that bare thee shall rejoyce:* God saith also by the mouth of his Prophet, Ezekiel 16.6 *and when I passed by thee, and saw thee polluted in thine own bloud, I said unto thee, when thou wast in thy bloud, live; yea, I sayd unto thee, when thou wast in thy bloud, live.* Here he dips his finger into the Cup full of Wine […] into which he had vented the bloud which he suckt out […] and anoints the lips of the child three times therewith, hoping that according to the fore-mentioned saying […] his dayes shall be more […] and that he shall live in the bloud of his circumcision. *David* also saith, Be ye mindful always of his covenant; the word which he commanded to a thousand generations.[6] **Then he proceeds to pray unto God, that he would defend them that are present, as being such men who would eftsoons confirm his covenant by the fulfilling of it. Furthermore, that he would vouchsafe to grant a long life to the Father and Mother of the child; and also to bestow a blessing on the Babe. [...] he reatcheth the Cup [...] to every one of the yong men, and invites them to drink thereof.** To conclude, all they return home with the young little Jew, **restoring him into the arms of the Mother**, and thus concluded the circumcision. As I noted, **Some of the upright Jews take the little Infant, and both before and after his circumcision lay him upon the bolster or cushion of** *Elias* for a little while so that Elijah himself **may touch** and bless him. **To proceed, the casting of the fore-skin into the sand, signifies that their seed shall be like the sand upon the sea shore.**[7] **[...] If an Infant be sickly, they [...] defer** circumcision **until the time of his recovery. If any Infant dye [...] then he is ci[r]cumcised in the Church-yard, over his grave, yet so that no Prayers be said for him.** Instead a gravestone is erected, so that prayers are said for him. When they return home from the synagogue, **great provision is made, to which [...]** at least **ten men are invited,** and at least one or two **Rabbines,** who deliver **a long Grace, and make a kind of Sermon, to which the hearers giving but lean little attention.** This is what happens with girls: when they are six weeks old, **some certain number of young girls seat themselves around about the Cradle, in which the infant lies wrapp'd in fine linnen [...] embroidered with silver, who heave the Infant together with the cradle, many times aloft into the aire, and at length name the child, she that stands at the head of the Cradle being the Godmother,** afterwards they too have a banquet.

On the Women's Baths[8]

I was also shown several tanks of water constructed under their temple, in which the women often purified themselves, as follows. **Sometimes they are compelled to dive so deep, that not so much as one hair doth appear above the water, [...] they stretch out their arms and fingers [...] that by this means the water may come unto every part, and so enrich the whole body with an exact cleanesse.** This was often very hazardous, especially in the winter, as where there are no warm springs, they are not[9] permitted to mix in warm water, as is described in detail, together with further customs of the women, in a **little book written in**

---

[6]   I Chronicles 16.15 (*King James Bible*). Here, Buxtorf instead quotes Psalms 105.8 (1603) or Psalms 105.5 (1663).

[7]   Genesis 32.11 (*King James Bible*).

[8]   Source of bold translations: Buxtorf 1663, 56–7 (Platter's original German language source: Buxtorf 1603, 130–1).

[9]   According to Buxtorf, this was permitted (1603, 131).

the *Germane* tongue and Hebrew Character, called *Frawen Buchlein*,[10] or the book of women.[11]

What the Jews do after Morning Prayer[12]

When they are returned unto their owne house, they lay aside their phylacteries and [...] garment of remembrance. They take breakfast before going to work. They believe that there are sixty three diseases of the Gall, which may all be cured by the eating of crust, and a [...] draught of [...] wine. [...] Honest wives [...] will in the meane time make ready [...] dinner so that their husbands can eat their midday meal promptly at eleven a clock otherwise they may fall into some disease. [...] It is necessary [...] to set downe to dinner [...] with an empty stomack and washed hands, and also considered very important to wash and dry hands thoroughly after eating. They also have many strange customs while eating, with the blessing, bread, [...] salt and wine. They must use a modest carriage, as if they were sitting in the presence of the Lord, should not cast the bones and finnes of fishes upon one hand or other, or behind themselves, lest they might touch [...] invisible creatures. After eating, one little piece of bread is left upon the table, that [...] something thereupon [...] may be the subject of blessing. Towards evening they say their evening and night prayers in their schools. And if two be at ods [...] one [...] steps unto the song book, out of which the Chanter sings [...], shuts it, and giving it a clap with his hand, saith *I conclude [...] this.* [...] And [...] it is not lawfull for them to say any more prayers until peace is reinstated. Thence it often fals out, that they retu[r]ne home without any praying; yet if the one party bee [...] refractory, there happens many times a surcease [....] of [...] prayer, for some whole dayes. In bed, they pray until they fall asleep. They undress as they dress.[13]

---

[10]   Keiser (294) identifies this as *Ein schön fruen büchlein* [1602].

[11]   There follow: 'On their child rearing'; 'How the Jews rise in the morning'; 'On the clothing of Jews and the characteristics of their laws and taboos'; 'Concerning the morning prayer of the Jews'.

[12]   Source of bold translations: Buxtorf 1663, 98*–9*, 101*, 106–7, 109, 111, 115, 120. (NB Duplicate paginations in the 1663 edition, here designated by asterisks: 97*–104*: after 104, 209*–10*: after 210. Additionally, 287 follows directly after 256). Platter's original German language source: Buxtorf 1603, 241–87.

[13]   There follow: 'On several matters in and carried out in their synagogues'; 'How the Jews prepare for their Sabbath'; 'How they keep the Sabbath'.

Easter feast of the Jews[14]

They spend several days preparing for this, and also celebrate for several days afterwards, so that it is observed even more thoroughly. But during the festival they all deem themselves **great Lords, [...] leane [...] upon their left sides** when they drink and **drinke** out four **consecrated [...] cups** of wine, one after the other, **curse all people which are not of Israel,** and finally pray **that God would** soon **build again** their **Temple.** Very often they say: **now build** up, **now build up [...] very quickly, very quickly,** etc. And they celebrate this festival very intensely, on 14 March for two days in a row.

Concerning the feast of Pentecost[15]

On the second night after Easter they begin to count when the stars rise, with a little prayer, and keep going in this way for seven nights, that makes a week. And on the eighth day they say today it is eight days. In this way they count **49 daies.** That is the eve **of Pentecost.** During this period **it is not lawfull [...] to use phlebotomy; for [...] there blowed a certaine [...] pestilent winde, which they call [...] butcher. [...] They keep this Feast for two daies together, [...] they** strew around grass mowings, **Sticking** up also **[...] green boughes.**

Feast of Tabernacles[16]

This festival is held in September, which is **the seventh month** or **the first,** because Adam was created during this month. And **this Feast, was as a signe** to **recall** that **God [...] sustained** his people **for the space of forty yeares in the desert,** in Tabernacles. And even though they say a lot of prayers during these festivities there is no real piety. Instead they just rattle their prayers out, and if they could say a thousand words in one breath, they would regard it as the highest art. **When,** in the school, **the Chanter hath proceeded [...] in his prayers [...] to [...]** *Give peace [...] O Lord;* **then every one taking a little bundle of palm, olive, and willow branches in his right hand, and** a lemon **in his left,** praises God, **[...] shakes the bundle,** and **shakes** it **towards** the four ends of the world, also up and down. **This they doe** seven times **for seven daies together, in remembrance that**

---

[14] Pesach. (Source of bold translations: Buxtorf 1663, 183, 187–8; Platter's original German language source: Buxtorf 1603, 414–40).

[15] Shavuot. (Source of bold translations: Buxtorf 1663, 196, 198; Platter's original German language source: Buxtorf 1603, 445–50).

[16] Sukkot. (Source of bold translations: Buxtorf, 200, 202; Platter's original German language source: Buxtorf 1603, 452–8).

the wals of Jericho being [...] compassed about seven times by them, fell flat unto the ground, and this is how the Christians will also fall.

On the Feast of the New Moon and etc.[17]

They also celebrate the new Moon, and are of the opinion, that at the beginning the Sun and Moon were equal in light. [...] But so soon as the Moon murmured against God, and would [...] be sole Monarch in the celestial Orbs, God made it smaller, takes away her own light, and caused her to borrow of the Sun. [...] God hearing the Moon complain of this [...] repented [...] and caused a propitiatory sacrifice to be offered [...] at every new Moon. They also believe that on New-years-day,[18] which falls in the first month of autumn, namely when the autumn moon is new, when Adam was created, God and his Angels sit in judgment over the sins of the Jews, so they also celebrate this day as a splendid festival. They also keep a feast of Reconciliation,[19] when they [...] humble themselves by abstaining from a five-fold kind of pleasure. Firstly they fast, excepting the sick, who are administred food by order of their Physitian. [...] Secondly, every one is bound to goe without shoes. [...] Thirdly, no man ought [...] to annoint himself with perfumed oyle. [...] Fourthly, no man must [...] wash. [...] Fifthly, they must not come at their wives.

On Jewish Fasting[20]

They have many fast days, even though in the law of *Moses* there is only one fast commanded to be kept [...] upon the tenth of September, [...] the feast of reconciliation. For example, because upon the ninth day of July [...] the temple was burnt, so that they regard it as an ominous month; Upon the eighth day they feed only upon lentiles, in signe of sorrow [...] but they will neither eat beans nor pease, because they have a certain black stroke in their upper parts much like unto a mouth: but [...] lentiles and egges, [...] have no such line [...] neither any representation of a mouth, and therefore do best decipher [...] a man ful of [...] sorrow, who [...] sayes nothing, as though he had no mouth.

---

[17]   Source of bold translations: Buxtorf 1663, 211, 223, 233–4 (Platter's original German language source: Buxtorf 1603, 473–527).

[18]   Rosh Hashanah.

[19]   Yom Kippur (Day of Atonement).

[20]   Source of bold translations: Buxtorf 1663, 246–7 (Platter's original German language source: Buxtorf 1603, 550–3).

On their Food Preparation and Diet[21]

Their kitchin boyling vessels are of two sorts, the one whereof is appointed for the seething of flesh, the other for milke. [...] A Jew continually carries about him two knives, one for flesh and another for cheese and fish, which have also [...] stamps upon them. [...] Flesh and milke must not be boiled together at the same time over the same fire: neither are they to be set on the table [...] against another. [...] He that eates [...] flesh, he may not be allowed for a whole houres space, to eat [...] any milke-meats. [...] It is a hainous offence to set fish and flesh at the same time upon one table, as also [...] to eat them together, for the leprosie follows. Jewish **Butchers** have to be very experienced and have a **testimonial letter** from **the Rabbines**, otherwise they are not permitted to practice this trade, because it is governed by numerous unusual written **Rules, [...] which he must therefore bestow great paines to study. [...] They eat not any thing which hath the least drop of blood in it [...] They likewise do not eat the hinder parts [...] because** *the Angel* injured *Jacobs thigh*. Genesis 32.[22] **They sell the hinder parts [...] to the Christians: [...] and defile them, causing their children to pisse upon them: they themselves pronouncing a curse upon them, that the Gentile that buyes them may eat up [...] death itself.** This is confirmed by the joynt testimony of so many Iews as have been converted to the Christian faith.

On Jewish Weddings[23]

While I was in Avignon, I saw a Jewish wedding held there, and also went to their dance. Around half a dozen Jews stood in one corner of the hall and with very loud voices sung all sorts of dance tunes, galliards and branles; they were not permitted any musical instruments. After **the handfasting [...] of the espousals** by both parties **many Iews both young and old are called together into some** room, **every one of the younger sort carrying a pot in his hand,** then the marriage **Letter** was read, also what **dowry** he should give them and when the wedding should take place. Then they wished them **good fortune,** and they **throw their [...] pots upon the ground, [...] saying that it is a token of good luck [...] and abundance.** While **every one departs,** they are given **sweetest wine** and confection. The **Bride upon the day before the marriage must wash her self in cold water [...] so that her whole body be hid in the water. She is led** by women with bells, so **that every one** hears it. The bridal pair send each other girdles, one

---

[21]   Source of bold translations: Buxtorf 1663, 251–2, 254, 287 (Platter's original German language source: Buxtorf 1603, 560–72).

[22]   Genesis 32.25 (*King James Bible*).

[23]   Source of bold translations: Buxtorf 1663, 288–94 (Platter's original German language source: Buxtorf 1603, 573–84).

with **gold** studs from **the Bridegroom,** and one with **silver studs** from the **Bride.** [...] **Upon the day whereon** she is **to receive a blessing, she** is dressed **as finely as** possible, her hair is daintily plaited and decorated with a beautiful bonnet. They **put a vail over her** eyes to prevent her from looking at the groom. While they thus prepare her, they cheer her by singing various entertaining **Bridal-Ballads.** Following this, she is blessed in front of the church in the street under the open sky, as I have seen. First, **the bridegroom** came, **attended with** several **men.** Then **followes the bride and her damsels.** And then **the Bride** was led [...] **about her bridgegroom three several times.** [...] **Then the bridegroom takes his bride and leads her once about** [...], **the people in the mean time casting** [...] **grain upon** them, **signifying that** [...] fruitfulness and **riches** [...] **shall befall them.** [...] **The bride** stands **upon the right hand of the Bridegroom,** with her face **towards the South,** as they position their beds in order to bear sons. **The Rabbine who marries** [...] **them** puts **the skirt of the hair-cloth** [...] **which the Bridegroom wears about his neck,** [...] **upon the head of the Bride.** Then the Rabbi **takes a glass of wine,** and after **giving thanks unto God** allows **the Bride and the Bridegroom** [...] **to drink thereof.** And the mother of the bride, who was standing behind her, wiped her mouth with a handkerchief. And because she tried to wipe it too soon, the bride was rushed, and spilled wine onto herself. She was completely dressed in white satin and her mother chastized her severely in front of everyone. Even though it was really her own fault, no-one was allowed to blame her. I was also told that because she was a virgin, this was her first visit to the church, because no unmarried women are permitted into the church before they are married, to prevent romantic complications which would distract from their prayers. During the blessing, **if the Bride be a virgin, then the cup must have a narrow mouth, if a widow a large one.** [...] **After that** [...] **The Rabbine takes the wedding-ring from the Bridegroom,** [...] **of pure gold, yet having no jewel in it,** shows it to the people for approval, **and then puts it upon the Brides second finger,** publicly **repeating the letters of contract.** Then, from a second **glass,** the Rabbi lets them drink as before, **giving thanks unto God that** they, already betrothed, **have mutually accepted one of another.** And the Bridegroom **takes the** first **Cup and throws it against the** ground **in remembrance of the ruinated temple. When the marriage is ended they sit down to dinner, the Bridgroom** [...] **is bound to sing a long prayer,** [...] **others are calling for the hens to be brought.** Then the bride is given **an henn and egge,** and with hearty laughter, they pull **in pieces the hens.** This lets **her know that she shall bring forth her children easily, without pain** [...] **even as a hen bringeth forth an egge, with** [...] **her cockling voice of joy.** Only after these amusing diversions is the wedding meal set up, at which they dance and sing with great joy. At the end of the wedding they dance a branle.[24] The groom leads the men, one after another, and the bride the women, and they all dance with each other, or **the chief man** [...] **takes the Bridegroom,** and **the chief matron** [...] **the Bride,** and they dance as

---

[24]   Buxtorf: 'Mitzuah', 'marriage *pavin*'.

described. **Their marriage rites [...] commonly endure for the space of eight dayes together.**[25]

On Jewish Illnesses[26]

Like **Christians**, they too have **many diseases**. They use many **Characters** and cabalistic arts, also supernatural and magical arts, against serious illnesses. All their books are filled with these matters.[27]

During the time of my stay in Avignon, I saw the Jews practice some of what I have described above. Some I heard from them and read about in their books, as they frequently came to our inn and brought the two brothers all sorts of lovely, precious goods to buy, or simply to look at, of which they bought little from them. Even so they came to us nearly every day. They are staunchly protected by the authorities, who ensure that nobody does them any harm, because they have to pay the Pope high taxes.

On the Actors[28]

Throughout my stay in Avignon, I often saw many unusual comedy players, mostly Italians, (*agieren*) perform there, notably (*Zan Bragetta*) Hans Latz.[29] For several weeks, on a stage in a tennis court, he presented many extremely amusing, entertaining comedies, with two women and four men, to which I too went several times. They generally lasted into the night and had to be finished by torchlight. Among others, I can still recall that once, one of his people was able to imitate all sorts of animal and bird noises with a single little whistle in his mouth, just by manipulating the whistle in his mouth with his tongue, without using his hands.[30] Item, on another occasion he hacked one young woman's head off behind the curtain, which he then drew aside, and there stood the head on its own in a bowl on the bench, and she stretched both arms down across the bench, so that one could

---

[25] There follow: 'On the divorce of the Jews'; 'How Jewish widows divorce their late husband's brother'.

[26] Source of bold translations: Buxtorf 1663, 303 (Platter's original German language source: Buxtorf 1603, 598).

[27] There follow: 'On several Jewish punishments'; 'On Jewish death'; 'On the coming of the Messiah'.

[28] Comœdianten.

[29] As here, Platter often supplements a term or name that he has translated literally into German, with its parenthesized and italicized original wording.

[30] Grimmelshausen's fictional sometime wandering quack Simplicius attracts a crowd of 600 customers for his wares by imitating animal and bird noises on his violin ('Springinsfeld [1670]', *Werke* I.2, 194–5).

see the stump at the neck very realistically. Anyone who didn't know this trick would not have suspected any irregularity, because of course it does not involve magic. They also performed (*pastorelle*) shepherd comedies most gracefully, and they could act Pantalone as well as Zanni most skilfully, not only with words, but also with dancing, mime and acrobatics, so that everyone had enough to laugh about, and watched with enjoyment. They spoke Italian, and sometimes mixed in some Occitan. They also had good musicians among them, who could accompany their own singing so pleasingly on the lute, harp and viola that it amazed many. When they noticed that not many people were coming to their comedies any more, even though they still had to pay a high rent for the tennis court, they set up a long table in the public square, called the Place du Change. After the midday meal, they all stood together on this same table, one next to another. They had placed a large locked chest next to them on the table, and when they had played an amusing comedy on this same table for a couple of hours or so, and saw that a large crowd had gathered, between 100 and 500, or even 1000 people, then Zanni, who was their leader, unlocked the chest. One of his companions, standing next to him in the costume of a doctor, asked him excessively loudly what sort of wares he had there. At that, he stood up again and started giving an impressive speech: that he had come from Turkey, where he had bought expensive medicines and learned many secret skills. But as a sign of his gratitude, because he had heard so many good reports of this town, and held it in such high regard, and had also had many good experiences here, he wanted to share his skill and medicines for the benefit of the inhabitants.

He took out a little tin, apparently full of (*pomata*) unguent, opened it, spread it on his hands, his face and elsewhere, smelt it, and gave it to his companions, all costumed and neatly masked, to examine and smell. They all gave him a good report of it, that it was very excellent, excluding the doctor, who argued with him, calling him an itinerant quack, it was just made of butter, etc., greatly belittling it. Then Zanni started again, and refuted all his arguments with solid reasons, and in this way they disputed most amusingly with each other for a good while, until at last the doctor had to be quiet and Zanni won the argument. Then they played something delightful together on their instruments, to which they sung delightfully. Meanwhile, he put out around a couple of 100 little tins which he has in stock and intends to sell. He resumes shouting about and praising his unguent again. Even though it cost him many 100 crowns excluding his labour, he is willing to part with each tin for only 10 crowns. This was indeed an excellent price, because he was not seeking a profit. Some paid a lot of money, he could save them a lot. Whoever wanted one should throw the money to him in their handkerchief, and he would give it to them. Meanwhile, they played music again, just a few verses. Then the doctor said that he wanted too much for a tin, and he in turn replied that he would take half, that is 5 crowns. He paused briefly, each time reducing the price by half, until he got to a steuber, the sixtieth part of a crown or half a Swiss batzen. At that point, he raised his voice and said that although he had hoped to make a good profit, and the pomade was well worth it, as a favour to the townspeople, he would charge not 10 crowns, not 5, not two, not one, not a half, not 10 steubers, not 5 not 2, but just one steuber for a tinful. Those who wanted it, should throw over their handkerchiefs, and he would give it to the first for nothing.

Immediately, the spectators were throwing their handkerchiefs by the heap to those on the table, each with a steuber knotted into it. Taking out the steuber and knotting the tin into it, they threw everyone back their own handkerchief again, and sometimes, when the women suggested it, they added a note to the tin, detailing where they could be met, and at what hour, as many such practices are also carried out.

And in this way they all have tasks which make fools of people. If he sells a couple of 100 and more keep throwing, he brings out more. Finally he warns them once more that anyone wanting it should throw now, as he is down to his last dozen and won't be getting any more. Because tomorrow he wants to sell another product. The following day, after the midday meal, the same seven again climb (en banque) onto their table and start by performing a lovely comedy. Then he brings out the product, perhaps a pleasantly-smelling toothpowder of which only the wrapping paper would actually be perfumed, or something for warts or sties, or Venetian soap, or something for toothache or wound herbs, or pleasantly-smelling powder or water or the like. And after the Doctor and Zanni have argued at length with each other, he displays the wares and sells them, generally for a steuber a piece.

Sometimes they also offer for sale several printed pictures on a broadsheet, demonstrating the most amusing ones to the crowd. Zanni says that if the text is too difficult for anyone who buys it for a steuber, and they can't understand or read it, they should come and meet him in his inn. He will explain it to him, and also show him other beautiful, secret prints, for a fee of one penny. With these and similar practices, they try to make a profit, which seldom happens, because they gamble, eat and drink away so much. And when they see that their skills start to count for nothing anymore, they pack up and move on to another city. In this way, they travel the world and save no money, because however much they want to save, time and again they can waste so much. They often perform many similar and different wonderful spectacles and dances, not all of which can be written down.

Journey to Montpellier

On 24 December, riding with the nobleman Johannes Escher, I journeyed away from Avignon and the two brothers, the noblemen Christoffel Lasser von Lasseregg and Wolff Dietrich.

Chapter 18

Hippolytus Guarinonius's *Grewel*: 35 Commedia dell'Arte Lazzi[1]

Lazzi no.1[2]

When humans gain pleasure through the five physical senses, there is no difference between them and the ass and all beasts, because they also gain delight in those things that entertain their eyes, ears, taste, etc. When, however, humans divert themselves inwardly with a clear conscience, through reason alone, that cannot be imitated by beasts. This is only appropriate to humans; it is the fitting human pleasure, while the other is completely false. However, the trait and tendency of bestial humans is to seek and wish their physical pleasures in all that is most beautiful and diverting, so that not just their eyes and ears, but if at all possible all five of their senses are always continually entertained, without ever stopping, to make them feel satisfied and satiated. As did that Zanni in an Italian comedy who was so devoted to his taste and gluttony that he wished and desired that his neck and gullet could be stretched from Padua to Constantinople, so that the fat macaroni, dumplings or noodles, of which he had swallowed one fistful after another at that time in the public square, would not slither down into his stomach so quickly, so that the pleasure of their taste would last all the longer. So this same Zanni, unable to rid himself of his wish, forcibly held up the swallowed macaroni and chunks in his gullet with his hand as long as he could, in order to prolong his enjoyment of them for longer.

---

[1]   These translations are not based on one continuous passage; each individual extract is separately referenced. Book, chapter and page references are to the 1610 published edition of Guarinonius's *Grewel*, the original German-language source of these passages. Also provided are volume and folio references to pre-publication versions of lazzi nos.1–21, in the treatise's incomplete manuscript (Innsbruck, UL Cod.110 vols. I and II, on which see Chapter 3, this volume). Also indicated, where available, are titles under which these lazzi are indexed in *Grewel*, and their associated sins.

[2]   2 [On the human mind], VII (On the other imperfect attributes of the mind from which joy and amusement are derived), 179–80 / I,f.273ᵛ, '*Zane* Wunsch' [Gluttony].

Lazzi no.2[3]

Tyrannical fathers [...] think that children should issue from their mothers' wombs exactly as their often really mad reasons lead them to wish them to be. This is no different from the Zanni in the Italian comedy who ordered his pregnant wife to heed that she did not deliver the young Zanni into the world until he could emerge from the womb ready to run around everywhere. Item, that she dress him, by bringing him into the world with breeches, doublet, shoes, hat, shirt and coat. Additionally, he supplied her with a man-sized measure as a guide to the height at which she should bear him, otherwise he would not accept or feed him. Just like those enraged madmen who instantly want to have grown-up, well bred, educated and intelligent children, without doing any of the things needed to achieve this.

Lazzi no.3[4]

This is to be understood concerning the nonsensical and unwise love practiced by almost all people. Not only do they boast to their acquaintances about everything that happens, but they make more than half of it up. This is like the *Magnificus* of the Italian comedy who rejoiced and jumped for joy, and boasted in what high favour he was with his beloved. But when his servant Zanni asked him 'Why?', *Magnificus* answered that when he was passing by yesterday, his beloved had opened her front door for him. Zanni said that maybe someone was going in or out. 'Yes of course', says *Magnificus*, 'the maid certainly came out'. Zanni laughed heartily at his master. Similarly, love robs many of their wit and reason, so that they consider all they see, hear, yes, even convince themselves to imagine, to be real gold and love. Out of happiness, they cannot hide it, but think that everyone should know about it, which leads to many later disagreements and arguments. Through this much love is broken apart and ended.

Lazzi no.4[5]

But the others, who seek their keep through regular manual work and must earn a daily wage as craftsmen, peasants, etc., often do not suffer much through love. Indeed, they marry a second, third and fourth time, raise many children, live together for many years, but still have nothing to say about love. Mostly,

---

[3]   2.XXV (On the terrifying abomination of partly tyrannical and coarse and partly far too lenient parents, against their children), 249 / I,ff.355–6, '*Zane* gebott an seinem schwangern Weib' [Sloth, wrath].

[4]   2.XXIX (A lovely secret about how to love honestly and without harm, with a happy ending), 284–5 / I,f.416, '*Zane* verlacht seinen verliebten Herrn' [Lechery].

[5]   2.XXIX, 285 / I,f.417, '*Zane* dient einem verliebten' [Lechery (Gluttony)].

their greatest ambition is a little jug of cool and blissful wine. In this way, Zanni thoroughly mocked his lovesick young master for not eating or drinking when he had such delicious food, not sleeping despite his soft featherbed, and for nourishing and sustaining himself solely with idle thoughts of love; so tyrannizing himself with love that it had diminished and withered away his body as well as his wits. Therefore Zanni made a public announcement that no position as servant is better than one like this, because the tasty, well-prepared meals, which through vain love the lovesick master will not eat, are much-appreciated meals for Zanni. If then frivolous humans were to love the creator himself as much as his creations, if they were willing to suffer for God's sake only the hundreth part of what they often tolerate, with great general loss and damage, for the sake of a vicious snake:

> What sort of reward from God?
> What sort of crown in heaven?
> Would then await them?

Lazzi no.5[6]

Occasionally, old fools engage in such illusions of vain love, which suit them most comically and pleasingly. In fact, actors have no better and more effective way of encouraging laughter than to bring forth a lovesick old man, who is standard to the Italian Comedy these days. Thus they prove that, as I noted previously, all those who treat love like this are foolish. Because young people are in any case not particularly wise, it is more acceptable in them. But to see this madness in those who are meant to be the wisest of all is completely disgraceful and shameful. As the old proverb says:

> Turpe senex miles, turpe senilis amor.
> It ill becomes the old to engage in war or love.[7]

They are not only harmful and damaging to themselves but, through their bad example, also to already thoughtless young people.

---

[6]   2.XXIX, 285–6 / I,f.418, 'Deren alte verliebte Tiltappen' [Lechery].

[7]   Here translated (as for lazzi nos.6, 7, 11, 14, 25, 34), is Guarinonius's German translation of the original quotation.

Lazzi no.6[8]

What is it, if not this godless and insufferable pride and ambition, that forces many in our time to descend into public disgrace and ridicule, poverty and eternal misery? It makes every fool want to be highly regarded, everyone want to strut and parade the public alleys displaying their fine feathers like an Indian peacock, to gain more respect in people's eyes. Through their outward appearance and clothing, everyone wants the eyes of others to judge them as more respectable and greater than they are, which is why such fellows end up over their ears in debt, because pride requires much. When one of this type stands in the middle of the square amongst eminent people who greatly respect him, then one merchant after another comes forward to deliver him a credit note here, a credit note there, for him to pay here, and pay there as well, and almost nowhere is safe for him. It was like this in the Italian comedy, when a proud aristocrat stood in a public garden, basking in his reputation and bragging of his refinement. When the cobbler approached him, offering him the credit note for his shoes and requesting money, he began to blush with embarrassment, saying he should visit him at home. The cobbler replies 'Well, Master, I am glad to have found you here for once, as I can never find you at home'. He ordered the cobbler to leave. He didn't want to give up, but demanded his due, until Zanni joined them and spun the cobbler such a yarn that the gallant got away with his honour intact. Thus the worldly shame of losing their reputation and good name causes the greatest misery to mad worldly people, especially those with great debts, great eminence and empty houses. But how can misery help them in this? Not at all, according to the Italian:

> Fastidi, non pagano debiti
> Misery does not repay debts.

Lazzi no.7[9]

Just see how often many an envious person, who has forced himself into the position and reputation from which he has pushed a good, honest man, suits that position and its duties. How many such people perform such strange, not to say foolish and mad tricks that they move more people to laugh at them than respect them. What is the cause of this? None other than only that he envied, and forcefully sought, something for which God had not created him and for which he was not suited, and thus is none other than:

---

[8]   2.XXXI (On the abomination of the remaining worry, fear, sadness, remorse, grief, suffering, impatience, shame, inconstancy), 296–7 / I,ff.435–7, '*Zane* hilfft eim stoltzen Juncker auß Noth' [Pride].

[9]   2.XXXV (On the monstrous abomination of envy), 356 / I,ff.514–16, '*Zane* wirdt zum Herrn / und ist nit zu neiden' [Sloth (envy, inquisitiveness)].

Asinus ad lyram,
The ass at the harp

It was like this in the Comedy, when Zanni, envying his master's power, developed an exceptional desire to know what it is like to be a master, because he had been a servant from childhood. His master, who was a student, noticed this. Pretending to be in despair, and even ready to disown himself through love, he asked his servant Zanni for his clothes, and put his own on Zanni, for whom this was in accordance with his wishes. He hung his rapier and dagger at his side, his gold chain around his neck and ordered him to step forward and be the master. He gave Zanni all his possessions, asking only that he should feed, protect and house him, as was fitting for a master. Zanni agreed to everything. Now, when Zanni strutted out and presented himself everywhere, his master's enemies approached and, from his clothing, could only assume that he was the right one. The 'servant' runs away, leaving his appointed 'master' in the lurch. The enemies draw their weapons and sand-filled sacks (with which minor debts are customarily paid off in Italy) and attacked Zanni. Zanni started shouting: 'Masters, masters, I am not the master; I am only the servant; I am only Zanni.' But nothing helped, and they beat him black and blue until he was almost half dead. Only when the enemies became tired did they realize that he was not the right one, and that they had trapped an innocent man. When Zanni noticed this he began moaning that he had been treated violently and unjustly. One of them replied: 'This serves you quite right, because you deceived us, and even though your master has escaped us this time, for now we are content and satisfied that at least we beat his clothes and let off steam on you, his servant.' Zanni had had enough, more than enough, of the position of master. He ran after his master and wanted nothing more than to reclaim his old clothes, job and position. Thus it often happens in this foolish world that, with envy and inappropriate ambition, we vigorously pursue that which is the most likely to break our necks.

Lazzi no.8[10]

Item: their curiosity to look at forbidden things has led many to the greatest corruption of body and soul. [...] Like the Zanni of the comedy who, in order to look at a ghost high above, climbed up a ladder to a window. When he got up there, a fiery flame and a young Devil shot out of the window at him, and one firework after another belched forth into his beard. When, frightened and screaming 'murder', he tried to jump back down the ladder, another ghost, with fire, appeared behind him on the ladder, and set alight his breeches. This drove him up again but the ghost above drove him down again, for a long time, until he was

---

[10]   2.XXXVII (On the abomination of curiosity), 375 / I,f.545, '*Zane* wirdt vom Fŭrwitz gestochen unnd gestrafft' [Inquisitiveness].

rescued. This demonstrates how curiosity leads the curious so strangely astray, that it is as if they are wandering aimlessly around a maze to which they can find neither entrance nor exit to get themselves out.[11]

Lazzi no.9[12]

Curiosity for nibbling also affects the aged and fully grown, especially those in unfaithful marriages. Because of all their nibbling, gobbling and gnawing, an honest woman must leave nothing standing or lying around into which such pig-mouths could stick their snouts, who don't merely satisfy their needs with their own food, but always eat to excess. This is amusingly demonstrated by the Italian comedy in which the master sent his servant Zanni to his beloved with a hot pie, and for greater safety instructed him to carry it on his head. On the way, however, perceiving the good smell, Zanni began salivating copiously. Unable to resist his curiosity, he had to find out what he was carrying, then what was in it, further how it tasted, then on top of all that, how it must feel to satisfy one's hunger with such food? So, out of curiosity, he ate up the whole pie. Immediately afterwards, his back was encouraged to greater strength.

Lazzi no.10[13]

The time has come to enjoy ourselves together for once, and talk about something towards which we are strongly inclined and motivated, namely eating and drinking. Whenever we hear talk of a banquet, or of any past, let alone future, opportunity to eat or drink, it is natural for our minds and likewise our entire bodies, to be moved with desire by it. This happened to the Zanni of the comedy. While listening to his master discuss well-roasted capons and similar tasty morsels with one of his friends, he completely forgot the big, heavy load he was unwillingly carrying on his shoulders. As if enchanted, he listened with eager attentiveness. Every time he heard the name of a dish or tasty morsel, the words alone delighted him so much that he would take a great, long and deep downward gulp, as if he already had the morsel in his mouth.

---

[11]   Guarinonius's schoolboy memories include chasing around the neglected maze gardens of the ruined old Prague castle with fellow boarders (*Grewel*, 1232).

[12]   2.XXXVII, 377 / I,ff.547–8, '*Zane* büßt sein Fürwitz an ein Pasteten' [Gluttony (inquisitiveness)].

[13]   4 [On food and drink], I (On the nature, necessity, form and regulation of human food), 520 / II,ff.176–7, '*Zane* vergißt seiner Burd' [Gluttony].

Lazzi no.11[14]

I was at a court, seated at table next to another doctor, when one of several dishes brought in was a beautiful big fish, decoratively and well-presented in pastry. A distinguished man sitting opposite us offered the doctor a piece of it. 'No, no', the doctor says, 'The gout and all this gluttony are not for me. This is one of the slimy fishes, and as such no better than eels, snakes and suchlike'. He offered me the fish that had been offered to him, at which I, with laughter, quoted what Zanni had said in the comedy. His master had offered him a massive helping of well-greased macaroni or noodles covered with cheese, saying:

> Signori, quest é un bocon froll:
> Matto chi l'lassa, é l'cancar' á chil'tuol.

> My dear sirs, here is a splendidly tasty morsel.
> Whoever refuses it is a fool, and may the French pox get whoever eats it.

Quickly, Zanni spoke and reached for the morsel with his hand: 'Well then, dear master, so that you don't get the French pox, I'd better eat this morsel'. Thus I said to the doctor, 'Dear sir, so that you don't get the gout, I will eat this'.

Lazzi no.12[15]

Should one eat more at the morning or evening meal? [...] Gracious reader, I can hardly think of anything to say on this that could please you better than Zanni's recommendations to his master concerning this matter. Namely, because a person does not know which meal is his last, he should regard each meal, whether in the morning or evening, as his last. For this reason, each should be a farewell meal at which he eats as much as he would cram in if it were his last, so that if he had to fight death he would have nourishment in his body.

---

[14] 4.VI (On seven properties and differences of foods, and that they cannot properly be judged solely from the form in which they are commonly served; as well as an example of a commonly served dish), 536–7 / II,ff.201–3, '*Zane* Trewfråssigkeit gegen seim Herrn' [Gluttony].

[15] 4.XIII (Whether the morning or evening meal should be the more satisfying and complete), 571–3 / II,ff.252–3, '*Zane* Freβraht' [Gluttony].

Lazzi no.13[16]

When you sit at a table laden with all kinds of foods and you choose a good dish from amongst them all, such as a bowl of gudgeon, from which you wish to satisfy your desire and eat until you are full, because it is not like your daily bread and you are well aware that by nature such a meal can be less unhealthy than, for example, a calf's head, then this proverb can also have its place. You can be specially nourished by the food you enjoy eating most; like Zanni, when he mistook lampreys for young adders. He thought that they had been offered to his master to dispose of him. But when his master began heartily eating them, Zanni, out of pure loyalty, tore them from his master's hands and himself ate every last one in the bowl, saying that even though he would shortly have to die, at least he had enjoyed eating the poison. But when he realized that he would not die, he daily wished for young adders, and asked his master whether he did not want to eat them again?

Lazzi no.14[17]

Another argument: whether one could more easily do without food or drink? Which has caused much discussion, although one hears of very few who can do for long without food, and even fewer without drink, or who would be willing to put this to the test. When the Venetian Pantalone could not reach a decision on this, and gave his servant Zanni the task of settling the argument, he advised his master to send for food, since he was famished with hunger and could not believe that anything more difficult than hunger could befall humans. When this had been done and Zanni had filled his stomach, he shouted at his master that previously he had lied. The pangs of thirst far exceeded those of hunger. Now that his hunger was satisfied, he was finding out that he suffered more pain from thirst than he had previously done with both. After his master had called for a goblet of wine for him and he had drained it, he answered in his Italian:

> Patru' e' stag bé mi
> Master, now I cannot tell you
> Whether I am tormented more by hunger or thirst
> Because I now feel as I should
> And my body feels enormously satisfied.

---

[16]   4.XVI (Whether that which tastes best to humans also agrees best with them), 584 / II,ff.265–6, '*Zane* frißt junge Natern' [Gluttony].

[17]   4.XVIII (On the necessity of drink for humans, and whether they can more easily manage without food or drink), 593 / II,ff.273–4, *Zane* befindt sich gewaltig wol' [Gluttony].

Lazzi no.15[18]

It is disgusting to become unreasonable and absurd through wine, especially for Germans or the German nation [...] For the sake of a horrible, redundant, and unnecessary drink, they forget themselves to the extent of turning into absolute fools and filthy beasts: mocked and ridiculed in the street by children, the joke and butt of comedians, discredited and gossiped about the world over [...] The [drunkard's] eleventh excuse: But when the nobility becomes angry at banquets and will not be appeased with good words or pleas, even with threats, or cannot be brought to their senses with the blows customary amongst such bestial types, then how should one behave with them? Answer: Even the same as you would behave with vicious, harmful beasts—retreat, flee, seek escape [...] But if you can't do that either, perhaps because you are enclosed with them, then do what you would otherwise do in extreme peril, in combat with such beasts, because if you are sober you will quite easily escape such a beast [...] Or behave with them like those who find themselves with angry lions; they throw themselves to the ground and stay as still as if life has left them. So, if you see that you cannot escape such beasts with honour and that they only want to make a beast out of you, then remove yourself from them a little, as if you were not feeling well. This is how the Italian comedians behave when they represent a German drunkard. They act as if they were nothing else but drunken beasts, even though they are really sober. Such fitting responses are the easiest way to escape such beasts without sin or harm.

Lazzi no.16[19]

> Meat wants meat,
> meat makes meat,
> meat devours meat,
> all beasts are meat;
> therefore one beast devours the meat of another beast.

A very funny example of that happened in an Italian comedy, when Zanni fell into conversation with a parasite and carnivore. While this glutton told him about all sorts of meat and tasty animals he had eaten throughout his life, such as partridges, chickens, capons, calves, oxen, fawns, lamb, pigs, deer, etc., Zanni grew pale in front of him. His eyes rolled around in his head, and his hands and feet began to tremble, and he would have liked to run away, and could not trust him for

---

[18]   4.XLI (To the pious authorities of Germany, on the common, as well as crooked and lame abomination of drunkenness), 700 and XLIII (Response to several incompetent excuses of the coarse brotherhood of boozing drunkards), 717–18 / II,ff.461–2 [Gluttony].

[19]   4.L (The rooting out of several foul, carnivorous, and stinking meat teeth), 756 / II,ff.512–13, '*Zane* meynt es gelt seinen Halβ' [Gluttony].

sheer terror and fear. But when the parasite asked Zanni: 'why this unexpected change', and likewise: 'why this fearful fainting fit?', Zanni stepped away from him and was so extremely startled by his enquiry that, to the great laughter of the audience, he passed wind. But when the parasite approached, wanting to help the unconscious man, Zanni immediately began screaming terribly: *Misericordia* and *Mordio* – mercy and murder – until people came running. In their presence, Zanni was once more restored. But when they questioned him about why he had been overcome with such fear, Zanni responded with a fearful voice and gestures that this glutton had indicated to him that all his life he had eaten so many smaller and bigger, indigenous and wild beasts, that he could only think that it would be his turn next, because he had eaten deer and oxen, which were so much bigger than him, and wild boar, which were so much fiercer than humans. This is truly not without reason, because in truth it is no different. A long time ago, Theogenes was such a bestial beast-glutton, who ate an entire bull every day. Even worse than him was one named Phago or Glutton, who in one meal at Emperor Aurelianus' table ate a whole ram or wether, a young piglet or sucking pig and a whole wild boar. In front of him, no less than any carnivore of that time, Zanni would not simply have fainted, but even have been so afraid to see him that he would have died of shock.

Lazzi no.17[20]

Know first that there are not just one but several New-Gluttony-lands, in German: Gluttony-, or Guzzle- or Slovenly-lands. [...] Not for nothing is the fictional Land of Cockaigne or Gluttony-land honoured with a second nickname, namely Narragonia.[21] This indicates that all Gluttony-landers should take to heart that they will stray from the path very soon if they mean to live through this brief life, uncertain from one hour to the next and made even briefer and more uncertain by their gluttony, in such a Gluttony-landish way. They will, as the Italian *comicus* said: '*dar del capo nel matto*: bang their head on fools', and unknowingly enter the Land of Narragonia. The longer they stay there, the more they will not only weaken their wit and judgment, but also their physical health. Their mortal life will be shortened and snuffed out as if in a poisonous spider's hunting web. Then they will leave Narragonia and via neighbouring territories such as Colic-land, Ram-

---

[20]   4.LV (On the abomination of many well known and much practiced [...] but also unseemly, unchristian, inhuman, abominable and insufferable gluttonous feasts), 789–90 / ff.559–61, 'Schnarraffenlandt/ wo es warhafftig zu finden' [Gluttony].

[21]   The carnivalesque, mythical land of folly that took its name from the Utopian island destination of Sebastian Brant's *Ship of fools*. Explicating the connection with Schlaraffenland (the German Land of Cockaigne), Brant interchangeably refers to it as 'Das schluraffen schiff' (Brant, *Stultifera nauis*, second frontispiece and illustration 50 of original 1494 edition).

land, Gout-land, Crooked-land, reach another neighbouring country bordering them, namely Hell-land, which will accept them as citizens.

Lazzi no.18[22]

Of gluttony at celebrations I have to speak separately and with special respect, because of all types of gluttony, none other exacts and is paid such high respect as this, which people look forward to for days in advance and specially prepare for. And when, three days early, Zanni began to devour the well-greased noodles he was only supposed to eat over three days, he repeatedly grasped his gullet and neck to check whether anything was coming back up or was obstructing his gullet, or whether the passage was blocked, so that the morsels could slip down nice and smoothly without obstruction. Gluttony of this type is sometimes enthusiastic and sometimes secret, so that people don't notice it [...] Most gluttons themselves recognize their behaviour as unreasonable and ungodly [...] At celebrations, however, everyone considers and regards it honourable, appropriate, and laudable, because they take place in public and with such ceremony, in which guests are serenaded and flattered, and have gluttony forced on them with cunning and art.

Lazzi no.19[23]

Says a great lord: 'Doctor, you speak well on health, but how does our reputation and rank fit in with this? Overflowing tables are a matter of honour with us, even though we often dislike the dishes served, etc.'

Answer: 'So, just as a matter of honour, you will be carried to your grave earlier than others. If reputation consists in harming oneself, then the sooner you curse this reputation, the sooner you will heal your damage. Come on! You can keep it without changing the smallest aspect of your kitchen. Let your meals be prepared but not served. Place them in the nearest room to the dining room. From there let one, or at the most two be served to you, and the rest be sent to the hospital. Thus you will keep your rank and dignity, as well as your long-term health and life, and will additionally gain everlasting [life], which is of greatest importance. Obey this and be healthy. He who wants to taste and take pleasure in well-prepared, delicious, tasty dishes is permitted to do so without any health risk, as long as he copies that Spanish *Grandes*, or stage fool,[24] who stuck his nose into a kitchen

---

[22]   4.LVI (On the abomination of gluttony at festivals), 790 / II,ff.564–6, 'Grewl der hochzeitlichen fressereyen' [Gluttony].

[23]   4.LVIII (On the abomination of the monstrous and greedy mixing and confusion of diverse foods and different wines in the stomach), 807 [Gluttony].

[24]   'Jenem Spanischen *Grandes*, oder Großhansen'.

window. He drew in a good nose- or gobfull of roast and braised aromas, while holding a large piece of stale bread in his hands. And as often as he drew the good smells into his nostrils, he took a hefty bite of the bread and satisfied his gluttonous feelings with the bread, until, through the good smells, he had eaten all the bread, and, without any damage, satisfied his hunger in gluttony.'

Lazzi no.20[25]

I believe that if someone else addresses me without taking the trouble to notice when I have a morsel in my mouth, then one should not respond to such conversation or questions before reaching a convenient moment. Like Zanni in the comedy, who had the prior agreement of his master that while he eats, his master should neither give him work nor orders, let alone address him.

Lazzi no.21[26]

Among others I knew an eminent man, whom neither I nor other doctors could persuade to chew his food in his mouth. He swallowed it almost whole, and continuously suffered from a weak stomach and blockage of the arteries, until he choked in the flower of his 30-year-old youth. Such gluttonous greed stems from over-eating, and from an excessively unreasonable, coarse, greed for food. The gluttonous participant fears that others of his type who may be sitting at the table are coveting just the same food he desires, and might dig into it before him, leaving nothing or hardly any for him. Zanni plays a similar trick on his lovesick master. Because when Zanni was given a kind message from the beloved to his master, he saved it until his master sat down to table. Then he waited until the best dish had been served, a good tart, whose good smell made Zanni's nostrils itch. Then, deciding it was time to chase his master from the table, Zanni gave him the news, as if he had almost forgotten it, that he should immediately go to his beloved. And because this news meant more to the old fool than a hundred banquets, he ran from the table to his beloved, and Zanni ran to the tart. He swallowed it in a few bites, because he feared that if his master did not return contented from his beloved, he might eat the tart out of ill humour.

---

[25]   4.LXI (On the greedy gluttonous abomination of the swallowing of unmasticated food), 813 / II,ff.593–4, '*Zane* Pact mit seinem Herrn' [Sloth (envy)].

[26]   4.LXI, 814 / II,f.595, '*Zane* jagt sein Herrn vom gerichten Tisch' [Lechery, gluttony].

Lazzi no.22[27]

According to the common proverb:

> Necessity breaks iron
> as proven by the force of the bowels.

Among others, the comical Zanni of the Italian comedy portrayed these three latest calls of nature most amusingly and concisely when he got into an intense and vigorous discussion with his master, Master Pantalone, and presented his master with this question: 'Which is the greatest of all physical pleasures on earth, occurring with greatest benefit and causing the least damage?' To which his love-struck, 70-year-old master, the old fool, quickly responded that it was when someone could enjoy the favours of his beloved or mistress. However, Zanni loudly laughed at and ridiculed him for this, explaining that love affairs can neither be carried out with benefit, nor without damage. Not with benefit, because lovers become beggars; not without damage because it causes deception, [cuckold's] horns and the French pox. Having to search deeper into his philosophy to keep guessing, the old man said that a table loaded with the best foods and wines was the greatest pleasure. Zanni made even more fun of him: 'What would the old man do at the laden table when he no longer wanted to eat?' The old man spoke again, that of all things many bags of ducats were the most delightful and useful thing on earth. Zanni derided him, reminding him of his own enormous generosity, because he had lots of money and neither Zanni, nor anyone else, nor the old man himself, had any gain from it, saying that only fools gained pleasure from money, but little benefit, since lots of money had driven some to hang themselves. (At this point he loyally offered his master that if he desired this, he would supply the rope and effort.) So, instructed and taught by Zanni, old Heintz learned to identify the very greatest pleasure on earth as none other than the undoing of the codpiece laces, following lengthy suppression of a highly urgent need by anxious hopping, bodily contortions and wriggling around, and vigorous emptying of one's bowels. This provides the greatest relief of all to the constitution, and the pleasure of it makes its smelly steam seem like mere musk. This pleasure occurs without any harm and with great benefit to one's health and longevity. Whenever he, Zanni, wants to experience physical pleasure, he simply forcibly suppresses his bowel movements for a long while, hopping, running and fighting the urge with his hands and feet. Thus, he can experience the most extreme distress, and the consequent inexpressible pleasure. And so that I tell the entire story, the curious old man was overcome with a desire to try out this pleasure as well. He allowed Zanni to persuade him to suppress his bowel movements, like a man and a knight. When

---

[27]   5 [On physical elimination], VII (On elimination through bowel movements and urination), 881–2, '*Zanes* aller größte Wollust auff Erden' [Lechery (gluttony and incontinence, inquisitiveness, avarice, wrath)].

after over two hours the master complained to Zanni that he no longer wanted to hold back his bowel movements, Zanni strongly exhorted him to bravely resist by wriggling and running around. Then the old man pressed one hand in front and one behind, squeezing them firmly together, running up and down the stage with fright, sucking his breath in to control himself, rolling his eyes in his head, and stretching out his tongue stuck out as long as a finger. When he additionally repeatedly screamed: '*Misericordia, Zane! Zane, misericordia!*', and was practically done in, Zanni would still not permit him to allow his prisoner to escape. Meanwhile, Zanni unexpectedly summoned out the old man's beloved. When the old man became aware of her, he was shocked into relieving himself of the stew, with screams, into his breeches, making a mighty good stink for the beloved, and much hearty laughter for Zanni as well as the spectators. Afterwards, when Zanni asked him which had given him greater pleasure, the emptying of his bowels or the presence of his beloved, the old man shouted: '*Cancro Zane, tu sei grand frisoloso.* In all my life, I have never felt or experienced anything more pleasurable than the release of this burden, and it felt so wonderful that I do not know what I said to my beloved.' Zanni said: 'Master, what about your breeches?' The old man answered: 'Breeches. Of course, breeches! But even if they had been gilt and bejeweled, it would not have mattered, compared with the pleasure I experienced. For such pleasure one should wear nothing but gold and silver pieces or velvet breeches, because no garment is too valuable to be worthy of such lasciviousness.'

Lazzi no.23[28]

The fourth type of gas is of the fourth element, namely earth, and is no less harmful than frightening [...] Human digestive gases are comparable to these movements, which we call earthquakes. [...] Their behaviour causes the body extreme inconvenience. When they are violently imprisoned, they occasionally rage so stormily up and down and through the whole body that they make people very afraid and anxious, frequently causing pains and stomach aches. Such calls of nature are relieved by the crashing and banging of their escape from the body. Not without reason did Zanni faint when he, in full armour, marched into war with his master, Pantalone, and, overcome with fear, one such exceedingly strong body gas accidentally escaped his old master. Zanni fell to the ground, thinking he had already been shot at and hit by a cannon ball. Whereupon his master, by sending a second, similar banger flying past his ears, speedily frightened him into awakening from his dead faint.

---

[28]   5.IX (On the natural elimination of minor and benign bodily gases by yawning, burping and sweating, sneezing, laughing, crying, speaking, snuffling, singing, shouting, sighing, panting, as well as coarser, more embarrassing ones like rumbling and farting, etc.), 889, '*Zane* zeucht mit seinem Herrn in Krieg' [Gluttony (incontinence)].

Lazzi no.24[29]

Such gases originate mostly from those foods which incorporate a lot of wind. Item, from excess food-matter, which cannot be fully and completely digested by natural heat, but is turned into wind by excess moisture. Item, from certain special foods. As shown by a robust question Zanni posed his master: 'Which food delights nature most?' And when Master Pantaleon could not figure it out, Zanni responded that it was the radish, because the arrival of no other food is honoured in such lavish fashion by nature, with drumming, piping and the unleashing of cannon salutes.

Lazzi no.25[30]

Anyone who serves at court and is frequently in the company of great lords must often swallow such rather coarse chunks instead of breakfast, and may hardly breathe in their presence, not to mention spitting, let alone throat clearing. Nor can they even always step aside for such needs. Unless they wanted to make use of Zanni's politeness, who, feeling the need to spit while speaking to his master Pantalone, said in his own language to his master:

> Ste n' drec' patru, ch'uoi spudá mi.
> Master, move back a little from me
> because I need to bend over to spit.

Lazzi no.26[31]

There is no-one who does not know how amusingly womenfolk can talk their men into seeking motherhood (I nearly said seeking whoredom) at the hot springs [...] Any man who is and wants to stay honest, and doesn't want to be crowned with the biggest cuckold's horns, should check his fortifications carefully, and not thoughtlessly trust his wife. Neither should he allow her go there unless she is in dire need, or has the necessary prior advice of a specialist doctor [...] Mischievous

---

[29] 5.IX, 889, '*Zane* gibt seim Herrn ein uberauß subtile Frag auff' [Gluttony (incontinence)].

[30] 5.XXV (On the abomination of unmannerly natural elimination, and also of the holding back of phlegm, swallowing of snot, suppression of sneezing, burping and laughter, crying, sobbing, speaking, shouting, rumbling), 941, '*Zane* Höfligkeit' [Gluttony (incontinence)]. The 'coarse chunks' refer to this chapter title.

[31] 5.XXVII (On the cursed abomination of the horrible and unbearable common abuse of public baths and hot springs), 953–4, 'Bett: und Tagzeiten der Håußlichen Wildbadenden Weiber' [Lechery].

women [...] convince their husbands that to ensure fertility they should be allowed into the hot springs, to which come their gallants and lovers, or the nearest sturdy young lumberjacks from the surrounding forests. If they have them in their mind and hearts, then of course their fertility won't fail them, but will be successful [...] O pious utter fools, how much more foolish and mad you are than any cuckolded Venetian Pantalone, who represents a blind fool in the comedy, and his wife a vulgar strumpet. Because what is more typical at these hot springs than that after their baths, the womenfolk wander out into the greenery, and disappear with premeditated eagerness into the deep forests and valleys, where the casually lurking satyrs wait to transport them to ecstasy, and then lead them back close to the baths again? Or also, because everyone lives under one roof and house, even though their living quarters are in separate rooms they can get together at night quite easily, and without any obstacles.

Lazzi no.27[32]

The third type of movement of the human body is the one which intentionally moves either the whole body, or one of its parts or limbs, or several simultaneously. And because this movement originates in the brain and thus in human will, it follows that it can be mobile or immobile, according to human will. This sixth book is concerned with and examines this final type of physical movement of the body or limbs, undertaken or neglected according to human will. Now this third type of physical movement is in turn very varied, because although all movements are initiated by human will and choice, there are still many which humans cannot control, in which, as it were, necessity forces their limbs to move and exercise. Accordingly, Zanni once desired that his master grant him his request that just for once, he, Zanni, could be freed from all work and movement for eight days, and totally rest all his bodily limbs. This the master granted with all his heart, but with one strong condition, that if Zanni stirred a single limb, he, his master, would bruise and beat him on it. And when Zanni heartily agreed to this and lay quite motionless onstage in his bed, quite blissfully dozing, with drooping eyelids, his master arranged for a bowl filled with the best and greatest macaroni, well-buttered and covered with cheese, to be placed in front of his bed and his eyes, allowing their steam to rise to his nostrils. Then Zanni, losing his taste for his wished-for rest, jumped swiftly out of bed and toward the noodles, for which his master, however, thrashed his back, forcing him to rest again. But then, when Zanni began complaining of the pact he had entered, his master hit him again, around his mouth, because he had moved it to speak. When he was not allowed to

---

[32]   6 [On exercise], II (On two types of physical movement that are natural and eternal, and three types that are both calming and exercised by human choice, and on the difference between movement and exercise), 1158, '*Zanes* seltzame Bitt an sein Herrn' [Sloth (envy, wrath, gluttony)].

talk either, he began to swallow the delicious, steaming vapour, smell, and steam: his master beat him on his throat because he was moving it, then bashed his nose because he was inhaling the smell. Then Zanni, with a heavy heart, turned his eyes to the macaroni, so that he could at least fed on the appearance of what he would rather have gobbled up. At that, his master bashed him on the eyes, because he was moving them, in contravention of their pact. Zanni wanted to be free of their contract again, but his master would not agree to this. So, when after two hours, Zanni, forced by another need, wanted to rise from his rest, his master beat him down again, until he released both his lower calls of nature into his breeches. Upon this, his master released him from his wished-for rest. Accompanied by the hearty laughter of the spectators, he, however, walked homeward with downcast eyes and contorted, slow strides, because of the warm brew he had produced. From these comic pranks, it seems that many body parts cannot be kept still at their appointed time without great physical damage: such as the mouth and tongue while talking, the eyes while seeing, the teeth while chewing the indispensable daily nourishment, the gullet while swallowing, the bowels while eliminating superfluity, the bladder while emptying out urine, the hands while transporting food to the mouth, or the feet while transporting the body to places and destinations required either by calls of nature or by business demands, etc.

Lazzi no.28[33]

Concerning differences in exercises […] The third difference is only of the body and limbs, or only the mind, or both together […] Body and mind together, as when a lute player also sings, dances, etc. with his beloved (even if she is an old gossip of 80 years) before his eyes. Thus, for example, the Magnificus danced for his beloved, whom he thought was at the window, while Zanni accompanied him on the violin. But only after enjoying this pleasure did he find out that it had not been his beloved, but the gruesome 80-year-old bawd for whom he, the old fool, had performed such an entertaining exercise.

Lazzi no.29[34]

Here, I do not wish to describe all manner of idle street-players' and other jumps, but those which are capable of doing most people good. Well known amongst these is the back-jump, which is commonly practiced by adolescents. It is carried out by two teams equal in number and strength, the members of one of which, chosen by drawing lots, offer their backs by bending over and supporting themselves one

---

[33]   6.IV (On the difference between exercisers and exercises), 1163–4 [Lechery].

[34]   6.XI (On back-, shoulder-, head-, coat-, ditch-, stream-, air-, and round-jumping), 1187–8, '*Zane* springt mit seinem Herrn, I' [Sloth (wrath)].

against the rear of the other. However, the first must brace himself tightly with his arms and shoulders against a wall, tree, or something stable. Meanwhile, the others take 30 or 40 strides back, in order to be able to take a run-up. The first has to travel furthest after running, over all the backs in front, swinging and jumping right on to the one at the front, where he has to remain seated. Then the second must jump onto the second, the third onto the third, and the fourth onto the fourth back. In the event that the first to jump is weak or lazy, and gets stuck on the end back, those who jump after him have to clear the height of two backs, in order to swing themselves onto those at the front. When they are thus stably seated on top, they give a signal with both hands, hop or tumble off again, and start the jump afresh. If one falls off before the end, then as a forfeit, he and his companions must offer their backs to the opposing team, and etc. Once, the Venetian Pantalone and his servant Zanni were practicing this jump together. While Zanni offered his back, and his master ran towards him from behind in his toga and slippers, Zanni put out a foot against which his master tripped up, and fell head over heels. Because of this, he made his servant lift him onto his back and carry him for a good while.

Lazzi no.30[35]

Concerning the shoulder- or head-jump, which is very amusing and entertaining to watch, and additionally requires almost uninterrupted running. When several acrobats get together for this, one of them takes several strides forward, so that all those behind have a run-up to him. He plants one foot in front of the other firmly on the ground, and braces both hands and arms on his forward thigh so that he tilts his body sideways, his head lowered a little. Then the first jumps over him, and runs a few more paces before stopping in the same position for the following jumper, so that the last has to jump over all those who have already jumped in this way. Then the very first to take the standing position also jumps over all the others, and offers his back again after a few more paces. In this way, jumping and running with great entertainment and laughter, one can cover a long distance in a short space of time. This exercise is very strong and swift, and exercises almost the entire body, the feet, thighs, arms, shoulders, back, etc. And whoever is well trained in it can jump effortlessly from behind a horse all the way up into, or even beside, its saddle [...] This jump is also useful in many short plays, of which I will say nothing, except that Zanni, when he wanted to jump over his master, remained stuck on his master's shoulders, and did not want to come down again, because he felt exceedingly comfortable, and no different (he told his master), than if he were riding the most excellent miller's ass.

---

[35]   6.XI, 1188, '*Zane* springt mit seinem Herrn, II' [Sloth].

Lazzi no.31[36]

Round fencing- and dancing-jumps, while closer to jugglers' tricks and curiosities than useful exercise, are also suitable for hard exercise. [...] The grotesque jugglers' tricks practiced by our German fencers in their fencing schools similarly serve as good exercises. They do not just move their feet but even more their arms, in that they reach around, up and down, and to and fro in the air with their hands and arms and grapple around no differently than, for example, Zanni. While he was supposed to be catching midges for his master Pantalone in the air, he punched his master's nose with his fist, etc.

Lazzi no.32[37]

In Italy, wrestling schools have been maintained to the present day, in which youths exercise, and learn the benefits associated with this. It is also considered very popular and laudable by the nobility, especially students, in many German towns. This was among the sports in which the nobleborn baron and knight, Niclaus von Firmion of blessed memory, was trained beyond measure. Kneeling, he could bring down the strongest wrestlers [...] Item: The epitome of excellent wrestling was once also demonstrated by the old Venetian Pantalone in the comedy, when he wanted his beloved to to see in what good shape he was. And when he asked his servant Zanni for advice on how to gain the advantage over his opponent in order to win, carry away fame, and reap honour, Zanni persuaded him to make himself as heavy as possible, so that his opponent would never be able to overcome him or bring him down. And after Zanni had distributed a hundredweight between his two shoulders, and left him staggering around the stage for a good while waiting for his rival, Zanni made off. He left his master stuck with the attached weights, whose sheer weight alone, without any other wrestler, dragged him to the ground.

Lazzi no.33[38]

Regarding horse-jumping, this is an exemplary, excellent exercise for young people, during which, as they exercise their horse in all sorts of ways [...] now by trotting, then by galloping, soon by jumping, they themselves are exercised by the trotting, galloping and jumping. In particular, the spine, the whole back, stomach, kidneys (as I previously indicated with reference to Galen), hips, thighs and feet, especially by those who splay these last out and apart while riding, so

---

[36]   6.XI, 1189–90 [Sloth (envy, wrath)].

[37]   6.XII (On wrestling, fencing, and dancing), 1190–1 [Lechery].

[38]   6.XX (On riding, horse-jumping, running at the ring, tournaments and quintain jousting), 1221–2, '*Zane* lehret seinen Herrn reitten' [Lechery (pride)].

that one foot points to the orient, the other to the occident. Thus, for example, rode the Venetian master Pantalone. When his servant Zanni was teaching him to ride, he mounted him facing backwards on his ass, giving him its tail in his hands for reins, and lifting both his legs as high as possible. He made him ride to the door of his beloved like this, so that he would earn her favour and love through this fine, chivalrous athleticism.

Lazzi no.34[39]

Human laziness is a dissolute abomination, which makes humans inhuman […] A special breed of these are the house-, window- and stove keepers, who gain their greatest exercise and work in moving from their bed to the warm stove, from stove to window, from window to table, and from table back to bed. This exceedingly intense and incomparable work exercises the mind in vices and sins, and the body into an overweight, fat paunch. All actions are aimed at protecting the paunch from any disagreeable experiences, so that even if everything else goes to rack and ruin, they can, with that Italian sponging glutton and comedian, daily address their huge paunchy fat bellies:

> O Panza, mia Panza
> Guardami di febre, ti guardarò di lanza.

> O you my paunch, balmy, fat, and soft
> Guard me against illness, then I will guard you against blows.

Lazzi no.35[40]

Because riding is an *exercitatio passiva*, that is, an exercise stemming not from one's own energy but from that of another, the horse, it is an exercise proper to the weak and old, and mere vain laziness in the young and strong, except perhaps for long journeys or bad roads […] Thus it is almost always the case that the young and strong, who exercise through walking and running, ought to be ashamed to the bottom of their stinking, lazy hearts at acquiring horses for riding, let alone sitting. These days, everyone just rides and drives, and even, for the most part, prefers to be carried and driven even for a few steps from the house by a creature or beast and by unreasonableness, rather than on their own sensible feet. How Zanni ridiculed his ass-riding master, Pantalone! Seeing him riding towards him,

---

[39]   6.XXVI (On the abomination of lazy couch potatoes, stove guardians, curtain twitchers, mosquito breeders and idle window shoppers), 1242–3 [Gluttony, sloth].

[40]   6.XXVII (On the abomination of pride and laziness in riding and driving, and of the spreading inertia), 1244–5 [Sloth].

he yelled: 'Look here, good people, see how my master approaches on bestial feet!' He wanted to show that even though his master had two sensible human feet for walking, he walked by using the bestial feet of a brute animal. And then, when his master dismounted the ass and commanded Zanni to ride the ass to the trough, he could not be persuaded by any means to mount the ass, because he would not consider trusting an irrational beast with his body and life. This in itself demonstrates reason, because everyone moved by others is either crippled in their limbs, like the crooked and lame, or weak like small children and the very old, or requires long, distant journeys of many days, etc.

Diagrams and Plates

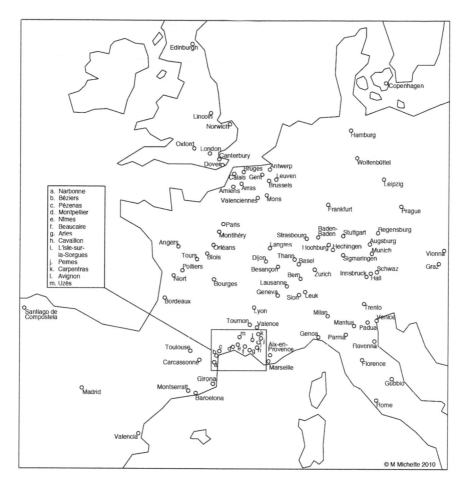

a. Narbonne
b. Béziers
c. Pézenas
d. Montpellier
e. Nîmes
f. Beaucaire
g. Arles
h. Cavaillon
i. L'isle-sur-
   la-Sorgues
j. Pemes
k. Carpentras
l. Avignon
m. Uzès

Diagram 1   Early modern Europe, showing principal locations cited

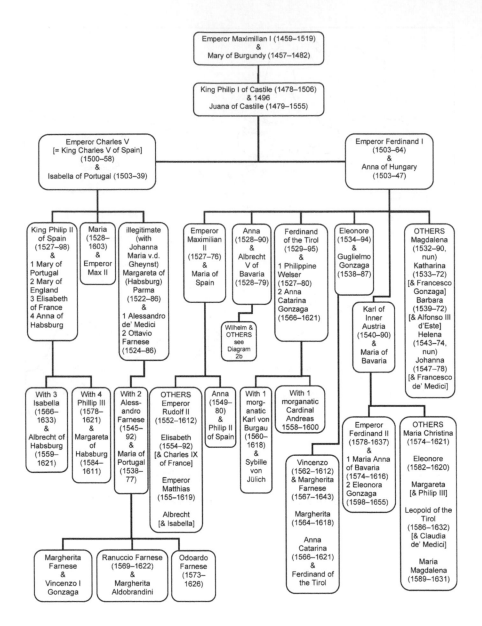

Diagram 2a   Family tree, showing some relationships between the Habsburg and Bavarian dynasties

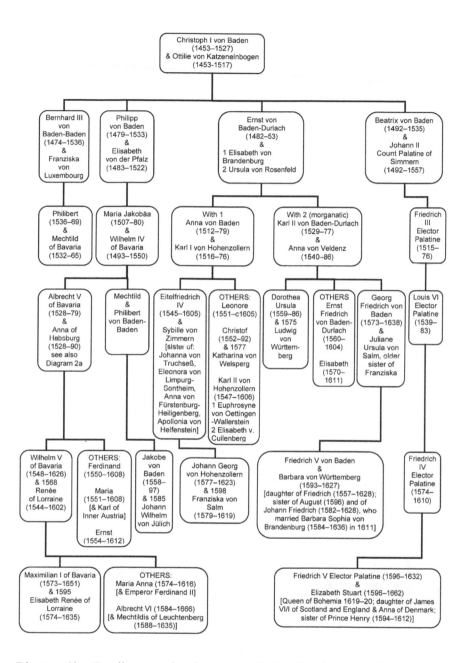

Diagram 2b   Family tree, showing some relationships between the Habsburg, Bavarian, Baden, Hohenzollern and Stuart dynasties

Diagram 3 Some plays noted by Felix Platter

Date	Page ref.	Place (Basle unless otherwise noted)	Play	
c.1541	FP[1] 93	In garden of Truchsess house	Unidentified play acted at 2nd wedding of the alchemist Hans Rüst, a neighbour of Thomas Platter the Elder	Fool = Jacob Truchsess (who cut such comic capers that Oswald Geisshüsler ('Myconius') later revealed that he had laughed so much he almost wet his breeches)
23 May 1546	FP 83	On the Fishmarket	Sixtus Birk, Susanna[2]	Director = Ulrich Coccius ('Koch'); Susanna = Margaretha Merian (fiancée of Koch); Daniel = Ludwig Ringler (glass painter)
6 June 1546	FP 82-3, 85	On the Cornmarket	Valentin Boltz, The Conversion of St Paul[3]	Paul = Hans Felix Irmy; God the Father = Balthasar Han; Captain = Hans Rudolf Frey
c.1546	FP 81-2, 84	Obern Kollegium (secularized Augustinian Monastery)	The resurrection of Christ (possibly 'Macropedius' (Georg von Langenfeldt), Passio Christi)	Maria = Johann Heinrich Ryhiner; Fools = Jacob Truchsess (was the best of them); Devils = unspecified
c.1546	FP 83-4	Thomas Platter the Elder's school (outdoor)	'Gnaphäus' (Willem van de Voldersgroft), Hypocrisis (1544)	Hypocrisis = Johann von Schallen ('Scalerus'); Gratia = Felix Platter; Psyche and/or Cupid = Theodor Zwinger[4]
c.1546	FP 84	Obern Kollegium (indoor)	Heinrich Pantaleon, Zacheus	Unspecified roles = Heinrich Pantaleon (director); daughters of Sebastian Häsli ('Lepusculus')
c.1546	FP 84-5	Obern Kollegium	'Naogeorgus' (Thomas Kirchmayer), Hamanus	Haman = Isaac Keller ('Cellarius'); Haman's son = Gamaliel Gyrenfalck; Executioner = Hans Ludwig Hummel
c.1546	FP 85	Haus 'zur Mücke'	Plautus, Aulularia	Director: Hans Ludwig Hummel Lycondes = Felix Platter; Strobilus = Hans Martin Huber[5]
1540s	FP 85-6	Thomas Platter the Elder's courtyard	Valentin Boltz, The Conversion of St Paul	Paul = Gavin de Beaufort, Baron de Rolles ('Roll'); God the Father = Felix Platter

Date	FP ref	Location	Play	Roles / Notes
	FP 86	Amandus Langbaum's house	Pamphilus Gengenbach, *The ten ages of man* (1515)	Unspecified roles = Felix Platter, Langbaum, Simon Colroß, Lucas Just, Gavin de Beaufort
	FP 86-7	Thomas Platter the Elder's student boarding house	Terence, *Phormio*	Crito = Sigmund von Andlau
c.1546	FP 94	House of Hieronymus Frobenius	Virgil, *Eclogues*	Shepherds = Felix Platter (feigned illness to get out of this role) & Gavin de Beaufort
24 Dec 1552	FP 152	Not performed	Plautus, *Amphytrion*	[Read in Montpellier by Felix Platter]
Nov 1553	FP 85, 188-9	Thomas Platter the Elder's boarding house	Thomas Platter the Elder, *The innkeeper of "The Withered Branch"*	Bromius the innkeeper (part originally written for Felix Platter) = Gilbert Catelan
Feb 1554	FP 194	Unspecified	*The doctor of the watering can* (Basle carnival farce)	'Gilbert and others wrote and told me that Dr Pantaleon had been given the nickname "doctor of the watering can", which came from the fact that he had advised a woman that in order to encourage sleep, she should try letting water drip onto her head at night from a watering can, or, according to others, let it drip into a beaker. This was made the subject of a carnival farce'.[6]
9 May 1566	FP 448	Collegio comoediam	'Macropedius' (Georg von Langenfeldt), *Hecastus* (1539)[7]	
26 May 1566	FP 448	Cornmarket	*Helisaeus*[8]	Civic play

[1] Page references are to *Felix Platter Tagebuch*. [2] These 1546 productions of *Susanna* and *The Conversion of St Paul* are also noted in the Basle preacher Johann Gast's Latin diary (Bücking, *Kultur und Gesellschaft in Tirol*, 96n266). [3] See previous footnote. [4] In Felix Platter's speech at the doctoral ceremony of Jacob Zwinger, he recalls his old friend, his student's father, 'acting the role of Cupid so well and fittingly in the comedy *Hypocrisis* that he was praised by all the others' (quoted, Hochlenert, 'Das "Tagebuch" des Felix Platter', 130). [5] 1536–64. This school friend of Felix Platter and son of the distinguished Basle physician and university professor Johannes Huber (1506–71) qualified as a lawyer and died in a Basle plague epidemic. [6] *Felix Platter Tagebuch*, 194. For a discussion of Platter's implied criticism of Pantaleon in this passage, see Hochlenert, 'Das "Tagebuch" des Felix Platter', 176–7. [7] This adaptation of the traditional morality play *Everyman* was in turn adapted by Hans Sachs (1549). [8] Possibly related to the lost play of *The prophet Elisaeus* condemned in the anti-theatrical writings of Gerhoh of Reichersberg (1093–1169). ('De spectaculis theatricis in ecclesia', c.1161, quoted by Chambers, *Medieval stage* II, 98–9).

Diagram 4   Some annual fixed and movable feasts and fasts noted by Felix Platter, Thomas Platter and Hippolytus Guarinonius

Event	Type	Date	FP	TP	HG
Epiphany (Three Kings; Twelfth Night)		6 January	1550s		
St Sebastian	Fixed	20 January		1599	Procession
Purification of the Blessed Virgin Mary (Candlemas)	Fixed	2 February		1599	Procession
CARNIVAL Shrove Tuesday (Mardi Gras)	Pre-Easter movable feasts	Variable length festival 40 days before Palm Sunday and last day of carnival	1540s 1550s 1560s	1596 1597 1599	1606
LENT Ash Wednesday Palm Sunday Maundy Thursday Good Friday	Pre-Easter movable feasts	40-day fast Day after Shrove Tuesday Last Sunday before Easter Last Thursday before Easter Last Friday before Easter		1599 1599	
Easter Sunday	Movable			1599	
Quasimodo Rogation Sunday Ascension Day Whitsun (Pentecost) Trinity Corpus Christi	Post-Easter movable feasts	First Sunday after Easter Fifth Sunday after Easter 40 days after Easter 50 days (seventh Sunday) after Easter Eighth Sunday after Easter First Thursday after Trinity		1599 1599 1599 1599 1598	1609 NB Corpus Christi was often celebrated three days later, on the ninth Sunday after Easter
St George	Fixed	23 April		1599	FAIR
St John Baptist	Fixed	24 June		1590s 1600	Various; FAIR
St Theobald	Fixed	1 July	1558		Procession
St Magdalen	Fixed	22 July	1556	1597	Various; FAIR

Feast	Type	Date					Category
St James	Fixed	25 July				1610	
Assumption of the Blessed Virgin Mary	Fixed	15 August			1599		Religious
St Bartholomew	Fixed	24 August		1553	1597		FAIR
Triumph of Cross	Fixed	14 September		1598			Pilgrims
Nativity of the Blessed Virgin Mary	Fixed	8 September					FAIR
St Firmin	Fixed	25 September			1597		FAIR
St Simon & Jude	Fixed	27 October	1536, 1540s, 1557				FAIR
All Saints' / or All Hallows'	Fixed	1 November					
All Soul's	Fixed	2 November		1552	1595		Procession
St Martin	Fixed	11 November			1599		FAIR
St Andrew	Fixed	30 November			1598		FAIR
First to fourth Advent Sundays	Movable	The four Sundays before Christmas Day					
St Nicholas	Fixed	6 December		1540			
Christmas Eve	Fixed	24 December		1552	1595, 1597, 1598	1580s	
Christmas Day	Fixed	25 December			1599		Ritual ceremony
St John Evangelist	Fixed	25 December				1604	
Holy Innocents	Fixed	28 December				1580s	

Diagram 5   Selective summary table of some court festivals referred to or described by Felix Platter, Thomas Platter and Hippolytus Guarinonius

Date	Author/ eyewitness	Place	Festival
8–9 January 1563	FP	Basle	Entry of Emperor Ferdinand I[1]
8–26 August 1577	FP	Sigmaringen	Wedding of Christof, Count of Hohenzollern & Katharina von Welsperg[2]
20/30 September 1595	TP / no	Lyon	Entry of King Henri IV of France[3]
3 October 1595	TP	Tournon	Entry of Henri duc de Montmorency, Connétable de Tournon & Louise de Budos[4]
28 February to 2 April 1596	FP	Stuttgart	Christening of Prinz August von Württemberg[5]
15 March 1596	TP	Montpellier	Entry of Anne de Lévis, duc de Ventadour and Marguerite de Montmorency[6]
February 1597	TP	Marseille	Carnival celebrations of Charles de Lorraine, duc de Guise[7]
9 June 1597	TP	Uzès	Coming of Age entry of Emanuel de Crussol, duc d' Uzés[8]
October 1598	FP	Hechingen	Wedding of Johann Georg von Hohenzollern and Franziska von Salm[9]
January 1599	TP / no	Barcelona	Formal reception of Don Giovanni de' Medici into Barcelona[10]
28 January 1599	TP / no	[relocated from Barcelona to Valencia]	Entry and wedding of Philip III and Archduchess Margareta of Habsburg[11]
24 August and 2 November 1599	TP / no	Antwerp	Entry of Archduke Albrecht and Archduchess Isabella of Habsburg[12]
September 1599	TP	Brussels	Entry of Albrecht and Isabella[13]
January 1600	FP	Hochburg	Christening (possibly of Juliane Ursula v. Baden-Durlach)[14]
November 1609	HG / no	Stuttgart	Wedding of Johann Friedrich von Württemberg and Barbara Sophia von Brandenburg[15]

[1] *Felix Platter Tagebuch*, 392–400. [2] *Felix Platter Tagebuch*, 456–66. [3] *Thomas Platter d.J*, 36–7. (See also Watanabe-O'Kelly & Simon, *Festivals and Ceremonies*: no.1672). [4] *Thomas Platter d.J*, 48, 52–4. [5] *Felix Platter Tagebuch*, 467–483. [6] *Thomas Platter d.J*, 145. [7] *Thomas Platter d.J*, 187–196. [8] *Thomas Platter d.J*, 221–7. [9] *Felix Platter Tagebuch*, 484–513. English translation: see Chapter 16, below. (See also Watanabe-O'Kelly & Simon, *Festivals and Ceremonies*: no.238). [10] *Thomas Platter d.J*, 341–2. [11] *Thomas Platter d.J*, 343. (See also Watanabe-O'Kelly & Simon, *Festivals and Ceremonies*: nos.2330 *et ff*). [12] *Thomas Platter d.J*, 675, 874. (See also Watanabe-O'Kelly & Simon, *Festivals and Ceremonies*: nos.2688–9). [13] *Thomas Platter d.J*, 690, 704–743. (See also Watanabe-O'Kelly & Simon, *Festivals and Ceremonies*: no.2689). [14] *Felix Platter Tagebuch*, 514–516. [15] Guarinonius, *Grewel*, 1195–1203. (See also Watanabe-O'Kelly & Simon, *Festivals and Ceremonies*, nos.354–5).

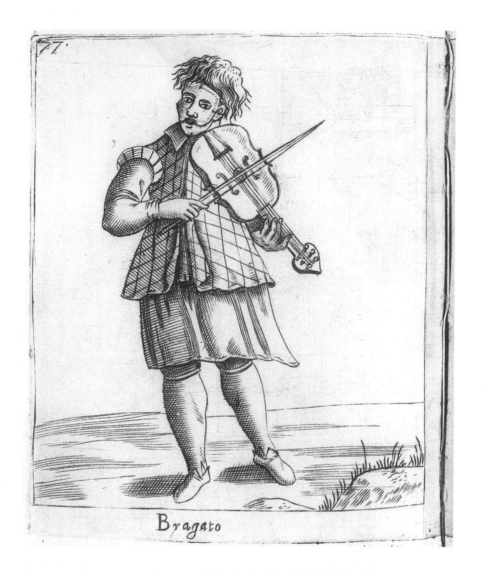

Plate 1   Jacopo Franco, *Bragato*, 1591, engraving. Pietro Bertelli, *Diversaru[m]
nationum habitus, iconibus in ære incisis* (Patavii: Aliatum Alcia et B Bertellium,
1589, 1591, 1596), 3 vols, II, plate 77. Berlin, Kunstbibliothek.

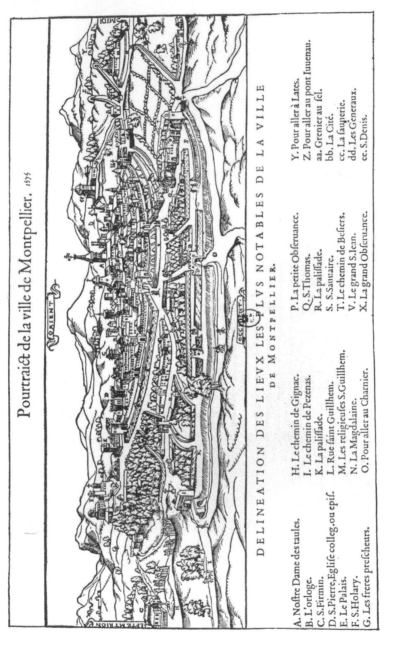

Plate 2 François Belleforest, *View of Montpellier*, 1575, 10x31cm, woodcut. Sebastian Münster (translated by Belleforest), *La cosmographie universelle de tout le monde* (Paris: Nicolas Chesneau, 1575), 330–1. Archives de Montpellier, Inventaire général du Languedoc.

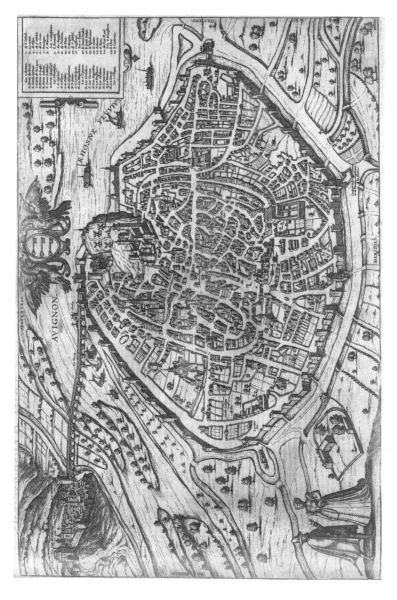

Plate 3 Franz Hogenberg, *Aerial view of Avignon and Villeneuve*, 1575, 31x47cm, engraving. Georg Braun and Franz Hogenberg, *Civitates Orbis Terrarum* (Cologne: Georg Braun, 1572–1617), II. Paris, Bibliothèque Nationale, 78c 89312 Va.84 t.3.

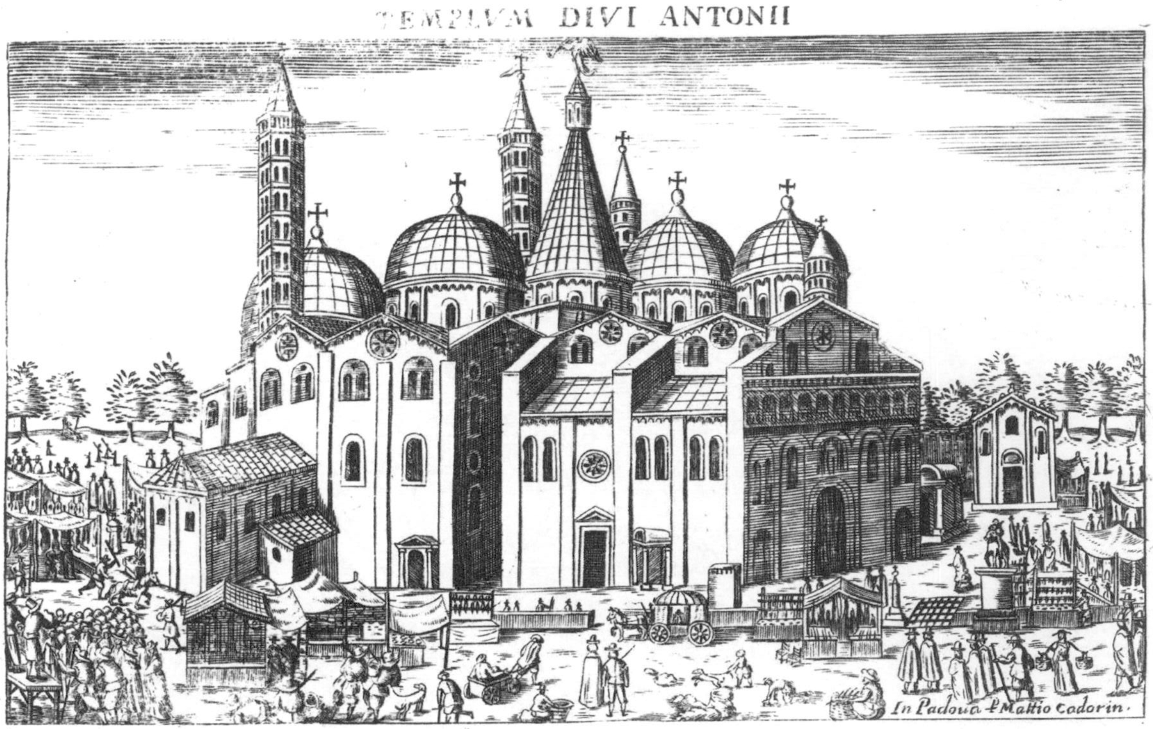

Plate 4 *Snake-charmers on a trestle stage at a fair at the Church of St Anthony, Padua*, fold-out engraving. Francesco Scoto, *Itinerario, o vero nova descrittione de' viaggi principali d'Italia* (Padoa: Mattio Cadorin, 1670), between pp.38–9. Wolfenbüttel, Herzog August Bibliothek, Gh 255.

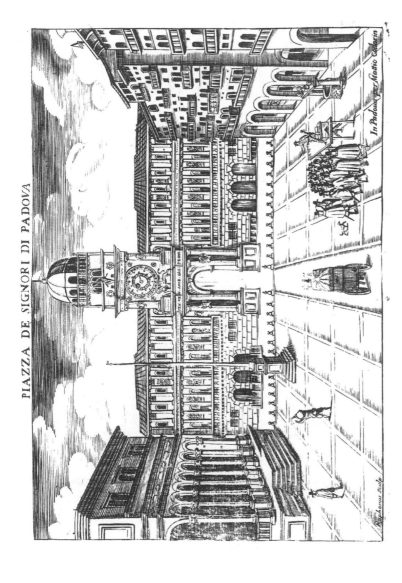

Plate 5 *A mountebank in Harlequin costume performing in the Piazza dei Signori, Padua*, fold-out engraving. Francesco Scoto, *Itinerario, o vero nova descrittione de' viaggi principali d'Italia* (Padoa: Mattio Cadorin, 1670) between pp.30–1. Wolfenbüttel, Herzog August Bibliothek, Gh 255.

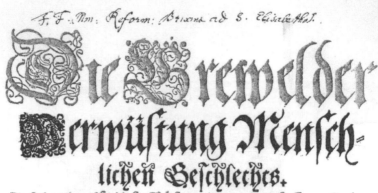

Die Grewelder
Verwüstung Mensch-
lichen Geschlechts.

In sieben unterschiedliche Bücher und unmeidenliche Hauptstucken /
sampt einem lustigen Vortrab / abgetheilt.

Neben vor: mit: und nachgehenden / so wol Natürlichen / als Christlich: und Politischen / dartwider streittbaren Mitteln.

Allen / so wol Geist: als Weltlichen / Gelehrt: und Ungelehrten / hoch und nidern
Stands Personen / überauß nutz und sehr notwendig / wie auch gar kurtzweilig zu lesen.

Zu sondern Nutz / Glück / Heil / Wolfahrt / langen Gesondt / Zeitlich: und ewigen
Leben / gantz Hochlöblicher Teutscher Nation / newlich ist gestellt

Durch

Hippolytum Guarinonium, Art. & Med. Doctorem, deß Königlichen Stiffts
Hall im Ynthal / und daselbst F. F. Durchl. Durchl. Ertzhertzoginen zu Oesterreich / ic.
Steyr / Cärnten / ic. Leib / und gemainer Stätt beställten Physicum.

MATTHÆI XXIIII. Wann ir den Grewel der Verwüstung sehen werdet / ic.

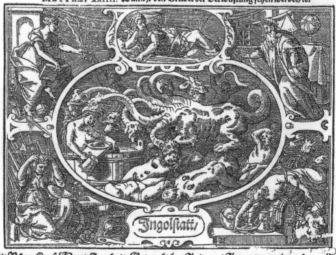

Ingolstatt /

Mit Röm. Keys. Mayt. Freyheit / Getruckt bey Andreas Angermayr / im 1610. Jar.

Plate 6   *Titlepage*, 1610, engraving. Hippolytus Guarinonius, *Die Grewel der Verwüstung menschlichen Geschlechts* (Ingolstadt: Angermayr, 1610). Bressanone-Brixen, Biblioteca del Seminario Maggiore.

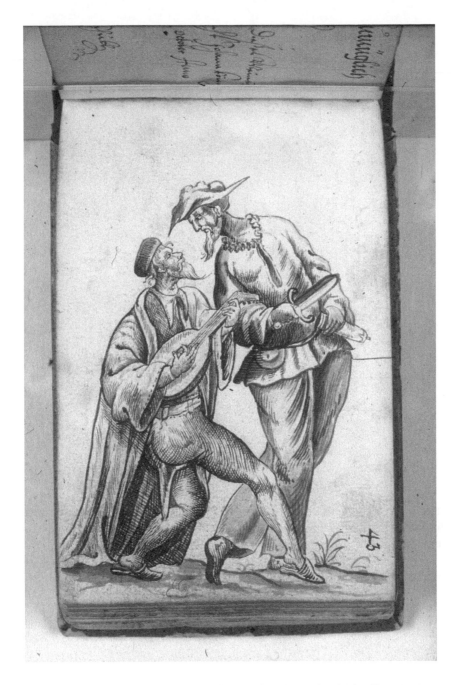

Plate 7   *Zanni and Pantalone*, ink and wash drawing. Friendship album (c.1647–
53) of Johann Koenig (b.1586), accompanying inscription dated 1648. Weimar,
Herzogin Anna Amalia Bibliothek, Stiftung Weimarer Klassik, Stb.112, f.43^r.

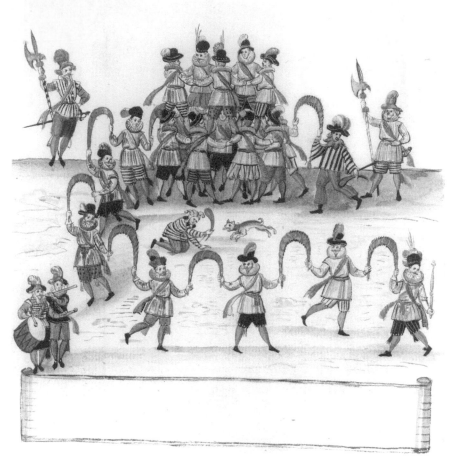

Plate 8   *A hoop dance*, c.1596, coloured drawing. Friendship album of Adam Pusch of Breslau (Wrocław). Munich, Bayerische Staatsbibliothek, cod. germ.8349, f.102ᵛ.

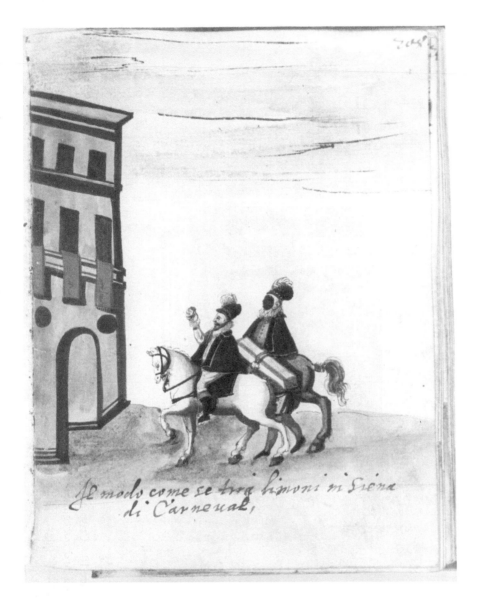

Plate 9 *Two mounted carnival revellers throwing lemons*, coloured drawing.
Friendship album. Munich, Bayerisches Nationalmuseum, Bibl.3659, f.208ʳ.

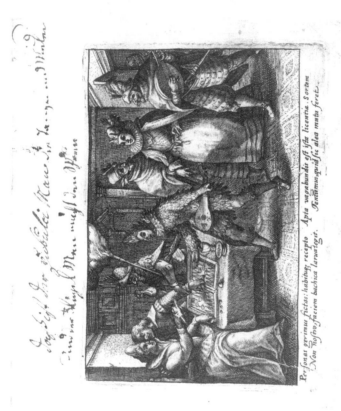

Plate 10   Crispin de Passe after Sebastian Vrancx, *Interior with five masked figures and two backgammon players*, dimensions of engraving 9.5x13.5cm, inscribed printed page. Friendship album (1615–33) of Hans Wilhelm Wolf. Weimar, Herzogin Anna Amalia Bibliothek, Stiftung Weimarer Klassik, Stb.434, f.2.

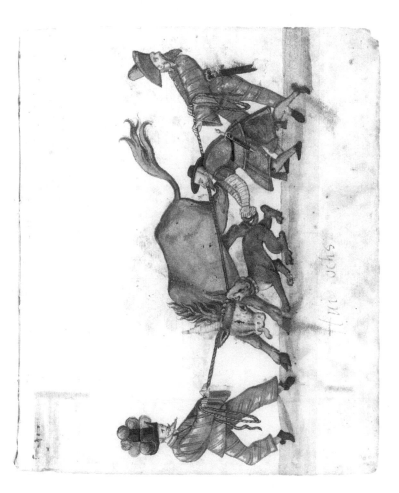

Plate 11   Carnival bullfight ('Un bel morire tutta la vita honora'), 1606, coloured drawing from friendship album. Munich, Bayerische Staatsbibliothek, Cgm.8930, f.359ᵛ.

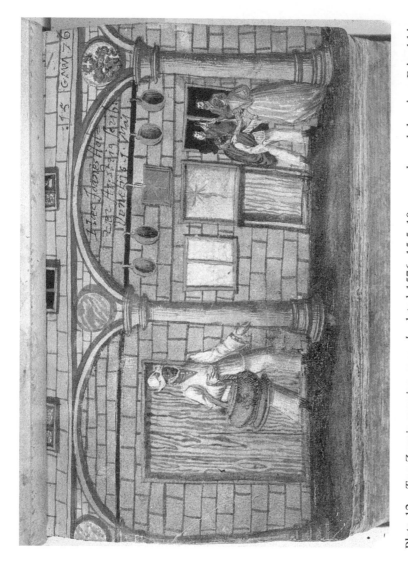

Plate 12 *Two Zannis running errands*, dated 1576, 15.5x10 cm, coloured drawing. Friendship album (1570–84) of Onophrius Berbinger. Nürnberg, Germanisches Nationalmuseum, Bibl. Hs.461, f.61r.

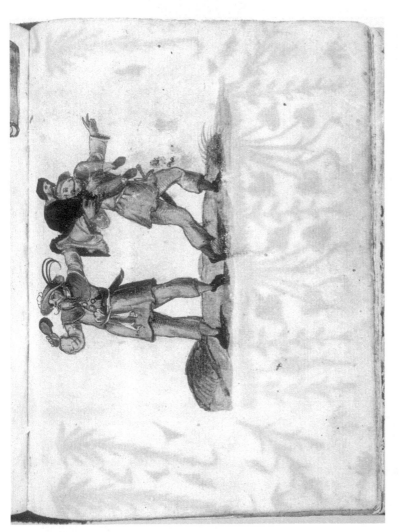

Plate 13   *Pantalone with two Zannis*, 16x12 cm, coloured drawing. Friendship album (1582–1617) of Ulrich Reuter. Nürnberg, Germanisches Nationalmuseum, Bibl.Hs.121.165, f.130^v.

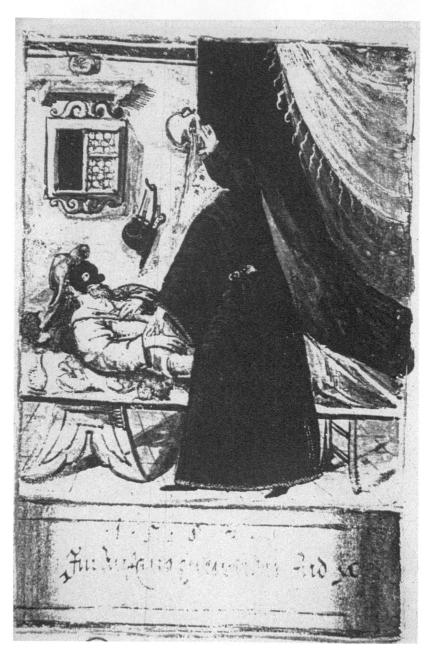

Plate 14   *Zanni and Pantalone ('Im Anfang gedenke das End')*, dated 1583, 15x10 cm, coloured drawing. Friendship album (1583–1601) of Hans Jakob Wintholz. Vienna, Österreichische Nationalbibliothek, Cod.Ser.nov.2968, f.8ᵛ.

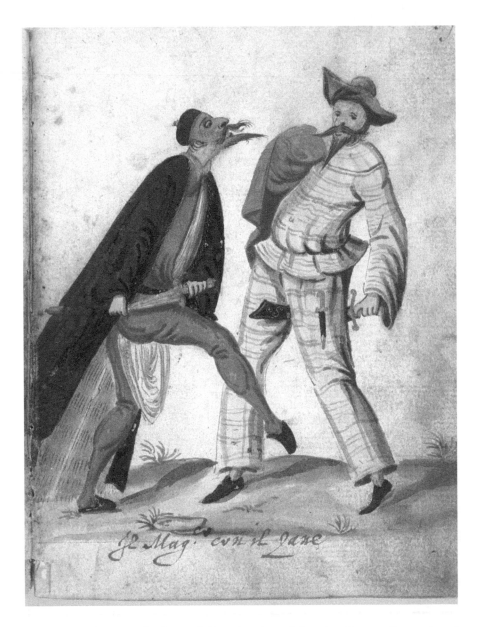

Plate 15   *'Il Mag[nifico] con il Zane'*, coloured drawing from a dismembered friendship album or costume book. Munich, Bayerisches Nationalmuseum, Kostümbuch Bibl.3659, f.39.

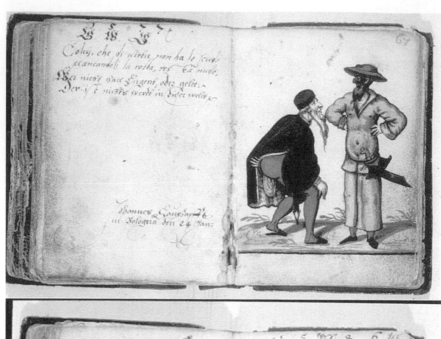

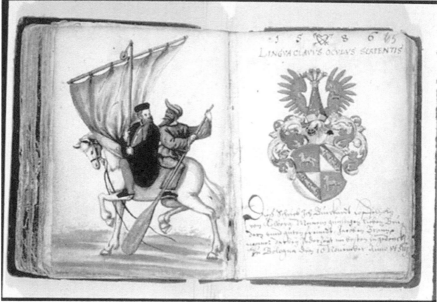

Plates 16a and b *Zanni and Pantalone*, accompanying inscriptions dated 1577 and 1586, coloured drawings from friendship album of Jacob Praun (1558–1627). Nürnberg, NStB, Solg.Ms.14. 8°, ff.64ᵛ–65ʳ and 66ᵛ–67ʳ.

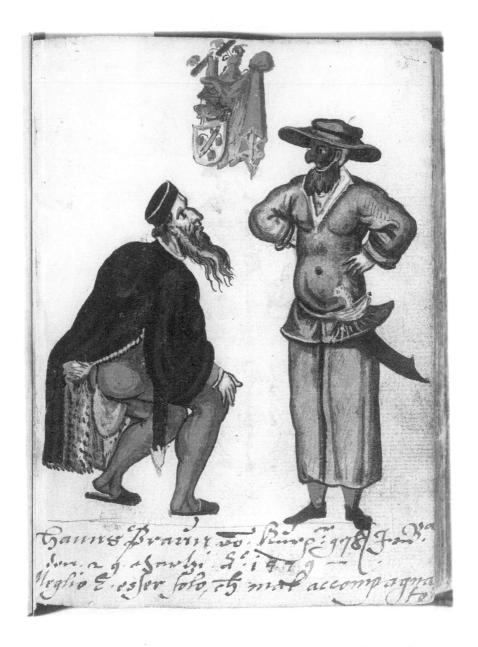

Plate 17 *'Meglio d'esser solo, ch' mal accompagnato' (it is better to be alone than in bad company)*, 1579, 13x9.5cm, coloured drawing. Friendship album (1579–1618 and 1649–60) of Wolfgang Harsdorfer and Wolfgang Carl Harsdorfer. Nürnberg, Germanisches Nationalmuseum, Bibl.Hs.32900, f.38ʳ.

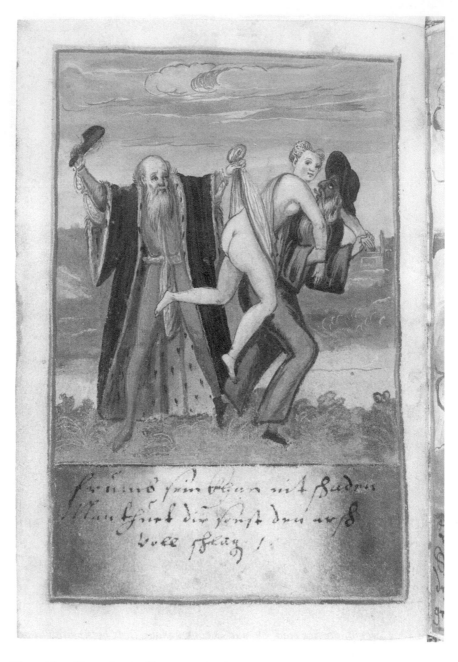

Plate 18 *'Freund sein khan nit schaden' (it can't hurt to be friends)*, c.1583, 15x10cm, coloured drawing. Friendship album (1583–1601) of Hans Jakob Wintholz. Vienna, Österreichische Nationalbibliothek, Cod.Ser.nov.2968, f.4ᵛ.

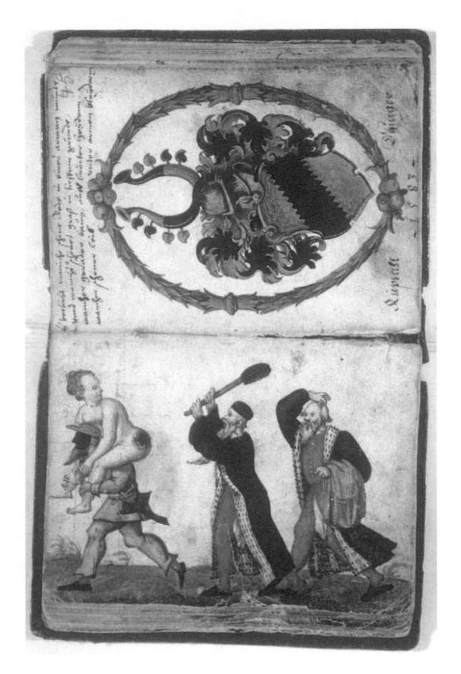

Plate 19 *Two Pantalones chasing a Zanni carrying a nude woman on his shoulders*, c.1583, coloured drawing from friendship album of Jacob Praun (1558–1627). Nürnberg, NStB, Solg.Ms.14. 8°, ff.44ᵛ–45ʳ.

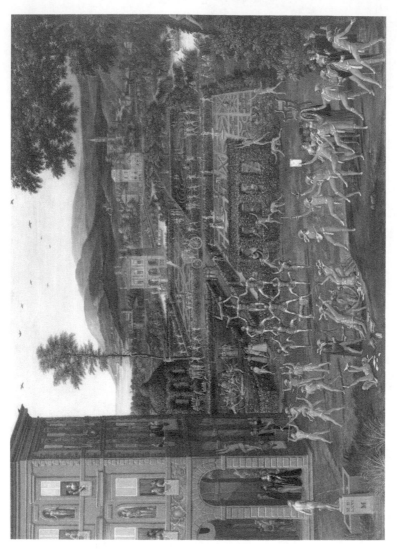

Plate 20 Monogramist MO (unidentified French, Netherlandish or German artist), *A court festival set in the garden of an Italian villa (featuring a mattacino dance and the Labours of Hercules)*, dated 1566, 169x235cm, oil on canvas. London, Netherlands and New York art markets (1998, 2010).

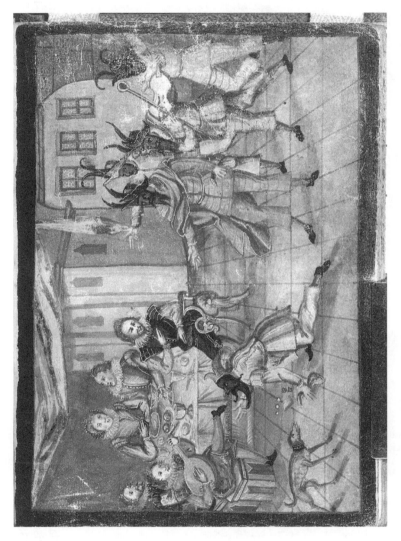

Plate 21 *Five mummers in an indoor setting*, c.1603, coloured drawing from friendship album. London, The British Library, Add.17025, f.26ᵛ.

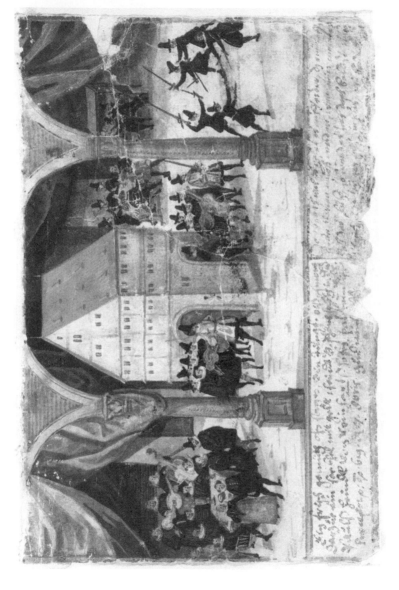

Plate 22 *Courtly pursuits: banqueting, dancing, music-making and fencing*, coloured drawing from dismembered friendship album. Stuttgart, Württembergisches Landesbibliothek, cod.hist.2° 888–11, f.38ʳ.

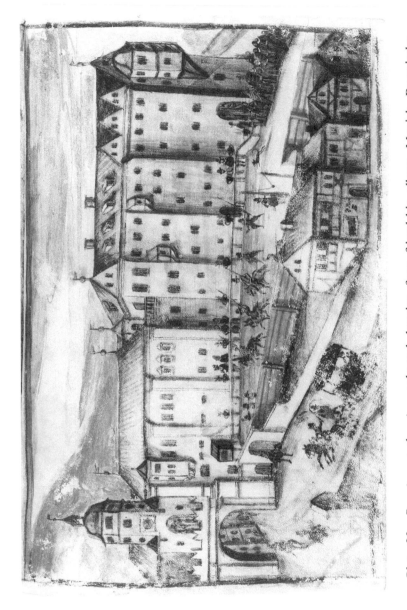

Plate 23 *Running at the ring*, coloured drawing from friendship album. Munich, Bayerische Staatsbibliothek, cod. germ.8189, f.108^{r}.

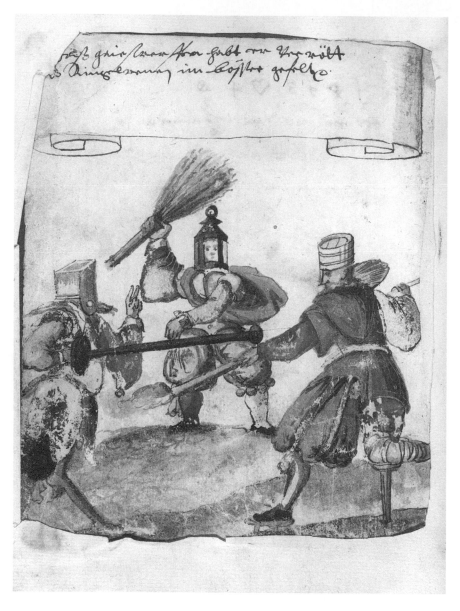

Plate 24 *Unmounted burlesque combat*, coloured drawing from dismembered friendship album. Stuttgart, Württembergisches Landesbibliothek, cod.hist.2° 888–15, f.187ᵛ.

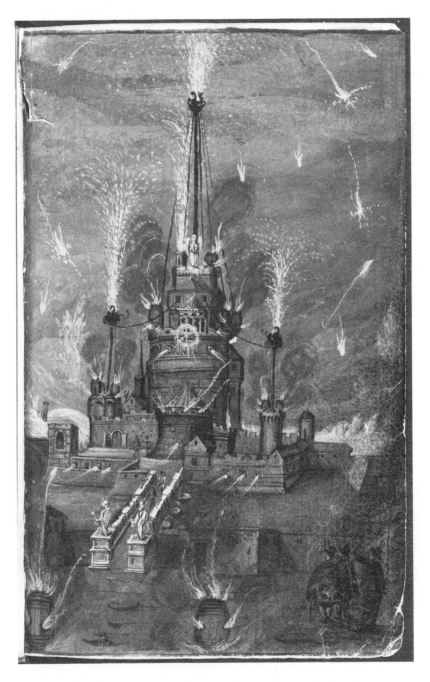

Plate 25 *Firework display*, coloured drawing from friendship album. Stuttgart, Württembergisches Landesbibliothek, Cod.Don.906, f.121ʳ.

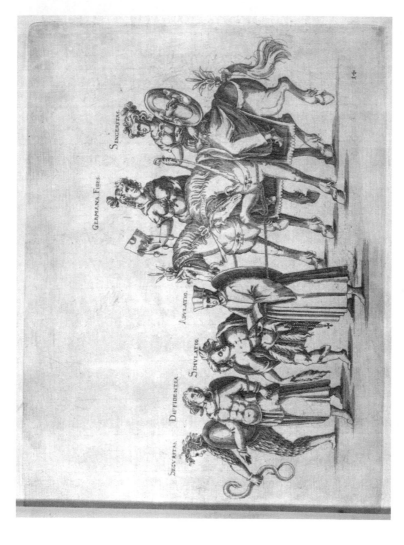

Plate 26 Balthasar Küchler, *Adulatio, Germana Fides and Sinceritas*, 1611. Küchler, *Repraesentatio*, plate 14. Wolfenbüttel, Herzog August Bibliothek, Gm 1152 4°.

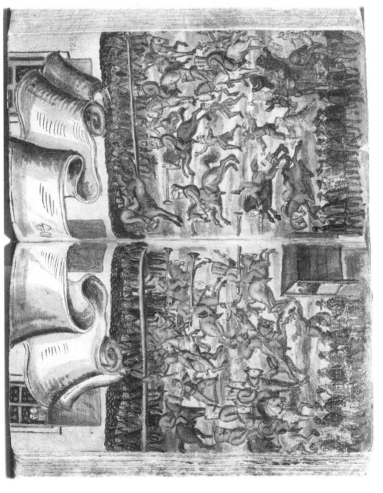

Plate 27 *Mounted burlesque tournament with unmounted referees, including two in Zanni costume, in attendance,* coloured drawing from friendship album. Nürnberg, Germanisches Nationalmuseum, Bibl.Hs.461, ff.122ᵛ–123ʳ.

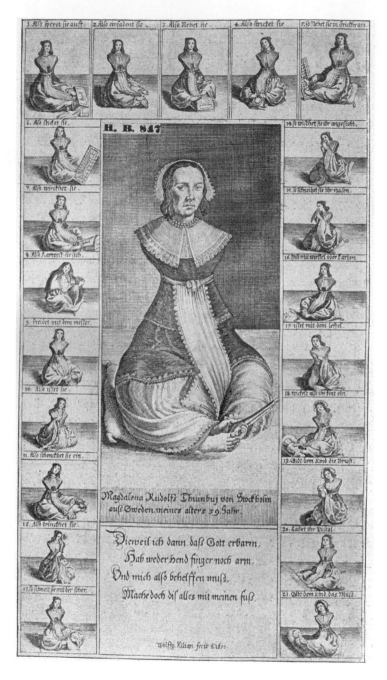

Plate 28   Wolfgang Kilian, *Magdalena Rudolfs of Stockholm in Sweden, aged 39 years*, 1651, engraving. Nürnberg, Germanisches Nationalmuseum HB.847.

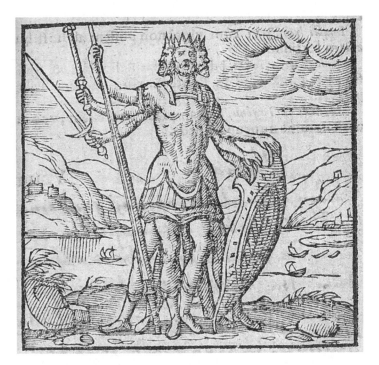

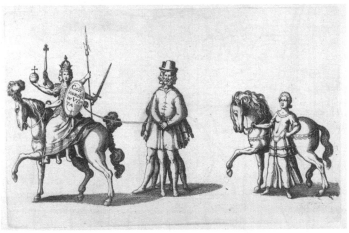

Plates 29a and b *Concordia Insuperabilis (Geryon)*. Andreas Alciatus, *Emblemata*, Antwerp: Christophe Plantin, 1584, 101, Emblem no.40. Wolfenbüttel, Herzog August Bibliothek, Li.62; Matthaeus Merian the Elder, *Concordia Invicta*, 1616. Hulsen et al., *Repræsentatio*, f.41^r. Wolfenbüttel, Herzog August Bibliothek, 36.17.3 Geom.2° (1).

To cut off ones head, and to laie it in a platter,
which the iugglers call the decollation of Iohn Baptiſt.

The forme of ẙ planks, &c.

The order of the action, as it is to be ſhewed.

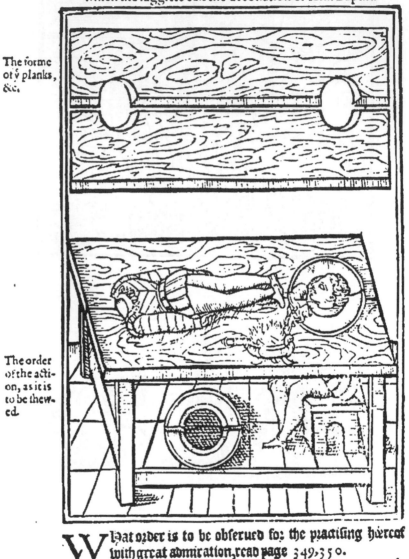

VVhat order is to be obſerued fo: the pꝛactiſing hẏerof with great admiration, read page 349,350.

¶ The

Plate 30 *Stage decapitation*, woodcut. Reginald Scot, *The discoverie of witchcraft* (London: William Brome, 1584), plate opposite p.353. Oxford, Bodleian Library.

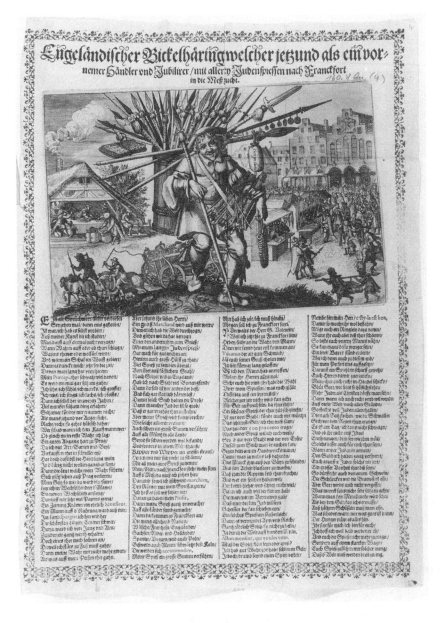

Plate 31 Matthaeus Merian the Elder, *Engeländischer Bickelhäring / welcher jetzund als ein vornemer Händler und Jubilirer / mit allerley Judenspiessen nach Franckfort in die Meß zeucht (English Pickelhering travelling as a merchant to the Frankfurt Fair)*, 1621, broadsheet. Wolfenbüttel, Herzog August Bibliothek, 160.8 Quodlibet (4).

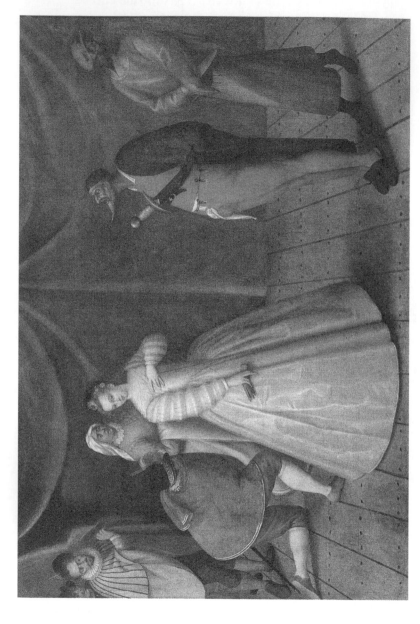

Plate 32 Anonymous French or Flemish artist, *Commedia dell'arte scene*, 96x138cm, oil on canvas. Avignon, Musée Calvet.

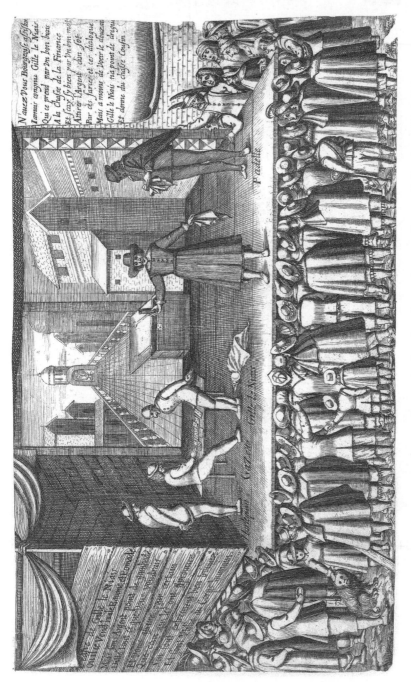

Plate 33   *Teatre de Gille le Niais*, 20x34cm, print. Oxford, Ashmolean Museum, Douce Collection, E.1.4 (76).

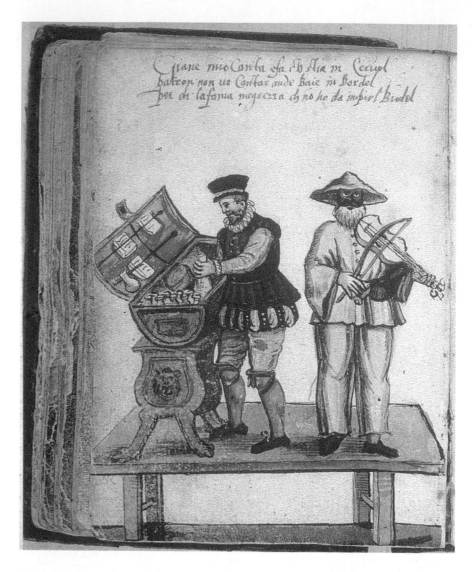

Plate 34 *Two mountebanks on a trestle stage*, c.1584, coloured drawing from friendship album of Jacob Praun (1558–1627). Nürnberg, NStB, Solg.Ms.14. 8°, f.57ᵛ.

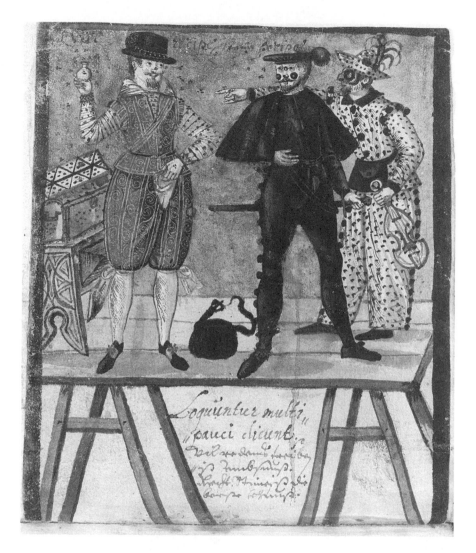

Plate 35   *Three mountebanks on a trestle stage*, coloured drawing. Friendship album of Michael Mailinger, 1615–31 (associated inscription on f.147^r is dated 1618). Vienna, Österreichisches Nationalbibliothek, Cod.Ser.nov.2608, f.146^v.

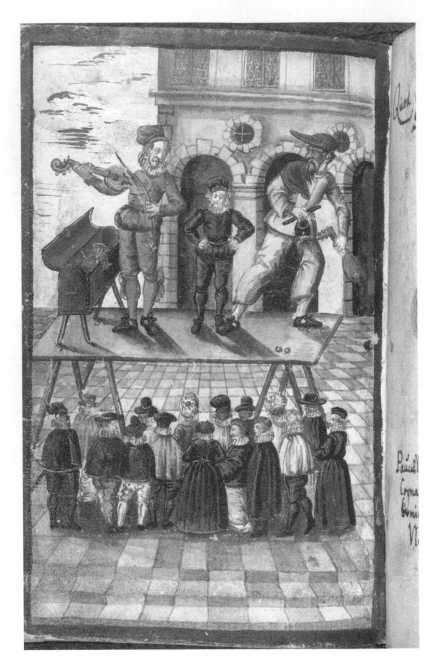

Plate 36 *Three mountebanks on a trestle stage*, coloured drawing. Friendship album of Hans Eitel Neupronner 1619–25, facing page (f.8ʳ) dated 1622. London, British Library, Add.17969 f.7ᵛ.

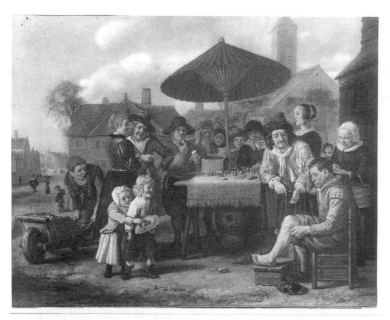

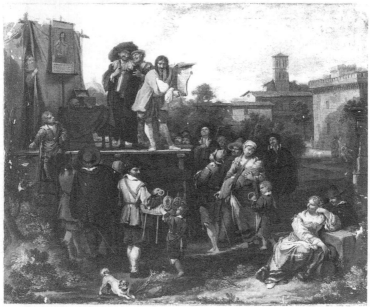

Plates 37a and b Jan Victors, *Market scene with a quack at his stall*, c.1650, 79x99cm, oil on canvas. Budapest Museum of Fine Arts. Dirk Helmbreker, *The quacksalver*, c.1660, 59x73cm, oil on canvas. Gemäldegalerie Kassel.

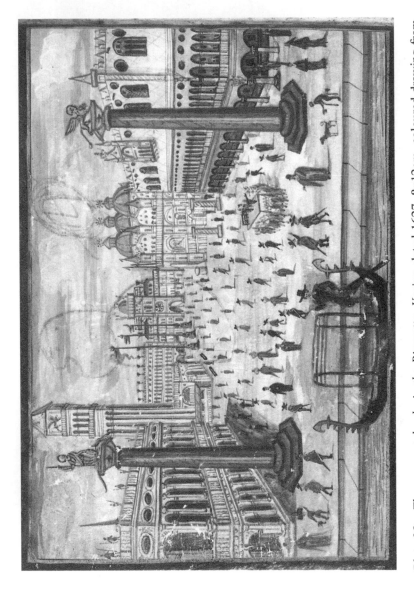

Plate 38   *Three mountebanks in the Piazzetta, Venice*, dated 1627, 8x12cm, coloured drawing from friendship album. Berlin, Kupferstichkabinett, 79.A.10, unfoliated.

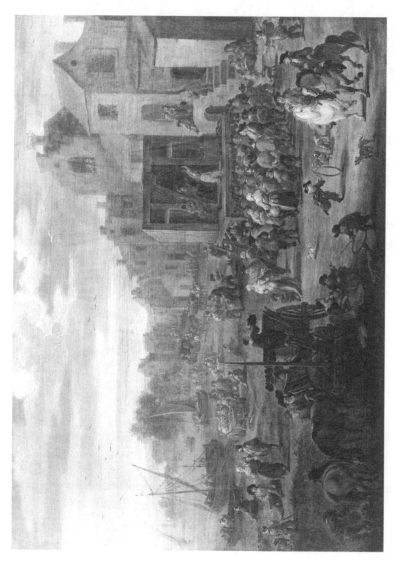

Plate 39 Mathys Schoevaerdts, c.1680s, *Commedia dell'arte quack troupe entertaining a crowd with music and acrobatics*, oil on canvas. Private collection.

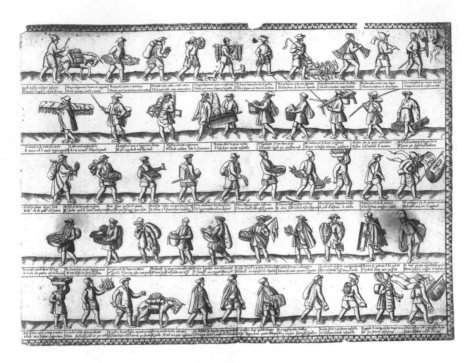

Plate 40 *Italian 'street cries'*, engraving, 48x35cm. Oxford, Ashmolean Museum, Douce Collection, 139 (534).

Bibliography

Principal Collections Cited

Basle
Universitätsbibliothek (UL)
   Frey-Grynaeum I, 8
   Codex A 1 III.3
   MS.A 1 V.7–8
   MS.A 1 V.9

Berlin
Kupferstichkabinett (KK)
   77.B.2
   79.A.10

Dijon
Archives Municipales (AM)
   I.134 (Liasse) unfoliated

Frankfurt
Stadt Archiv (StA)
   Burgermeister Bücher (BMB) 1592

Innsbruck
Tiroler Landesmuseum Ferdinandeum
   Botanik nr.01
Universitätsbibliothek (UL)
   Cod.110, I-IV

London
British Library (BL)
   551.a.32
   MS.Add.17025
   MS.Add.17969
   MS.Harley 5133

Milan
Biblioteca Teatrale Livia Simone (Teatro alla Scala)
   CR.U.119

Munich
Bayerisches Hauptstaatsarchiv (BHStA)
   Fürstensachen 426/I
   Jesuitica 513/III
Bayerisches Hauptstaatsarchiv, Geheimes Haus Archiv (BHStA.GHA)
   Korr.Akt 606
   Korr.Akt 609
   Korr.Akt 924
Bayerisches Nationalmuseum (BNM)
   Kostümbuch Bibl.3659
Bayerische Staatsbibliothek (BSB)
   Cod.germ.8189
   Cod.germ.8349
   Cgm.8930

Nürnberg
Germanisches Nationalmuseum (GNM)
   Bibl.Hs.121
   Bibl.Hs.461
   Bibl.Hs.32900
   Bibl.Hs.137321
   HB.847
Stadtbibliothek (NStB)
   Solg.Ms.14. 8°

Oxford
Ashmolean Museum
   Douce Collection
Corpus Christi College (CCC)
   MS.CCC94

Paris
Bibliothèque Nationale (BN)
   78c 89312 Va.84

Sigmaringen
Stadtarchiv (StAS)
   FAS HH1-50 T1-5 A696

Stuttgart
Württembergische Landesbibliothek (WLB)
  Cod.Don.899
  Cod.Don.906
  Cod.hist.2° 888

Weimar
Herzogin Anna Amalia Bibliothek (HAAB)
  Stb.112
  Stb.434

Wien
Österreichische Nationalbibliothek (ÖNB)
  Cod.Ser.nov.2608
  Cod.Ser.nov.2968

Wolfenbüttel
Herzog August Bibliothek (HAB)
  21.2 Ethica
  36.17.3 Geom.2°
  128.3 Med
  Gh 255
  Gm 1152 4°
  A:57.8 Pol
  160.8 Quodlibet
  550.12 Quodlibet

Printed Works

The cited German language printed primary sources were mostly consulted at the Herzog August Library, Wolfenbüttel. The cited English language printed primary sources were mostly consulted on the EEBO (Early English Books Online) database, and checked as necessary in London, Oxford or Cambridge.

Aaron, Melissa D., 'The Globe and Henry V as business document'. *Studies in English Literature 1500–1900* 40.2 (2000): 277–92.
Ady, Thomas, *A candle in the dark: shewing the Divine Cause of the distractions of the whole Nation of England, and of the Christian World [...]*. London: Robert Ibbitson, 1655.
Aker, Gudrun, *Narrenschiff: Literatur und Kultur in Deutschland an der Wende zur Neuzeit*. Stuttgart: Hans-Dieter Heinz Akademischer Verlag (Stuttgarter Arbeiten zur Germanistik, nr.216), 1990.

Albertinus, Ægidius, *Der Landtstörtzer Gusman von Alfarche oder Picaro genannt [...]*. München: Nicolaus Henricus, 1615.

Amann, Klaus and Max Siller (eds), *Hippolytus Guarinonius. Akten des 5. Symposiums der Sterzinger Osterspiele (5.-7.4.2004). 'Die Greuel der Verwüstung menschlichen Geschlechts'. Zur 350. Wiederkehr des Todesjahres von Hippolytus Guarinonius (1571–1654)*. Innsbruck: Wagner (Schlern-Schriften 340), 2008.

Anon., *A merry wedding; or, o brave Arthur of Bradly*. London: W O & A M, c.1695.

Anon., *A myraculous, and Monstrous, but yet most true, and certayne discourse, of a Woman (now to be seene in London) of the age of threescore yeares, or there abouts, in the midst of whose fore-head (by the wonderfull worke of God) there groweth out a crooked Horne, of foure ynches long*. London: Thomas Orwin, 1588.

Anon. ('Well-willer'), *The women's petition against coffee*. London: A W, 1700.

Anon., 'Witchcraft'. *The North American Review* 106.218 (1868): 176–232.

Anon., *The wonderfvl discoverie of the witchcrafts of Margaret and Phillip Flower, daughters of Ioan Flower neere Beuer Castle*. London: J. Barnes, 1619.

Austern, Linda Phyllis, '"Art to enchant": musical magic and its practitioners in English renaissance drama'. *Journal of the Royal Musical Association* 115.2 (1990): 191–206.

Baader, Berndt Ph., *Der bayerische Renaissancehof Herzog Wilhelms V. (1568–1579)*. Leipzig and Strassburg: Heitz, 1943.

Bailey, Michael D., 'From sorcery to witchcraft: clerical conceptions of magic in the later Middle Ages'. *Speculum* 76.4 (2001): 960–90.

Baillie, William M., '"Henry VIII": a Jacobean history'. *Shakespeare Studies* 12 (1979): 247–66.

Balme, Christopher, 'Cultural anthropology and theatre historiography: notes on a methodological rapprochement'. *Theatre Survey* 35.1 (1994): 33–53.

Barbieri, Nicolò, *Discorso famigliare*. Venetia: Antonio Pinelli, 1628.

Barbieri, Nicolò, *La supplica discorso famigliare a quelli che trattano de' comici [Venice, 1634]*, edited by F. Taviani. Milan: Il Polifilo, 1971.

Barclay, John, *Repliqve av sievr Coeffeteav, svr sa response à l'Aduertissement du Roy aux Princes & Potentats de la Chrestienté*. Londres: I. Norton, 1610.

Baretti, Joseph, *An account of the manners and customs of Italy, with observations on the mistakes of some travellers, with regard to that country*, 2 vols. London: Davies, Davis & Rymers, 1768.

Bartels, Max, 'Ueber abnorme Behaarung beim Menschen'. *Zeitschrift für Ethnologie* 8 (1876): 110–29, 11 (1879): 145–94, 13 (1881): 213–33.

Bartoli, Adolfo, *Scenari inediti della commedia dell'arte*. Florence: Arnaldo Forni, 1880.

Baschet, Armand, *Les comédiens italiens a la cour de France sous Charles IX, Henri III, Henri IV et Louis XIII*. Paris: Plon, 1882.

Battafarano, Italo Michele, *L'Italia ir-reale. Descritta dai tedeschi negli ultimi cinque secoli e raccontata agli italiani dal loro punto di vista*. Taranto: Scorpione, 1995.

Battafarano, Italo Michele, 'Literarische Skatologie als Therapie literarischer Melancholie: Johann Beers "Der Berühmte Narren-Spital"'. *Simpliciana* 13 (1991): 191–210.

Battafarano, Italo Michele, 'Zettelkraut statt Zitronen. Nationaler Stolz aus defensiver Kritik an Ausländerei und Exotismus bei Hippolytus Guarinonius'. *Simpliciana* 17 (1995): 141–53.

Baumann, Werner, 'Ernst Friedrich von Baden-Durlach, Felix Platter und Polan'. *Theologische Zeitschrift* 59 (2003): 335–41.

Bawcutt, N. W., 'William Vincent, alias Hocus Pocus: a travelling entertainer of the seventeenth century'. *Theatre Notebook* 54.3 (2000): 130–8.

Beaumont, Francis and John Fletcher, *Comedies and tragedies*. London: Humphrey Robinson & Humphrey Moseley, 1647.

Beer, Johann, *Weiber-Hächel, Jungfer-Hobel, Bestia-Civitas, Narren-Spital. Sämtliche Werke*, V, edited by Ferdinand van Ingen and Hans-Gert Roloff. Bern: Peter Lang, 1991.

Behringer, Wolfgang, 'Arena and pall mall: sport in the early modern period'. *German History* 27.3 (2009): 331–57.

Behringer, Wolfgang, *Shaman of Oberstdorf: Chonrad Stoekhlin and the phantoms of the night*. Charlottesville: University Press of Virginia, 1998.

Beijer, Agne and Pierre Louis Duchartre, *Recueil de plusieurs fragments des premières comédies italiennes qui on ésté représentées en France sous le règne de Henry III*. Paris: Duchartre et Van Buggenhoudt, 1928.

Bell, Dean Phillip and Stephen G. Burnett (eds), *Jews, Judaism, and the Reformation in sixteenth-century Germany*. Leiden: Brill, 2006.

Benedict, Barbara M., *Curiosity: a cultural history of early modern inquiry*. Chicago: University of Chicago Press, 2001.

Bergerac, Cyrano de, *Satyrical characters and handsome descriptions in letters written to severall persons of quality*. London: Henry Herringman, 1658.

Bertelli, Franc[esc]o, *Il carnevale italiano mascherato, oue si veggono in figura varie inueutioni di Capritii*. [Venetia], 1642.

Bertelli, Pietro, *Diversaru[m] nationum habitus, centum et quattor iconibus in ære incisis*, 3 vols. Patavii: Alciatum Alcia et P. Bertellium, 1589, 1591, 1596.

Bever, Edward, 'Witchcraft, female aggression, and power in the early modern community'. *Journal of Social History* 35.4 (2002): 955–88.

Bibiena, Jean Galli De (edited by Francesca Pagani), *La nouvelle Italie*. Bergamo: Sestante, 2008.

Biggins, Dennis, 'Sexuality, witchcraft, and violence in "Macbeth"'. *Shakespeare Studies* 8 (1975): 255–77.

Biggs, Robert, 'Medicine in Ancient Mesopotamia'. *History of Science* 8 (1969): 94–105.

Binz, Gustav, 'Londoner Theater und Schauspiele im Jahre 1599'. *Anglia* 22 (1899): 456–64.

Blackburn, Bonnie and Leofranc Holford-Strevens, *The Oxford companion to the year*. Oxford: Oxford University Press, 1999.

Bochius, Joannes, *Historica narratio profectionis et inavgvrationis Serenissimorvm Belgii Principvm Alberti et Isabellæ Austriæ Archidvcvm, et eorum optatissimi in Belgium aduentus*. Antwerp: Jan Moretus, 1602.

Bodin, Jean, *De la demonomanie des sorciers*. Paris: Iacques de Puys, 1580.

Bondeson, Jan, *The two-headed boy and other medical marvels*. Ithaca: Cornell University Press, 2000.

Boos, Heinrich, *Thomas und Felix Platter. Zur Sittengeschichte des XVI Jahrhunderts*. Leipzig: Hirzel, 1878.

Bowers, John Z. and Robert W. Carrubba, 'Drug abuse and sexual binding spells in seventeenth century Asia: essays from the "Amoenitatum Exoticarum" of Engelbert Kaempfer'. *Journal of the History of Medicine and Allied Sciences* 33.3 (1978): 318–43.

Brand, Peter, 'Der englische Komödiant Robert Browne'. Heidelberg University (unpublished MA dissertation), 1978.

Brandauer, Christine, 'Die poetischen Teile im ungedruckten zweiten Teil von "Die Greuel der Verwüstung menschlichen Geschlechts" des Hippolytus Guarinonius (1652)'. *Hippolytus Guarinonius*, edited by Amann and Siller, 15–23.

Brandstätter, Klaus, 'Hall in der Zeit von Hippolyt Guarinoni'. *Hippolytus Guarinonius*, edited by Amann and Siller, 25–38.

Brant, Sebastian (tr. Jacob Locher: Latin, Alexander Barclay: English), *Stultifera nauis, Narrenschiff*. London: Richard Pynson, 1509.

Brantôme, [Pierre Bourdeille de], *Recueil des Dames, poésies et tombeaux*, edited by Etienne Vaucheret. Paris: Gallimard, 1991.

Breuer, Dieter, 'Hippolytus Guarinonius als Erzähler'. *Die österreichische Literatur. Ihr Profil von den Anfängen im Mittelalter bis ins 18. Jahrhundert (1050–1750)*, edited by Herbert Zeman with Fritz Peter Knapp, Teil 2. Graz: Akademische Druck, 1986, 1117–33.

Breuer, Dieter, '"Schöne des Leibs". Gesichtspunkte zum Auffinden "vergessener Kulturleistungen" der frühen Neuzeit am Beispiel der "Grewel der Verwüstung Menschlichen Geschlechts" des Hippolytus Guarinonius'. *Gegenwart als kulturelles Erbe: ein Beitrag der Germanistik zur Kulturwissenschaft deutschsprachiger Länder*, edited by Bernd Thum. München: iudicium, 1985, 123–30.

Brockliss, Laurence and Colin Jones, *The medical world of early modern France*. Oxford: Clarendon Press, 1997.

Brouwer, Francesco de Simone, 'Due scenari inediti del secolo XVII'. *Giornale storico* 18 (1891): 277–90.

Browe, Peter, SJ, *Beiträge zur Sexualethik des Mittelalters*. Breslau: Müller & Seiffert, 1932.

Brown, Iain Gordon, 'Water, windows and women: the significance of Venice for Scots in the age of the Grand Tour'. *Eighteenth-Century Life* 30.3 (2006): 1–50.

Brückle, Wolfgang and Jürgen Müller, '"Die unzimblichen *Gemåhl* sein Lehrmeister *und Zeyger*": Kunsttheoretische Splitter bei Hippolyt Guarinoni'. *Hippolytus Guarinonius im interkulturellen Kontext*, edited by Locher, 97–116.

Brüggemann, Romy, *Die Angst vor dem Bösen: Codierungen des* malum *in der spätmittelalterlichen und frühneuzeitlichen Narren-, Teufel- und Teufelsbündnerliteratur.* Würzburg: Königshausen & Neumann, 2010.

Brun, Pierre, *Pupazzi et statuettes. Études sur le XVIIe siècle.* Paris: Édouard Cornély, 1908.

Bücking, Jürgen, 'Hippolytus Guarinonius (1571–1654), Pfalzgraf zu Hoffberg und Volderthurn. eine kritische Würdigung'. *Österreich in Geschichte und Literatur* 12.2 (1968): 65–80.

Bücking, Jürgen, *Kultur und Gesellschaft in Tirol um 1600. Des Hippolytus Guarinonius' "Grewel der Verwüstung menschlichen Geschlechts" (1610) als kulturgeschichtliche Quelle des frühen 17. Jahrhunderts.* Lübeck and Hamburg: Matthiesen (Historische Studien 401), 1968.

Bujok, Elke, 'Ethnographica in early modern *Kunstkammern* and their perception'. *Journal of the History of Collections* 21.1 (2009): 17–32.

Bujok, Elke, *Neue Welten in europäischen Sammlungen: Africana und Americana in Kunstkammern bis 1670.* Berlin: Reimer, 2004.

Bumiller, Casimir, 'Die Brüder Frischlin und ihre Beziehungen zu den Grafen von Zollern'. *Zeitschrift für Hohenzollersche Geschichte* 27 (1991): 9–28.

Bumiller, Casimir, 'Die "Selbstanalyse" des Arztes Felix Platter (1534–1614)'. *Die Psychohistorie des Erlebens*, edited by Ralph Frenken and Martin Rheinheimer. Kiel: Oetker-Voges, 2000, 303–24.

Burnett, Mark Thornton, *Constructing 'monsters' in Shakespearean drama and early modern culture.* Basingstoke: Palgrave Macmillan, 2002.

Burnett, Stephen G., 'Distorted mirrors: Antonius Margaritha, Johann Buxtorf and Christian ethnographies of the Jews'. *Sixteenth Century Journal* 25.2 (1994): 275–87.

Burnett, Stephen G., *From Christian Hebraism to Jewish Studies: Johannes Buxtorf (1564–1629) and Hebrew learning in the seventeenth century.* Leiden: Brill, 1996

[Burton, Robert], *The anatomy of melancholy, what it is. With all the kindes, cavses, symptoms, prognostickes, and severall cvres of it.* Oxford: Henry Cripps, 1621.

Butterworth, Emily, 'The work of the devil? Theatre, the supernatural, and Montaigne's public stage'. *Renaissance Studies* 22.5 (2008): 705–22.

Butterworth, Philip, 'Brandon, Feats and Hocus Pocus: jugglers three'. *Theatre Notebook* 57.2 (2003): 89–106.

Butterworth, Philip, *Magic on the early English stage.* Cambridge: Cambridge University Press, 2005.

Buxtorf, Johannes, *The Jewish Synagogue, or an historical narration of the state of the Jewes*. London: H. R. & T. Young, 1663.

Buxtorf, Johannes, *Synagoga Ivdaica: Das ist / Jüden Schul*. Basle: Sebastian Henricpetrus, 1603.

'C', I., *A pleasant comedie, called the two merry milke-maids [...] As it was acted before the King [...] by the Companie of the Reuels*. London: Lawrence Chapman, 1620.

Calabi, Donatella, 'Les quartiers juifs en Italie entre 15ᵉ et 17ᵉ siècle. Quelques hypothèses de travail'. *Annales HSS* 52.4 (1997): 777–97.

Campion, Thomas, *The description of a maske*. London: Laurence La'sle, 1614.

Campos, Giulia, 'L'"Arlichino" di Giorgio Maria Raparini'. *Giornale storico della letteratura italiana* 102 (1933): 165–223.

Capozza, Nicoletta, *Tutti i lazzi della commedia dell'arte: un catalogo ragionato del patrimonio dei Comici*. Rome: Dino Audino, 2006.

Chambers, E[dmund] K[erchever], *The Elizabethan stage*, 4 vols. Oxford: Clarendon Press, 1923.

Chambers, E[dmund] K[erchever], *The mediaeval stage*, 2 vols. Oxford: Clarendon Press, 1903.

Chambrier, Pauline, 'La relation de voyage de Thomas Platter en Angleterre: ou comment re-visiter les plus remarquables châteax anglais du XVIᵉ siècle'. *Journal de la Renaissance* 4 (2006): 173–87.

[Chapman, George], *The shadow of night: containing two poeticall hymnes*. London: William Ponsonby, 1594.

Clark, Stuart, 'Inversion, misrule and the meaning of witchcraft'. *Past & Present* 87 (1980): 98–127.

Clark, Stuart, *Thinking with demons: the idea of witchcraft in early modern Europe*. Oxford: Clarendon Press, 1997.

Collins, David J., *Reforming saints: saints' lives and their authors in Germany, 1470–1530*. Oxford: Oxford University Press, 2008

Collins, Samuel, *The present state of Russia in a letter to a friend at London*. London: Dorman Newman, 1671.

Comenius, J. A., *Joh. Amos Comenii orbis sensualium picti denuò aucti pars secunda [...] Der Neu=Vermehrten Sichtbaren Welt Anderer Theil / mit 150. Figuren versehen und erläutert*. Nürnberg: Martin Endter, 1719.

Coryate, Thomas, *Coryats crudities hastily gobled vp in fiue moneths trauells in France, Sauoy, Italy, Rhetia commonly called the Grisons country, Heluetia alias Switzerland, some parts of high Germany and the Netherland*. London: W[illiam] S[tansby], 1611.

Cowley, Abraham, *Poems*. London: Humphrey Moseley, 1656.

Craik, Katharine A., 'Reading *Coryats Crudities* (1611)'. *Studies in English Literature* 44.1 (2004): 77–96.

Cranefield, Paul, 'Little known English versions of the *Praxis* and *Observationes* of Felix Platter'. *Journal of the History of Medicine and Allied Sciences* 17.2 (1962): 309–11.

Creizenach, Wilhelm, *Das englische Drama im Zeitalter Shakespeares.* (*Geschichte des neueren Dramas, IV*). Halle: Niemeyer, 1909.

Creizenach, Wilhelm, 'Verloren gegangene englische Dramen aus dem Zeitalter Shakespeares'. *Jahrbuch der deutschen Shakespeare Gesellschaft* 54 (1918): 42–7.

Crull, J., *The antient and present state of Muscovy.* London: A. Roper & A. Bosvile, 1698.

Daston, Lorraine and Katharine Park, *Wonders and the order of nature, 1150–1750.* New York: Zone, 2001.

Davis, Natalie Zemon, 'Ghosts, kin and progeny: some features of family life in early modern France'. *Dædalus* 106.2 (1977): 87–114.

Davis, Natalie Zemon, 'The reasons of misrule: youth groups and charivaris in sixteenth-century France'. *Past and Present* 50 (1971): 41–75.

Day, Cyrus L., 'Knots and knot lore'. *Western Folklore,* 9.3 (1950): 229–56.

Deierkauf-Holsboer, S. Wilma, *L'histoire de la mise en scène dans le théatre français a Paris de 1600 à 1673.* Paris: Nizet, 1960.

Deierkauf-Holsboer, S. Wilma, 'La vie théâtrale a Paris de 1612 a 1614'. *Modern Language Notes* 63.1 (1948): 10–19.

Deierkauf-Holsboer, S. Wilma, *Le Théatre de l'Hotel de Bourgogne, I, 1548–1635.* Paris: Nizet, 1968.

Deierkauf-Holsboer, S. Wilma, 'Les représentations bilingues á l'Hôtel de Bourgogne en 1612'. *Modern Language Notes* 62.4 (1947): 217–22.

Deierkauf-Holsboer, S. Wilma, *Vie d'Alexandre Hardy, Poète du roi 1572–1632. 47 documents inédits. Nouvelle édition revue et augmentée.* Paris: Nizet, 1972.

Deierkauf-Holsboer, S. Wilma, 'Vie d'Alexandre Hardy, Poète du roi: quarante-deux documents inédits', *Proceedings of the American Philosophical Society* 91.4 (1947): 328–401.

Del Cerro, Emilio, 'Lazzi inediti della commedia dell'arte'. *Rivista d'Italia,* 17 (1914): 589–99.

Deutsch, Yaacov, '"Von der Iuden Ceremonien": representations of Jews in sixteenth-century Germany'. *Jews, Judaism, and the Reformation,* edited by Bell and Burnett, 335–56.

Deutscher, Thomas, 'The role of the Episcopal Tribunal of Novara in the suppression of heresy and witchcraft, 1563–1615'. *Catholic Historical Review* 77.3 (1991): 403–21.

Deutschländer, Gerrit, '"Allein auß begirdt, ettwaß zesehen". Die Englandreise des jüngeren Thomas Platter von 1599'. *Entdeckung und Selbstentdeckung. Die Begegnung europäischer Reisender mit dem England und Irland der Neuzeit,* edited by Otfried Dankelmann. Frankfurt: Peter Lang, 1999, 51–69.

Diemerbroeck, Ysbrand van, *The anatomy of human bodies.* London: W. Whitwood, 1694.

Diemling, Maria, 'Anthonius Margaritha on the "whole Jewish faith": a sixteenth-century convert from Judaism and his depiction of the Jewish religion'. *Jews, Judaism, and the Reformation,* edited by Bell and Burnett, 303–33.

Dörrer, Anton, 'Guarinoni als Volksschriftsteller'. *Hippolytus Guarinonius (1571–1654)*, edited by Dörrer et al., 137–85.

Dörrer, Anton, 'Quellen- und Schrifttumsweiser'. *Hippolytus Guarinonius (1571–1654)*, edited by Dörrer et al., 205–14.

Dörrer, Anton, Franz Grass, Gustav Sauser and Karl Schadelbauer (eds), *Hippolytus Guarinonius (1571–1654). Zur 300. Wiederkehr seines Todestages*. Innsbruck: Wagner (Schlern-Schriften 126), 1954.

Drexel, Kurt, 'Hippolyt Guarinonis "Die Grewel der Verwüstung Menschlichen Geschlechts" als Quelle zur Musikgeschichte Tirols im frühen 17. Jahrhundert'. *Hippolytus Guarinonius*, edited by Amann and Siller, 49–60.

Driesen, Otto, *Der Ursprung des Harlekin*. Berlin: Duncker, 1904.

Dulieu, Louis, *La médecine a Montpellier Tome II: La Renaissance*. Avignon: Presses universelles, 1979.

Dulieu, Louis (ed.), *La médecine à Montpellier du XIIᵉ au XXᵉ siècle*. Paris: Editions Hervas, 1990.

Egan, Gabriel, 'The Lords Howard's Men at the Rose and on tour in 1599'. *Notes and Queries* 46.2 (1999): 234–6.

Egan, Gabriel, 'NTQ book reviews'. *New Theatre Quarterly* 18.3 (2002): 290.

Egan, Gabriel, 'Thomas Platter's account of an unknown play at the Curtain or the Boar's Head'. *Notes and Queries* 47.1 (2000): 53–6.

Entin-Bates, Lee R., 'Montaigne's remarks on impotence'. *Modern Language Notes* 91.4 (1976): 640–54.

Evelyn, John (edited by E. S. de Beer, intro. Roy Strong), *The diary of John Evelyn*. London: Everyman, 2006.

Ewinkel, Irene, *De monstris: Deutung und Funktion von Wundergeburten auf Flugblättern im Deutschland des 16. Jahrhunderts*, Tübingen: Niemeyer, 1995.

Eyre, Mary, *A lady's walks in the south of France in 1863*. London: Richard Bentley, 1865.

Feinberg, Anat, 'Quacks and mountebanks in Stuart and Caroline drama'. *Ludica* 5–6 (2000): 116–26.

Ferrone, Siro, *Attori mercanti corsari: la commedia dell'arte in Europa tra cinque e seicento*. Torino: Einaudi, 1993.

Ferrone, Siro, Claudia Burattelli, Domenica Landolfi and Anna Zinnani (eds), *Comici dell'arte. Corrispondenze, G B Andreini, N Barbieri, P M Cecchini, S Fiorillo, T Martinelli, F Scala*, 2 vols. Firenze: Le Lettere, 1993.

Fischart, Johann (edited by Ute Nyssen and Hugo Sommerhalder), *Johann Fischart. Geschichtklitterung (Gargantua). Text der Ausgabe letzter Hand von 1590*. Düsseldorf: Karl Rauch, 1963.

Fischer, Alfons, 'Der Tiroler Arzt Hippolyt Guarinonius als Erzieher zur Gesundheitspflicht und Vorkämpfer für den Ausbau des Gesundheitsrechts'. *Geschichte des deutschen Gesundheitswesens*, I, Berlin, 1933, 282–92 (reprint edition used: Hildesheim: Olms, 1965).

Fournier, Édouard, *Chansons de Gaultier Garguille*. Paris: P. Jannet, 1858.

Fransen, J., 'Documents inédits sur l'Hôtel de Bourgogne'. *Revue d'histoire littéraire de la France* 34 (1927): 321–55.

Fransen, J., *Les comédiens français en Hollande au XVIIᵉ et au XVIIIᵉ siècles.* Paris: Honoré Champion, 1925.

Frenken, Ralph, *Kindheit und Autobiographie vom 14. bis 17. Jahrhundert. Psychohistorische Rekonstruktionen.* Kiel: Oetker-Voges, 1999.

Frey, Winfried, 'Hippolytus Guarinonius und die Tradition der Ritualmordbeschuldigungen'. *Hippolytus Guarinonius,* edited by Amann and Siller, 61–76.

Frischlin, Jakob (edited by Casimir Bumiller), *Jakob Frischlin, Drey schöne und lustige Bücher von der Hohenzollerischen Hochzeyt.* Konstanz: Isele, 2003.

Frischlin, Nicodemus, *De nuptijs illvstrissimi principis, ac Domini, D. Lvdovici, ducis Wirtembergici & Teccij [...] Libri septem, versu heroico conscripti.* Tubingæ: Georg Gruppenbach, 1577.

Fuhrmann, Joëlle, *Theorie und Praxis in der Gesetzgebung des Spätmittelalters in Deutschland am Beispiel der Ingelheimer Schöffensprüche.* Bern: Peter Lang, 2001.

Gambelli, Delia, *Arlecchino a Parigi,* 3 vols [I: *Dall'inferno alla corte del re sole,* II–III: *Lo scenario di Domenico Biancolelli, edizione critica, introduzioni e note,* Parte Prima (II) and Parte Seconda (III)]. Roma: Bulzoni, 1993 and 1997.

Garfein, Herschel and Mel Gordon, 'The Adriani Lazzi of the commedia dell'arte'. *The Drama Review* 22.1 (1978): 3–12.

Garzoni, Tomaso (edited by Giovanni Battista Bronzini), *La piazza universale di tutte le professioni del mondo,* 2 vols. Firenze: Olschki, 1996.

Gebhardt, Michael, 'Der "Gegenreformator" Hippolyt Guarinoni'. *Hippolytus Guarinonius,* edited by Amann and Siller, 77–105.

Gemert, Guillaume van, 'Tridentinische Geistigkeit und Moraldidaxis in Guarinonius' "Greweln": Der Arzt als geistlicher Autor'. *Hippolytus Guarinonius im interkulturellen Kontext,* edited by Locher, 45–63.

Gemert, Guillaume van, 'Übersetzung und Kompilation im Dienste der katholischen Rerformbewegung. Zum Literaturprogramm des Aegidius Albertinus (1560–1620)'. *Daphnis* 8.3–4 (1979): 123–42.

Gemert, Guillaume van, 'Medizinisches Naturverständnis und gegenreformatorisches Literaturprogramm. Zum Stellenwert des erzählerischen Moments in Hipplytus Guarinonius' "Grewel der Verwüstung Menschlichen Geschlechts"'. *Künste und Natur in Diskursen der Frühen Neuzeit,* edited by Hartmut Laufhütte. Wiesbaden: Harrassowitz, 1123–37.

Gennep, Arnold Van, *Manuel de Folklore français contemporain.* Paris: Picard, 1958.

Gentilcore, David, '"Charlatans, mountebanks and other similar people": the regulation and role of itinerant practitioners in early modern Italy'. *Social History* 20.3 (1995): 297–314.

Gentilcore, David, *Medical charlatanism in early modern Italy.* Oxford: Oxford University Press, 2006.

Gerster, C., 'Ueber einige Diätetiker des 16. und 17. Jahrhunderts'. *Deutsche medicinische Wochenschrift* 44 (1899): 727–9.

Geßler, Albert, *Felix Platters Schilderung der Reise des Markgrafen Georg Friedrich von Baden und Hochberg nach Hechingen zur Hochzeit [...] im Jahre 1598*. Basel: Werner-Riehm (Seperat-Abdruck, *Basler Jahrbuch* 1891), 1890.

Goodey, C. F., '"Foolishness" in early modern medicine and the concept of intellectual disability'. *Medical History* 48 (2004): 289–310.

Gordon, Mel, *Lazzi: the comic routines of the commedia dell'arte*. New York: Theatre Library Association, 1981.

Gothein, Marie, 'Die Todsünden'. *Archiv für Religionswissenschaft* 10 (1907): 416–84.

Goulart, Simon, *Admirable and memorable histories containing the wonders of our time. Collected into French out of the best authors. By I Govlart. And out of French into English. By Ed. Grimeston*. London: George Eld, 1607.

Gowland, Angus, 'The problem of early modern melancholy'. *Past and Present* 191 (2006): 77–120.

Graizbord, David L., *Souls in dispute: converso identities in Iberia and the Jewish diaspora, 1580–1700*. Philadelphia: University of Pennsylvania Press, 2004.

Granichstaedten-Czerva, Rudolf, 'Die Familie Guarinoni von Hoffberg'. *Hippolytus Guarinonius (1571–1654)*, edited by Dörrer et al., 19–20.

Grass, Franz, 'Dr Hippolytus Guarinonius zu Hoffberg und Volderthurn 1571–1654' and 'Hippolytus Guarinonius. Ein Vorkämpfer für deutsche Volksgesundheit im 17. Jhdt.'. *Hippolytus Guarinonius (1571–1654)*, edited by Dörrer et al., 9–17 and 57–90.

Graß, Nikolaus, 'Der Kampf gegen Fasnachtsveranstaltungen in der Fastenzeit. Nach Tiroler Quellen dargestellt'. *Zeitschrift für Volkskunde* 53 (1956/7): 204–37.

Greene, Robert, *The comicall historie of Alphonsus, King of Aragon*. London: Thomas Creede, 1599.

Greene, Robert, *The historie of Orlando Furioso, one of the twelue Pieres of France*. London: Cuthbert Burbie, 1594.

Grell, Ole Peter and Andrew Cunningham, 'Introduction: medicine and religion in seventeenth-century England'. *Religio medici: medicine and religion in seventeenth-century England*, edited by Ole Peter Grell and Andrew Cunningham. Aldershot: Scolar Press, 1996, 1–11.

Grimm, Jakob and Wilhelm Grimm, *Deutsche Sagen*, 2 vols. Berlin: Nicolai, 1816–18.

Grimmelshausen, Hans Jacob Christoffel von (edited by Dieter Breuer), *Hans Jacob Christoffel von Grimmelshausen Werke*, I.2. Frankfurt: Deutscher Klassiker Verlag, 1992.

Guarinonius, Hippolytus, *Chylosophiæ academicæ artis Æscvlapiæ nouis Astris*. Oeniponte: Michael Wagner, 1648.

Guarinonius, Hippolytus, *Die Grewel der Verwüstung Menschlichen Geschlechts. In sieben unterschiedliche Bŭcher und unmeidenliche Hauptstucken / sampt einem lustigen Vortrab / abgetheilt. Neben vor: mit: und nachgehenden / so wol Natŭrlichen / als Christlich: und Politischen / darwider streittbaren Mittlen. Allen / so wol Geist: als Weltlichen / Gelehrt: und Ungelehrten / hoch und nidern Stands Personen / ŭberaub nutz und sehr notwendig / wie auch gar kurtzweilig zu lesen. [...] MATTHÆI XXIIII. Wann ir den Grewel der Verwŭstung sehen werdet / etc.* Ingolstatt: Andreas Angermayr, 1610.

Guarinonius, Hippolytus, *Hydroenogamia trivmphpans ... Heillig vnd heilsamber Wasser vnd Wein Heurath.* Oeniponte: Michael Wagner, 1640.

Guarinonius, Hippolytus, [tr.; Italian original: J. P. Giussano], *In memoria æterna erit ivstvs. Prælaten Cron. Lebens und der gewaltigen Thaten deß H Caroli Borromæi, Weiland der H Röm[ischen] Kirchen [...].* Freyburg: Johann Strasser, 1618.

Guarinonius, Hippolytus, *Pestilentz Guardien / fŭr allerley Stands Personen / mit Săuberung der inficierten Hăuser / Beth-Leingewandt / Kleider / etc.* Ingolstadt: Andreas Angermayr, 1612.

Guarinonius, Hippolytus, (edited and translated by Sepp Mitterstiller), *Thomas von Bergamo, Kapuzinerlaienbruder.* Innsbruck: St Laurentius Druckerei, 1933.

Guazzo, Francesco Mario, *Compendium maleficarum. The Montague Summers edition, translated by E A Ashwin.* New York: Dover, 1988.

Hädge, Martina, 'Meß-Ärtzte in Leipzig im 17. und 18. Jahrhundert'. *Theaterkunst & Heilkunst. Studien zu Theater und Anthropologie*, edited by M. Hädge and G. Baumbach. Köln: Böhlau, 2002, 41–73.

Hallar, Marianne, *Teaterspil og tegnsprog. Ikonografiske studier i commedia dell'arte.* København: Akademisk, 1977.

Hansen, Günther (posthumously edited by Helmut G. Asper), *Formen der Commedia dell'arte in Deutschland.* Emsdetten: Lechte, 1984.

Happé, Peter, 'The vice and the folk-drama'. *Folklore* 75 (1964): 161–93.

Harsdörffer, Georg Philipp, *Der grosse Schau-platz Lust- und Lehrreicher Geschichte.* Franckfurt: Johann Georg Spörlin, 1664.

Hart, James, *Klinike, or the diet of the diseased.* London: Robert Allot, 1633.

Haslinger, Adolf, 'Die erste Schilderung einer Hochgebirgsbesteigung in Tirol'. *Tradition und Entwicklung, Festschrift Eugen Thurnher zum 60. Geburtstag*, edited by Werner M. Bauer, Achim Masser and Guntram A. Plangg. Innsbruck: Institut für Germanistik der Universität Innsbruck, 1982, 211–22.

Hastaba, Ellen, 'Theater in Tirol – Spielbelege in der Bibliothek des Tiroler Landesmuseums Ferdinandeum'. *Veröffentlichungen des Tiroler Landesmuseums Ferdinandeum* 75/76 (1995–6 [1997]): 233–343.

Hastaba, Ellen, 'Vom Lied zum Spiel. Das Anderl-von-Rinn-Lied des Hippolyt Guarinoni als Vorlage für Anderl-von-Rinn-Spiele'. *Literatur und Sprachkultur in Tirol*, edited by Johann Holzner, Oskar Putzer and Max Siller. Innsbruck: Ferdinandeum, 1997, 273 288.

Hattori, Natsu, *Performing cures: practice and interplay in theatre and medicine of the English Renaissance*. University of Oxford (unpublished doctoral dissertation), 1995.

Havers, G. (tr.), *A general collection of discourses of the Virtuosi of France, upon questions of all sorts of philosophy, and other natural knowledg, made in the assembly of the Beaux Esprits at Paris*. London: Thomas Dring & John Starkey, 1664.

Havers, G. and J. Davies (tr.), *Another collection of philosophical conferences of the French Virtuosi upon questions of all sorts; for the improving of natural knowledg, made in the assembly of the Beaux Esprits at Paris*. London: Thomas Dring & John Starkey, 1665.

[Hawker, Essex], *The country-wedding and skimington: a tragic-comi-pastoral-farcical opera*. London: W. Trott, 1729.

Heck, Thomas F., *Commedia dell'arte: a guide to the primary and secondary literature*. New York and London: Garland, 1988.

Henke, Robert, 'The Italian mountebank and the *commedia dell'arte*'. *Theatre Survey* 38.2 (1997): 1–29.

Henke, Robert, *Performance and literature in the commedia dell'arte*. Cambridge: Cambridge University Press, 2002.

Henke, Robert, 'Representations of poverty in the commedia dell'arte'. *Commedia dell'arte, annuario internazionale* 1 (2008): 141–60.

Henkel, Arthur and Albrecht Schöne, *Emblemata. Handbuch zur Sinnbildkunst des XVI. und XVII. Jahrhunderts*. Stuttgart: Metzler, 1996.

Hentzner, Paul (tr. Horace Walpole), *Paul Hentzner's travels in England during the reign of Queen Elizabeth*. London: Edward Jeffery, 1797.

Herrick, Robert, *Hesperides: or the works both humane and divine of Robert Herrick Esq*. London: John Williams & Francis Eglesfield, 1648.

Herrington, H. W., 'Witchcraft and magic in the Elizabethan drama'. *The Journal of American Folk-lore* 32.4 (1919): 447–85.

Hertel, Christiane, '"Der rauch man zu Münichen". Die Porträts der Familie Gonsalus in der Kunstkammer Erzherzog Ferdinands II. von Tirol'. *Sammler – Bibliophile – Exzentriker*, edited by Aleida Assmann, Monika Gomille and Gabriele Rippl. Tübingen: Gunter Narr, 1998, 163–91.

Heywood, Thomas, *Gynaikeion, or nine bookes of various history concerning women*. London: Adam Islip, 1624.

Heywood, Thomas and Richard Brome, *The late Lancashire witches*. London: Benjamin Fisher, 1634.

Highfill, Philip H., Kalman A. Burnim and Edward A. Langhans (eds), *A biographical dictionary of actors, actresses, musicians, dancers, managers and other stage personnel in London, 1660–1800*, 16 vols. Carbondale and Edwardsville: Southern Illinois University Press, 1973–93.

Hirn, Joseph, *Erzherzog Ferdinand II von Tirol. Geschichte seiner Regierung und seiner Länder*, 2 vols. Innsbruck: Wagner, 1885 and 1888

Hochenegg, Hans, 'Die Bildnisse Guarinonis'. *Hippolytus Guarinonius (1571–1654)*, edited by Dörrer et al., 21–6.

Hochlenert, Dieter, 'Das "Tagebuch" des Felix Platter: die Autobiographie eines Arztes und Humanisten'. Tübingen (Philosophische Dissertation, Neuphilologische Fakultät der Universität Tübingen, 1996).

Höchstetter, Hans Ludwig (edited and translated by John Kmetz), *Ein Brief vom 6. Februar 1551 an Felix Platter enthaltend 'ein Stückle auffs Clavicordium'*. Stuttgart: Cornetto, 2006.

Holeton, David R., 'Fynes Moryson's "Itinerary": a sixteenth century English traveller's observations on Bohemia, its reformation, and its liturgy'. *The Bohemian Reformation and Religious Practice*, vol. 5, edited by Zdeněk David & D. R. Holeton. Prague: Academy of the Sciences of the Czech Republic, 2005, part 2, 379–410.

Holinshed, Raphael, *The Chronicles of England, Scotlande, and Irelande*, II, 'The historie of Scotlande'. London: John Hunne, 1577.

Holländer, Eugen, *Wunder, Wundergeburt und Wundergestalt in Einblattdrucken des fünfzehnten bis achtzehnten Jahrhunderts*. Stuttgart: Ferdinand Enke, 1921.

Holmes, Christopher, 'Time for the plebs in "Julius Caesar"'. *Early Modern Literary Studies* 7.2 (2001): 2.1–32. Available at: http://purl.oclc.org/emls/07-2/holmjuli.htm [accessed 16 January 2008].

Homes, Nathanael, *Dæmonologie and theologie*. London: Thomas Roycroft, 1650.

Hoppe, Harry R., 'La circulation comique: acteurs français aux pays-bas espagnols: (?) Valleran le Conte (1613) et Valerand Dufour (1616)'. *Revue d'histoire du théatre* 6.3 (1954): 166–8.

Howarth, William D. (ed.), *French theatre in the neo-classical era, 1550–1789*. Cambridge: Cambridge University Press, 1997.

Howe, Alan, *Le Théâtre professionnel à Paris 1600-1649: documents du Minutier central des Notaires de Paris*. Paris: Centre historique des Archives nationales, 2000.

Howell, James, *Epistolæ Ho-Elianæ. Familiar letters, domestic and forren [...] The 6th edition*. London: Thomas Guy, 1688.

Howell, James, *Paroimiographia. Proverbs or, old sayed sawes & adages*. London: J G, 1659.

Hsia, R. Po-Chia, 'Christian ethnographies of Jews in early modern Germany'. *Problems in the historical anthropology of early modern Europe*, edited by R. P. Hsia and R. W. Scribner. Wiesbaden: Harrassowitz, 1997, 35–47.

Huber, Katharina, *Felix Platters 'Observationes': Studien zum frühneuzeitlichen Gesundheitswesen in Basel*. Basel: Schwabe, 2003.

Hulsen, Esaias van, Georg Donauer and Matthaeus Merian, *Repræsentatio der Fvrstlichen Avfzvg vnd Ritterspil. So der Dvrchleuchtig Hochgeborn Fvrst und Herr Herr Johan Friderich Hertzog zu Württemberg, vnd Teckh, Graue zu Montpellgart, Herr zu Haidenhaim. etc. beij Ihr Fl. Gl Neüwgebornen Sohn. Friderich Hertzog zu Württemberg etc. Fürstlicher Kindtauffen, denn 10 biss auff denn 17 Martij, Anno 1616. Inn der Fürstlichen Haupt Statt Stuetgarten, mit grosser solennitet gehalten*, [Stuttgart: Hulsen] 1616.

Iancu, Carol, 'The language, literary works and liturgy of the Pope's Jews in southern France'. *Studia Hebraica* 8 (2008): 81–95.

Immermann, Karl Leberecht (edited by Robert Boxberger), *Werke*, 8 vols (20 parts). Berlin: Gustav Hempel, [1883].

Ingram, Martin, 'Ridings, rough music and the "Reform of popular culture" in early modern England'. *Past & Present* 105 (1984): 79–113.

Irenæus, Christoph, *De monstris. Von seltzamen Wundergeburten*. Ursel: Henricus, 1584.

James VI/I, [King], *Daemonologie, in forme of a dialogue*. Edinburgh: Robert Waldegrave, 1597.

James VI/I, [King] (ed.), *The Holy Bible, conteyning the Old Testament, and the New: newly translated out of the Originall tongues: & with the former Translations diligently compared and reuised by his Maiesties speciall Comandement*. London: Robert Barker, 1611. [Here cited as *King James Bible*].

James, Robert, *Pharmacopœia universalis: or, a new universal English dispensatory*. London: T Osborne et al., 1764.

Jennett, Seán, *Beloved son Felix. The journal of Felix Platter a medical student in Montpellier in the sixteenth century*. London: Frederick Muller, 1961.

Jennett, Seán, *Journal of a younger brother. The life of Thomas Platter as a medical student in Montpellier at the close of the sixteenth century*. London: Frederick Muller, 1963.

Johnson, Eugene J., 'The short lascivious lives of two Venetian theaters, 1580–85'. *Renaissance Quarterly* 55.3 (2002): 936–68.

Jones, Colin, 'Pulling teeth in eighteenth-century Paris'. *Past and Present* 166 (2000): 100–45.

Jones-Davies, M. T., Ton Hoenselaars and John Jowett, 'Masque of Cupids'. Middleton, *Thomas Middleton*, 1027–33.

Jonson, Ben, *The sad shepherd: or a tale of Robin Hood, a fragment*. London: J. Nichols, 1783.

Jonson, Ben, *The workes of Beniamin Jonson*. London: W. Stansby, 1616.

Jonstonus, Joannes, *An history of the wonderful things of nature. Set forth in ten severall classes*. London: John Streater, 1657.

Joubert, Laurent and Jean Paul Zangmaister, *La pharmacopee*. Lyon: Anthoine de Harsy, 1581.

Jütte, Robert (guest ed.), 'The doctor on the stage'. *Ludica* 5–6 (2000): 61–261.

Katritzky, M. A., *The art of commedia: a study in the commedia dell'arte 1560–1620 with special reference to the visual records*. Amsterdam: Rodopi, 2006.

Katritzky, M. A., 'The autobiographical writings of Felix and Thomas II Platter. Court festivals and commedia dell'arte'. *Theaterwetenschap spelenderwijs. Theatre studies at play*, edited by P. Eversmann, R. van Gaal and R. van der Zalm. Amsterdam: Pallas, 2004, 34–56.

Katritzky, M. A., 'Comic stage routines in Guarinonius' medical treatise of 1610'. *Theatre Research International* 25.3 (2000): 217–32.

Katritzky, M. A., (guest ed.), 'The commedia dell'arte'. *Theatre Research International* 23.2 (1998): 99–178.

Katritzky, M. A., 'Franco Bertelli's "Carnevale Italiano Mascherato" of 1642 and other printed influences on theatrical pictures in alba amicorum'. *Klovićev Zbornik. Minijatura – crtež – grafika 1450–1700*, edited by Milan Pelc. Zagreb: Hrvatska akademija znanosti i umjetnosti – Institut za povijest umjetnosti, 2001, 216–29.

Katritzky, M. A., 'Guarinonius' *lazzi*: English comedians, Italian charlatans, and German quacks in a medical treatise of 1610'. *Hippolytus Guarinonius*, edited by Amann and Siller, 107–37.

Katritzky, M. A., 'Hippolytus Guarinonius' descriptions of commedia dell'arte lazzi in Padua, 1594–97'. *Quaderni Veneti* 30 (1999): 61–126.

Katritzky, M. A., 'I costumi della commedia dell'arte italiana negli *alba amicorum* tedeschi', *La ricezione della commedia dell'arte*, edited by Martino and De Michele, 461–509.

Katritzky, M. A., 'Images of "monsters" and performers: J A Comenius's *Orbis pictus* and *Aristotle's Masterpiece*'. *Practicing New Editions. Transformation and Transfer of the Early Modern Book 1450 – 1800*, edited by Hiram Kümper and Vladimir Simić. Nordhausen: Bautz (Bibliothemata 26), 2011, 77–118.

Katritzky, M. A., 'Italian comedians in renaissance prints', *Print Quarterly* 4.3 (1987): 236–54.

Katritzky, M. A., 'Mountebanks, mummers and masqueraders in Thomas Platter's diary (1595–1600)'. *The renaissance theatre: texts, performance, design I: English and Italian Theatre*, 2 vols, edited by Christopher Cairns. Aldershot: Ashgate, 1999, I, 12–44.

Katritzky, M. A., 'Was *commedia dell'arte* performed by mountebanks? *Album amicorum* illustrations and Thomas Platter's description of 1598'. *Theatre Research International* 23.2 (1998): 104–26.

Katritzky, M. A., *Women, medicine and theatre 1500–1750: literary mountebanks and performing quacks*. Aldershot: Ashgate, 2007.

Katritzky, M. A., 'Zan Bragetta a Jan Potage: divadelní kočovníci v raně novověké Evropě'. *Divadelní revue* 2 (2010): 48–61.

Kemp, Friedhelm, 'Hippolytus Guarinonuis als Schriftsteller: "Kunst/Tuegnt vnd nutz beysammen/sein viel künstlicher/dann Kunst allein" (Die Grewel der Verwüstung)'. *Hippolytus Guarinonius im interkulturellen Kontext*, edited by Locher, 9–19.

Kermode, Frank, 'Julius Caesar'. Shakespeare, *The Riverside Shakespeare*, 1146–50, 1164–5.

Kernan, Alvin B., *Shakespeare, the king's playwright: theater in the Stuart court, 1603–1613*. New Haven: Yale University Press, 1995.

Kerwin, William, *Beyond the body: the boundaries of medicine and English renaissance drama*. Amherst and Boston: University of Massachusetts Press, 2005.

King, Roger, *The making of the dentiste, c.1650–1760*. Aldershot: Ashgate, 1998.

Klaar, Karl, *Dr Hippolytus Guarinoni und die Bürger-Kongregation in Hall*. Innsbruck: marianische Vereinsbuchdruckerei, 1903.

Klinnert, Renate S., 'Von Besessenen, Melancholikern und Betrügern. Johann Weyers "De Praestigiis Daemonum" und die Unterscheidung der Geister'. *Dämonische Besessenheit: Zur Interpretation eines kulturhistorischen Phänomens / Demonic possession: interpretations of a historico-cultural phenomenon*, edited by Hans de Waardt, Jürgen Michael Schmidt, H. C. Erik Midelfort, Sönke Lorenz and Dieter R. Bauer. Bielefeld: Verlag für Regionalgeschichte, 2005, 89–105.

Knowles, James, '"Can ye not tell a man from a marmoset?": Apes and others on the early modern stage'. *Renaissance beasts: of animals, humans, and other wonderful creatures*, edited by Erica Fudge. Urbana and Chicago: University of Illinois Press, 2004, 138–163.

Koch, Karl, 'Guarinonis Anteil an der Erbauung der Karlskirche an der Volderer Brücke'. *Hippolytus Guarinonius (1571–1654)*, edited by Dörrer et al., 197–204.

Koelbing, M. F., 'Felix Platters Patienten'. *Felix Platter (1536–1614) in seiner Zeit*, edited by Ulrich Tröhler. Basel: Schwabe, 1991, 60–7.

Könneker, Barbara, *Satire im 16. Jahrhundert. Epoche – Werke – Wirkung*. München: Beck, 1991.

[Kramer, Heinrich and] Christopher S. Mackay, *The hammer of witches. A complete translation of the 'Malleus Maleficarum'*. Cambridge: Cambridge University Press, 2009.

Kranz, David L., 'The sounds of supernatural soliciting in "Macbeth"'. *Studies in Philology* 100.3 (2003): 346–83.

Kraus, Theodor, *Hekate: Studien zu Wesen und Bild der Göttin in Kleinasien und Griechenland*. Heidelberg: Carl Winter, 1960.

Kreuder, Friedemann, 'Flagellation of the Son of God and divine flagellation: flagellator ceremonies and flagellation scenes in the medieval passion play'. *Theatre Research International* 33.2 (2008): 176–90.

Kröll, Katrin, '"Kurier die Leut auf meine Art ..." Jahrmarktskünste und Medizin auf den Messen des 16. und 17. Jahrhunderts'. *Heilkunde und Krankheitserfahrung in der frühen Neuzeit. Studien am Grenzrain von Literaturgeschichte und Medizingeschichte*, edited by Udo Benzenhöfer and Wilhelm Kühlmann. Tübingen: Niemeyer, 1992, 155–86.

Kröll, Katrin, 'Spectacles de foire à Strasbourg de 1539 à 1618'. *Théâtre et Spectacles hier et aujourd'hui. Moyen Âge et Renaissance (Actes du 115ᵉ Congrès National des Sociétés Savantes, Avignon 1990)*. Paris: Comité des Travaux Historiques et Scientifiques, 1991, 245–59.

Küchler, Balthasar, *Repræsentatio der fürstlichen Auffzüg vnd Ritterspil. So bei des Durchleuchtigen Hochgebornen Fürsten vnd Herren Herrn Johann Friderichen Hertzogen zu Württenberg [...] Hochzeitlich. Ehrnfest.* Schwäbisch Gmund: Balthasar Küchler, [1611].

Kuefler, Mathew, 'Anderl of Rinn, the accusation of Jewish ritual murder, and the historical memory of childhood'. *Journal of the History of Childhood and Youth* 2.1 (2009): 11–36.

Kümper, Hiram, 'Das "Anderl von Rinn" – Unterrichtsmaterialien für einen historischen Längsschnitt zum Thema Judenhass und Ritualmordlegende'. *Neuzeit* (2007/8): 32–45.

Kurras, Lotte, *Zu gutem Gedenken. Kulturhistorische Miniaturen aus Stammbüchern des Germanischen Nationalmuseums 1570–1770.* München: Prestel, 1987.

Lancashire, Anne, '"The Witch": stage flop or political mistake?'. *'Accompaninge the players': essays celebrating Thomas Middleton, 1580–1980,* edited by Kenneth Friedenreich. New York (AMS), 1983, 161–82.

Lancaster, Henry Carrington, *A history of French dramatic literature in the seventeenth century, Part I: the pre-classical period 1610–1634,* 2 vols. Baltimore: Johns Hopkins, 1929.

Lanson, Gustave, 'Molière and farce'. *Tulane Drama Review* 8.2 (1963): 133–54 [reprinted from *Revue de Paris*, May 1901].

Laroque, François, *Shakespeare's festive world: Elizabethan seasonal entertainment and the professional stage.* Cambridge: Cambridge University Press, 1993.

Lea, Kathleen Marguerite, 'The bibliography of the commedia dell'arte: the miscellanies of the comici and virtuosi'. *The Library* fourth series, 11.1 (1930): 1–38.

Lea, Kathleen Marguerite, *Italian popular comedy, a study in the commedia dell'arte, 1560–1620, with special reference to the English stage,* 2 vols. Oxford: Clarendon Press, 1934.

Lebègue, Raymond, 'La Comédie Italienne en France au XVIe Siècle'. *Revue de littérature comparée* 24 (1950): 5–24.

Lederer, David, *Madness, religion and the state in early modern Europe: a Bavarian beacon.* Cambridge: Cambridge University Press, 2006.

Leigh, Edward, *Select and choyce observations.* London: John Williams, 1657.

Le Roy Ladurie, Emmanuel (tr. Arthur Goldhammer), *The beggar and the professor: a sixteenth-century family saga.* Chicago: University of Chicago Press, 1997.

Lewalski, Barbara Kiefer, 'Anne of Denmark and the subversions of masquing'. *Criticism* 35.3 (1993): 341–55.

Lietzmann, Hilda, 'Zu einem unbekannten Brief Heinrich Pantaleons aus dem Jahre 1576'. *Basler Zeitschrift für Geschichte und Altertumskunde* 94 (1994): 75–102.

Lima, Robert, *Stages of evil: occultism in western theater and drama*. Lexington: University Press of Kentucky, 2005.

Limon, Jerzy, *Gentlemen of a company: English players in central and eastern Europe 1590–1660*. Cambridge: Cambridge University Press, 1985.

Linke, Hansjürgen, 'Vom Sakrament bis zum Exkrement. Ein Überblick über Drama und Theater des deutschen Mittelalters'. *Theaterwesen und dramatische Literatur. Beiträge zur Geschichte des Theaters*, edited by Günter Holtus. Tübingen: Francke, 1987, 127–64.

Linke, Hansjürgen, 'Zwischen Jammertal und Schlaraffenland. Verteufelung und Verunwirklichung des saeculum im geistlichen Drama des Mittelalters'. *Zeitschrift für deutsches Altertum und deutsche Literatur* 100 (1971): 350–70.

Little, Lester K., 'Pride goes before avarice: social change and the vices in Latin Christendom'. *American Historical Review* 76.1 (1971): 16–49.

Locher, Elmar, 'Beglaubigungsstrategien als rhetorisch-topische Verfahren in den "Greweln der Verwüstung Menschlichen Geschlechts"'. *Hippolytus Guarinonius*, edited by Amann and Siller, 139–53.

Locher, Elmar, 'Von der Bewegung. Frühneuzeitliche Reflexionen zu Raum und Zeit in den *Greweln* des Hippolyt Guarinoni'. *Hippolytus Guarinonius im interkulturellen Kontext seiner Zeit. Acta der Tagung Neustift 1993*, edited by Locher. Bozen: Sturzflüge, 1995, 81–95.

Lötscher, Valentin, *Felix Platter und seine Familie*. Basel: Helbing & Lichtenhahn, 1975.

Lough, John, 'French actors in Paris from 1612 to 1614'. *French Studies* 9.3 (1955): 218–26.

Lough, John, *Paris theatre audiences in the seventeenth and eighteenth centuries*. London: Oxford University Press, 1957.

Lyly, John, *Euphves, the anatomy of vvyt, very pleasant for all gentlemen to reade*. London: Gabriell Cawood, 1578.

Lyly, John, *Mother Bombie. As it was sundrie times plaied by the Children of Powles*. London: Cuthbert Burby, 1594.

Magni, Maria, 'Il tipo dello zanni nella commedia dell'arte in Italia nei secoli XVI e XVII'. *Bergomvm, Bollettino della Civica Biblioteca* 20.3–4 (1926): 111–38, 163–84.

Maley, Uta, 'Hippolyt Guarinoni als Dichter'. *Literatur und Sprache in Tirol von den Anfängen bis zum 16. Jahrhundert. Akten des 3. Symposiums der Sterzinger Osterspiele (10.-12. April 1995)*, edited by Michael Gebhardt and Max Siller. Innsbruck: Wagner, 1996, 323–37.

Mann, David, 'Female play-going and the good woman'. *Early Theatre* 10.2 (2007): 51–70.

Mann, Gunter, 'Gesundheitswesen und Hygiene in der Zeit des Übergangs von der Renaissance zum Barock'. *Medizin historisches Journal* 2 (1967): 107–23.

Marescot, Michel, *A trve discovrse, vpon the matter of Martha Brossier of Romorantin pretended to be possessed by a deuill. Translated out of French into English, by Abraham Hartwell*. London: John Wolfe, 1599.

Marlowe, Christopher, *The tragicall history of D Faustus*. London: Thomas Bushell, 1604.

Marquardt, Patricia A., 'A portrait of Hecate'. *American Journal of Philology* 102.3 (1981): 243–60.

Marrone, Daniela, 'Ippolito Guarinoni: "Detti, fatti, profezie e segreti del frate cappuccino Tommaso da Bergamo"'. *Hippolytus Guarinonius*, edited by Amann and Siller, 163–5.

Marston, John, *Histrio-mastix, or the player whipt*. [London]: Th. Thorp, 1610.

Marston, John, *Iacke Drums entertainment: or The comedie of Pasquill and Katherine. As it hath bene sundry times plaide by the Children of Powles*. London: Richard Oliue, 1601.

M[artini], G[iovanni] S[imone], *Bragato, Comedia molto piacevole, et ridicolosa*. Vinegia: Altobello Salicato, 1607.

Martino, Alberto, 'Fonti tedesche degli anni 1565–1615 per la storia della commedia dell'arte e per la costituzione di un repertorio dei *lazzi* dello Zanni'. *La ricezione della commedia dell'arte*, edited by Martino and De Michele, 13–68

Martino, Alberto, 'Fonti tedesche degli anni 1585–1615 per la storia della commedia dell'arte e per la costituzione di un repertorio dei "lazzi" dello zanni'. *Aspetti dell'identità tedesca. Studi in onore di Paolo Chiarini*, edited by Mauro Ponzi and Aldo Venturelli, 2 vols. Rome: Bulzoni, 2003, II/2, 657–708.

Martino, Alberto and Fausto De Michele (eds), *La ricezione della commedia dell'arte nell'Europa centrale 1568–1769: storia, testi, iconografia*. Pisa: Fabrizio Serra Editore, 2010.

Marvell, Andrew, *The third part of the collection of poems on affairs of State*. London, 1689.

Mayr, Elfriede, 'Volksnahrung, Anbau und Wirtschaft in Guarinonis Werken'. *Hippolytus Guarinonius (1571–1654)*, edited by Dörrer et al., 119–36.

McDowell, John Huber, *An iconographical study of the early commedia dell'arte (1560–1650)*. University of Yale (unpublished doctoral dissertation), 1937.

McFadden, Megan, 'Reviews: "O let us howle some heavy note" by Amanda Eubanks Winkler'. *Women & Music* 13 (2009): 101–6.

McLaren, Angus, *Impotence: a cultural history*. Chicago: University of Chicago Press, 2007.

McManus, Clare, *Women on the renaissance stage, Anna of Denmark and female masquing in the Stuart court (1590–1619)*. Manchester: Manchester University Press, 2002.

McNeill, John T., 'Folk-paganism in the penitentials'. *The Journal of Religion* 13.4 (1933): 450–66.

Meissner, Johannes, *Die englischen Comoedianten zur Zeit Shakespeares in Oesterreich*. Wien: Konegen, 1884.

Meissner, Johannes, 'Die englischen Komödianten in Oesterreich'. *Jahrbuch der deutschen Shakespeare Gesellschaft* 19 (1884): 113–54.

410 HEALING, PERFORMANCE AND CEREMONY

Mellinkoff, Ruth, 'Riding backwards: theme of humiliation and symbol of evil'. *Viator* 4 (1973): 153–76.

Mengarelli, Stefano, 'The commedia all'improvviso pictures in the Corsini Manuscript: a new reading'. *Early Theatre* 11.2 (2008): 212–26.

Menzer, Paul, 'The tragedians of the city? Q1 *Hamlet* and the settlements of the 1590s'. *Shakespeare Quarterly* 57.2 (2006): 162–82.

Middleton, Thomas (edited by Gary Taylor and John Lavagnino), *Thomas Middleton the collected works*. Oxford: Oxford University Press, 2010.

Midelfort, H. C. Erik, *A history of madness in sixteenth-century Germany*. Stanford: Stanford University Press, 1999.

Millar, Peter, 'The gullible age'. *Sunday Times News Review* (5 August 2007): 1–2.

Moisan, Thomas, '"What's that to you?" or, facing facts: anti-paternalistic chords and social discords in "The taming of the shrew"'. *Renaissance Drama* ns.26 (1995): 105–29.

Montaigne, Michel de (tr. Donald M. Frame, intro. Stuart Hampshire), *The complete works, essays, travel journal, letters*. London: Everyman, 2003.

Montaigne, Michel de (tr. John Florio), *Essayes written in French by Michael Lord of Montaigne*. London: Edward Blount & William Barret, 1613.

Moro, Anna L., 'A semiotic interpretation of the *Lazzi* of the *commedia dell'arte*'. *Theatre Symposium* 1 (1993): 66–76.

Morris, Irene, 'A Hapsburg letter'. *Modern Language Review* 69 (1974): 12–22.

Mortoft, Francis (edited by Malcom Letts), *Francis Mortoft: his book, being his travels through France and Italy, 1658–1659*. London: Hakluyt Society, 1925.

Moryson, Fynes, *An Itinerary containing his ten yeeres travell throvgh the twelve domjnions of Germany, Bohmerland, Sweitzerland, Netherland, Denmarke, Poland, Jtaly, Turky, France, England, Scotland and Ireland*. London: John Beale, 1617.

Moryson, Fynes (edited by Charles Hughes), *Shakespeare's Europe. Unpublished chapters of Fynes Moryson's Itinerary*. London: Sherratt and Hughes, 1903.

Moser, Hans, 'Deutsche und Tiroler: Ethnische Stereotype im Weltbild Guarinonis'. *Hippolytus Guarinonius*, edited by Amann and Siller, 171–83.

Moss, Stephanie and Kaara L. Peterson (eds), *Disease, diagnosis, and cure on the early modern stage*. Aldershot: Ashgate, 2004.

Mueller, Sara, 'Touring, women, and the English professional stage'. *Early Theatre* 11.1 (2008), 53–76.

Murad, Orlene, *The English comedians at the Habsburg court in Graz 1607–1608*. Salzburg: Institut für englische Sprache und Literatur, Universität Salzburg, 1978.

Nada (=Langdon-Davies), John, *Carlos the bewitched: the last Spanish Hapsburg, 1661–1700*. London: Jonathan Cape, 1962.

Nagl, Johann Willibald and Jakob Zeidler (eds), *Deutsch-Österreichische Literaturgeschichte. Ein Handbuch zur Geschichte der deutschen Dichtung in Österreich-Ungarn, I. Von der Kolonisation bis 1750*. Wien: Fromme, 1898.

Naupp, Thomas, 'Über "Bad-Curen" und "Aderlass" bei den alten Georgenbergern'. *Veröffentlichungen des Tiroler Landesmuseum Ferdinandeum* 70 (1990): 161– 82.

Neuber, Wolfgang, 'Vom Grewel deb Trawrens: Hippolyt Guarinonis geschichtliche Stellung in der europäischen Melancholie-Tradition'. *Hippolytus Guarinonius im interkulturellen Kontext*, edited by Locher, 65–79.

Neuhauser, Walter, *Katalog der Handschriften der Universitätsbibliothek Innsbruck, Teil 2, Cod.101-200*. Wien: Verlag der Österreichische Akademie der Wissenschaften, 1991.

Neuhauser, Walter, 'Die Überlieferung der Schriften des Hippolyt Guarinoni unter besonderer Berücksichtigung der handschriftlichen Überlieferung in der Universitätsbibliothek Innsbruck'. *Hippolytus Guarinonius*, edited by Amann and Siller, 185–213.

Neuwirth, Markus and Theresa Witting, 'Die sprechende Architektur von Hippolytus Guarinoni'. *Hippolytus Guarinonius*, edited by Amann and Siller, 215–36.

Norbrook, David, '"The masque of truth": court entertainments and international Protestant politics in the early Stuart period'. *Seventeenth Century* 1.2 (1986): 81–110.

Nothegger, P. Florentin, 'Aus Guarinonis Freundeskreis'. *Hippolytus Guarinonius (1571–1654)*, edited by Dörrer et al., 31–40.

Nutton, Vivian (guest ed.), 'Medicine in the renaissance city'. *Renaissance Studies* 15.2 (2001): 101–228.

O'Connor, Marion, 'The witch'. Middleton, *Thomas Middleton*, 1124–8.

Oppenheimer, Jane M., 'Guillaume Rondelet', *Bulletin of the Institute of the History of Medicine* 4 (1936): 817–34.

Orgel, Stephen and Roy Strong, *Inigo Jones: the theatre of the Stuart court*, 2 vols. London: Sotheby Parke Bernet, 1973.

Ottonelli, Giovan Domenico, 'Della Cristiana Moderazione del Teatro'. *La commedia dell'arte e la società barocca, la fascinazione del teatro*, edited by F. Taviani. Roma: Bulzoni, 1969, 320–526.

Pandolfi, Vito, *La commedia dell'arte. Storia e testo*, 6 vols. Firenze: Sansoni, 1957–61.

Paré, Ambroise, *The workes of that famous chirurgion Ambrose Parey translated out of Latine and compared with the French by Th. Johnson*. London: Th. Cotes & R. Young, 1634.

Park, Katharine, 'Country medicine in the city marketplace: snakehandlers as itinerant healers'. *Renaissance Studies* 15.2 (2001): 104–20.

Parker, Patricia, 'Gender ideology, gender change: the case of Marie Germain'. *Critical Inquiry* 19.2 (1993): 337–64.

Pelling, Margaret, *Medical conflicts in early modern London: patronage, physicians, and irregular practitioners, 1550–1640*. Oxford: Clarendon, 2003.

Pelling, Margaret and Frances White, 'BUGGS, John'. *Physicians and irregular medical practitioners in London 1550–1640: Database (2004)*. Available at: www.british-history.ac.uk/report.aspx?compid=17281 [accessed 16 April 2010].

Pepys, Samuel (intro. Stuart Sim), *The concise Pepys*. Ware: Wordsworth Editions, 1997.

[Perron, Cardinal Jacques Davy Du], *Perroniana sive excerpta ex ore Cardinalis Perronii per F.F.P.P.* Genevæ: Petrus Columesius, 1669.

Pettigrew, Todd H. J., *Shakespeare and the practice of physic: medical narratives on the early modern English stage*. Newark: University of Delaware Press, 2007.

Piluland, Elias (tr.), *Vielvermehrter Hocus Pocus oder Taschen=Spieler*, [s.l.], 1668.

Pinkus, Assaf, *Workshops and patrons of St Theobald in Thann*. Münster: Waxmann, 2006.

Pizzinini, Meinrad, ‚Eine mittelalterliche Ritualmordlegende aus Lienz'. *Veröffentlichungen des Tiroler Landesmuseum Ferdinandeum* 70 (1990): 219–34.

Plank, Steven E., ‚"And now about the cauldron sing": music and the supernatural on the Restoration stage'. *Early music* 18.3 (1990): 393–407.

Platter, Felix, *De Corporis Hvmani Strvctvra et vsv*, 3 vols. [Basel]: Ambrosius Froben, 1583.

Platter, Felix (edited by Valentin Lötscher), *Felix Platter Tagebuch (Lebensbeschreibung) 1536–1567*. Basel and Stuttgart: Schwabe, 1976.

Platter, Felix, *Obseruationum, in hominis affectibus plerisq[ue], corpori & animo, functionum læsione, dolore, aliá ve molestiá & vitio incommodantibus, Libri Tres*. Basileæ: Ludovic König, 1614 [=*Observations*].

Platter, Felix, *Praxeos seu de cognoscendis, prædicendis, præcauendis, curandisq[ue] affectibus homini incommodantibus Tractatus*, 3 vols. Basel: Conrad Waldkirch, 1602, 1603, 1608 [=*Praxis medica*].

Platter, Felix and Thomas Platter the Younger, *Félix et Thomas Platter a Montpellier 1552–1559 – 1595–1599. Notes de voyage de deux étudiants balois, publiées d'après les manuscrits originaux appartenant a la bibliothèque de l'université de Bâle*. Montpellier: Camille Coulet, 1892.

Plat[t]er, Felix, Abdiah Cole and Nicholas Culpeper, *A golden practice of physick. In five books and three tomes. After a new, easie, and plain method of knowing, foretelling, preventing, and curing, all diseases incident to the body of man*. London: Peter Cole, 1662.

Plat[t]er, Felix, Nicholas Culpeper and Abdiah Cole, *Platerus histories and observations upon most diseases offending the body and mind*. London: Peter Cole, 1664.

Platter the Elder, Thomas (edited by Otto Fischer), 'Thomas Platters Lebensbeschreibung'. *Thomas und Felix Platters und Theodor Agrippa d'Aubignés Lebensbeschreibungen*. München: Martin Mörike, 1911, 18–168.

Platter the Younger, Thomas (edited by Rut Keiser), *Thomas Platter d.J: Beschreibung der Reisen durch Frankreich, Spanien, England und die Niederlande 1595–1600*. Basel and Stuttgart: Schwabe, 1968.

Platter the Younger, Thomas (edited by Hans Hecht), *Thomas Platters des Jüngeren Englandfahrt im Jahre 1599. Nach der Handschrift der Öffentlichen Bibliothek der Universität Basel*. Halle: Niemeyer, 1929.

Platter the Younger, Thomas and Emmanuel Le Roy Ladurie, *Le siècle des Platter, 1499–1628* (I: *Le mendiant et le professeur*; II: *Le voyage de Thomas Platter, 1595–1599*; III: *L'Europe de Thomas Platter, France, Angleterre, Pays-Bas, 1599–1600*). Paris: Fayard, 1995, 2000, 2006.

Porter, Roy, *Quacks, fakers & charlatans in English medicine*. Stroud: Tempus, 2000.

Powell, John S., *Music and theatre in France 1600–1680*. Oxford: Oxford University Press, 2000.

Prynne, William, *Histrio-mastix: the players scourge, or, actors tragœdie*. London: Michael Sparke, 1633.

Przybilski, Martin, *Kulturtransfer zwischen Juden und Christen in der deutschen Literatur des Mittelalters*. Berlin: De Gruyter (Quellen und Forschungen zur Literatur- und Kulturgeschichte), 2010.

Rabelais, François [tr. Sir Thomas Urquhart and Pierre Le Motteux, edited by Terence Cave], *Gargantua and Pantagruel*. London: Everyman, 1994.

Raparini, Giorgio Maria, *L'Arlichino, poema carnevalesco dedicato a Signori Accademici sfacendati* (sl, sd).

Raparini, Giorgio Maria, *L'Arlichino poema dedicato a Ss. Accademici Sfaccendati*, seconda edizione. Heidelberg: Müller, 1718.

Rapp, Ludwig, *Hippolytus Guarinoni, Stiftsarzt in Hall. Ein tirolisches Kulturbild aus dem 17. Jahrhundert*. Brixen: Weger, 1903.

Rastel, John, *The third booke, declaring by Examples out of Auncient Councels, Fathers, and Later writers, that it is time to beware of M Iewel*. Antverpiae: Ioannis Fouleri, 1566.

Rausse, Hubert, *Zur Geschichte des spanischen Schelmenromans in Deutschland*. Münster: Schöningh (Münstersche Beiträge zur neueren Literaturgeschichte, VIII. Heft), 1908.

Reinhardstöttner, Karl von, 'Aegidius Albertinus, der Vater des deutschen Schelmenromans'. *Jahrbuch für Münchener Geschichte* 2 (1888): 13–86.

Remshardt, Ralf Erik, 'The birth of reason from the spirit of carnival: Hans Sachs and "Das Narren-Schneyden"'. *Comparative Drama* 23.1 (1989): 70–94.

Richards, Kenneth and Laura Richards, *The commedia dell'arte. A documentary history*. Oxford: Blackwell, 1990.

Riewald, J. G., 'New light on the English actors in the Netherlands, c.1590–c.1660'. *English Studies* 41 (1960): 65–92.

Rigal, Eugène, *Alexandre Hardy et le théâtre français a la fin du XVIe et au commencement du XVIIe siècle*. Paris: Librairie Hachette, 1889.

Rigal, Eugène, *Hotel de Bourgogne et Marais, Esquisse d'une histoire des Théâtres de Paris de 1548 à 1635*. Paris: Dupret, 1887.

Rigal, Eugène, *Le Théatre Français avant la période classique (fin du XVIᵉ et commencement du XVIIᵉ siècle)*. Paris: Librairie Hachette, 1901.

Robbins, Kevin C., 'Magical emasculation, popular anticlericalism, and the limits of the Reformation in western France circa 1590'. *Journal of Social History* 31.1 (1997): 61–83.

Rolfe, W. J., 'Is the part of Hecate in "Macbeth" Shakespeare's?'. *Poet Lore* 11 (1899): 602–5.

Rowlands, Alison, 'Witchcraft and old women in early modern Germany'. *Past & Present* 173 (2001): 50–89.

Royce, Anya Peterson, 'The Venetian commedia: actors and masques in the development of the commedia dell'arte'. *Theatre Survey* 27.1–2 (1986): 69–87.

Salmon, William, *Medicina practica: or, practical physick, shewing the method of curing the most usual diseases happening to humane bodies*. London: T. Hawkins, J. Taylor, J. Harris, 1692.

Sanderson, James L., 'Poems on an affair of state – the marriage of Somerset and Lady Essex'. *Review of English Studies* n.s.17 (1966): 57–61.

Scala, Flaminio, *Il Teatro delle Fauole rappresentatiue, overo la ricreatione comica, boscareccia, e tragica: divisa in cinquanta giornate*. Venetia: Gio. Battista Pulciani, 1611.

Scaligero, Giulio Cesare, *Exotericarvm exercitationvm Liber XV. De subtilitate, ad Hieronymvm Cardanvm*. Francofvrti: Claudii Marnii hæredum, 1612 [1st edition: Paris 1557].

Schade, Richard Erich, *Studies in early German comedy 1500–1650*. Columbia: Camden House, 1988.

Schadelbauer, Karl, 'Von den kranken Menschen und der hohen Kunst der Arzneidoktoren. Aus den unveröffentlichten medizinischen Schriften des Dr Hippolyt Guarinoni'. *Hippolytus Guarinonius (1571–1654)*, edited by Dörrer et al., 91–111.

Schanzer, Ernest, 'Thomas Platter's observations on the Elizabethan stage'. *Notes and Queries* 3.11 (1956): 466–7.

Schennach, Martin P., 'Hippolyt Guarinoni, die Innsbrucker Zentralbehörden und der Innsbrucker Hof'. *Hippolytus Guarinonius*, edited by Amann and Siller, 237–42.

Schiendorfer, Max, 'Vorformen zu Guarinonis Lehre vom "Gesondt" in mittelalterlicher Dichtung und Heilkunde'. *Hippolytus Guarinonius*, edited by Amann and Siller, 243–60.

Schindler, Otto G., 'Zan Tabarino, "Spielmann des Kaisers". Italienische Komödianten des Cinquecento zwischen den Höfen von Wien und Paris'. *Römische Historische Mitteilungen* 43 (2001): 411–544.

Schindler, Otto G., '"Mio compadre Imperatore", Comici dell'arte an den Höfen der Habsburger'. *Maske und Kothurn* 38.2–4 (1997): 25–154.

Schmid, Ernst Fritz, *Musik an den schwäbischen Zollernhöfen der Renaissance: Beiträge zur Kulturgeschichte des deutschen Südwestens.* Kassel: Bärenreiter, 1962.

Schmitt, Natalie Crohn, '"Il finto negromante": the vitality of a *commedia dell'arte* scenario by Flaminio Scala, 1611'. *Text and Performance Quarterly* 29.4 (2009): 299–326.

Schnabel, Werner Wilhelm, *Das Stammbuch. Konstitution und Geschichte einer textsortenbezogenen Sammelform bis ins erste Drittel des 18. Jahrhunderts.* Tübingen: Niemeyer, 2003.

Schnabel, Werner Wilhelm, *Die Stammbücher und Stammbuchfragmente der Stadtbibliothek Nürnberg. Teil 1. Die Stammbücher des 16. und 17. Jahrhunderts (Die Handschriften der Stadtbibliothek Nürnberg: Sonderband).* Wiesbaden: Harrassowitz, 1995.

Schöner, Petra, 'Visual representations of Jews and Judaism in sixteenth-century Germany'. *Jews, Judaism, and the Reformation*, edited by Bell and Burnett, 357–91.

Schrickx, Willem, '"Pickleherring" and English actors in Germany'. *Shakespeare Survey* 36 (1983): 135–47.

Schupbach, William, 'A new look at "The cure of folly"'. *Medical History* 22 (1978): 267–81.

Scot, Reginald, *The Discouerie of Witchcraft, wherein the lewde dealings of witches and witchmongers is notablie detected.* London: William Brome, 1584.

Scott, Virginia, *The commedia dell'arte in Paris 1644–1697.* Charlottesville: University Press of Virginia, 1990.

Senn, Walter, *Aus dem Kulturleben einer süddeutschen Kleinstadt. Musik, Schule und Theater der Stadt Hall in Tirol in der Zeit vom 15. bis zum 19. Jahrhundert.* Innsbruck: Tyrolia, 1938.

Senn, Walter, *Musik und Theater am Hof zu Innsbruck. Geschichte der Hofkapelle vom 15. Jahrhundert bis zu deren Auflösung im Jahre 1748.* Innsbruck: Österreichische Verlagsanstalt, 1954.

Shadwell, Thomas, *The Lancashire-witches and Tegue o Divelly the Irish Priest: a comedy.* London: John Starkey, 1682.

Shadwell, Thomas, *The Sullen Lovers: or, the Impertinents.* London: Henry Herringman, 1668.

Shakespeare, William (edited by G. Blakemore Evans et al.), *The Riverside Shakespeare. Second edition. The complete works.* Boston: Houghton Mifflin, 1997.

Shesgreen, Sean, *Images of the outcast, the urban poor in the Cries of London.* Manchester: Manchester University Press, 2002.

Sidney, Philip, *The Covntesse of Pembrokes Arcadia.* London: William Ponsonbie, 1590.

Siller, Max, 'Ausgewählte Aspekte des Fastnachtspiels im Hinblick auf die Aufführung des Sterzinger Spiels "der scheissennd"'. *Fastnachtspiel – Commedia dell'Arte, Gemeinsamkeiten – Gegensätze. Akten des 1. Symposiums der Sterzinger Osterspiele (31.3-3.4.1991)*, edited by Max Siller. Innsbruck: Wagner (Schlern-Schriften 290), 1992, 147–59.

Siller, Max, 'Die Sprache des Hippolytus Guarinonius: linguistische Beobachtungen zu einem deutsch schreibenden Italiener der Frühneuzeit'. *Hippolytus Guarinonius im interkulturellen Kontext*, edited by Locher, 27–44.

Silvette, Herbert, *The doctor on the stage: medicine and medical men in seventeenth-century England*. Knoxville: University of Tennessee Press, 1967.

Simmons, J. L., 'Diabolical realism in Middleton and Rowley's "The Changeling"'. *Renaissance Drama* n.s.11 (1980): 135–70.

Simpson, Jacqueline, 'Witches and witchbusters'. *Folklore* 107 (1996): 5–18.

Slater, John and Mariá Luz López Terrada, 'Scenes of mediation: staging medicine in the Spanish interludes'. *Social History of Medicine* 24.2 (2011): 226–43.

Smith, Moira, 'The flying phallus and the laughing inquisitor: penis theft in the "Malleus Maleficarum"'. *Journal of Folklore Research* 39.1 (2002): 85–117.

Smith, Warren D., 'The Elizabethan rejection of judicial astrology and Shakespeare's practice'. *Shakespeare Quarterly* 9.2 (1958): 159–76.

Sohmer, Steve, '12 June 1599: opening day at Shakespeare's Globe'. *Early Modern Literary Studies* 3.1 (1997): 1.1–46 Available at: http://purl.oclc.org/emls/03-1/sohmjuli.html [accessed September 2009].

Spada, Stefania, *Domenico Biancolelli ou l'art d'improviser. Textes, documents, introduction, notes*. Naples: Institut universitaire oriental, 1969.

Speaight, George, 'A commedia dell'arte "Lazzo"'. *Theatre Research International* 18.1 (1993): 1–3.

Spong, Andrew, 'Bad habits, "bad" quartos, and the myth of origin in the editing of Shakespeare'. *New Theatre Quarterly* 12 (1996): 65–70.

Sprengel, Peter, 'Herr Pantalon und sein Knecht Zanni. Zur frühen Commedia dell'arte in Deutschland'. *Kleine Schriften der Gesellschaft für Theatergeschichte* 34/35 [*Wanderbühne. Theaterkunst als fahrendes Gewerbe*, edited by Bärbel Rudin] (1988): 5–18.

Staehelin, Martin, 'Felix Platter und die Musik'. *Felix Platter (1536–1614) in seiner Zeit*, edited by Ulrich Tröhler. Basel: Schwabe, 1991, 74–81.

Stephens, Walter, 'Witches who steal penises: impotence and illusion in "Malleus maleficarum"'. *Journal of Medieval and Early Modern Studies* 28.3 (1998): 495–529.

Stichler, Carl, 'Reisende Ärzte, Wunderdoktoren und Medizinhändler des 17. Jahrhunderts nach ungedruckten Originalberichten geschildert'. *Archiv für Geschichte der Medizin* 2 (1909): 285–300.

Stokes, James and Robert J. Alexander, *Records of early English drama: Somerset, including Bath*, 2 vols. Toronto: University of Toronto Press, 1996.

Stolberg, Michael, 'The decline of uroscopy in early modern learned medicine (1500–1650)'. *Early Science and Medicine* 12 (2007): 313–36.

Stroumsa, Guy G., *A new science. The discovery of religion in the Age of Reason*. Cambridge, MA: Harvard University Press, 2010.

[Tabarin], *Recveil general des rencontres, qvestions, demandes & autres œuures Tabariniques, auec leurs responses*. Paris: Anthoine de Sommaville, 1622.

Taylor, Gary and Inga-Stina Ewbank, 'The tragedy of Macbeth: a genetic text'. Middleton, *Thomas Middleton*, 1165–9.

Taylor, John, *Taylor his trauels: from the Citty of London in England, to the Citty of Prague in Bohemia*. London: Henry Gosson, 1620.

Terrada, María Luz López, 'Medical pluralism in a renaissance city: the case of Valencia'. *Ludica* 5–6 (2000): 216–32.

Theile, Verena, *Staging the occult: continental European influences on the literature of the English renaissance stage*. Washington State University (unpublished doctoral dissertation), 2006.

Thomas, Keith, *Religion and the decline of magic: studies in popular beliefs in sixteenth and seventeenth century England*. London: Weidenfeld & Nicolson, 1980.

Tiffany, Grace, 'Review: John Drakakis (ed), "New casebooks: Antony and Cleopatra"'. *Shakespeare Newsletter* 45.2 (1995): 42.

Tilg, Stefan, 'Die Popularisierung einer Ritualmordlegende im Anderl-von-Rinn-Drama der Haller Jesuiten (1621)'. *Daphnis* 33 (2004): 623–40.

Tomlinson, Sophie, *Women on stage in Stuart drama*. Cambridge: Cambridge University Press, 2005.

Trapp, Oswald, 'Hippolyt Guarinoni als Baukünstler'. *Hippolytus Guarinonius (1571–1654)*, edited by Dörrer et al., 189–92.

Trautmann, Karl, 'Deutsche Schauspieler am bayrischen Hofe', *Jahrbuch für Münchener Geschichte* 3 (1889): 259–430.

Trautmann, Karl, 'Französische Schauspieler am bayrischen Hofe'. *Jahrbuch für Münchener Geschichte* 2 (1888): 185–334.

Trautmann, Karl, 'Italienische Schauspieler am bayrischen Hofe'. *Jahrbuch für Münchener Geschichte* 1 (1887): 193–312.

Trinkler, Hedwig, *Aus der Geschichte der Pathologie und ihrer Anstalt in Basel*. Basel: Helbing & Lichtenhahn, 1973.

Troiano, Massimo, *Dialoghi di Massimo Troiano: Ne' quali si narrano le cose piu notabili fatte nelle Nozze dello Illustriss. & Eccell. Prencipe Gvglielmo VI. Conte Palatino del Reno, e Duca di Bauiera; e dell'Illustriss. & Eccell. Madama Renata di Loreno*. Venetia: Bolognino Zaltieri, 1569.

Valentin, Jean-Marie, 'Bouffons ou religieux? Le débat sur le théâtre dans l'Allemagne catholique au début du XVIIe siècle (A. Albertinus, H. Guarinonius)'. *Revue d'Allemagne* 12.4 (1980): 442–76.

Valentin, Jean-Marie, *Französischer 'Roman comique' und deutscher Schelmenroman*. Opladen: Westdeutscher Verlag: Rheinisch-Westfälische Akademie der Wissenschaften (Vorträge G315), 1992.

Valentin, Jean-Marie, 'Herr Pantalon und sein Knecht Zani: Zur Funktion und Bedeutung der *welschen comedi* in den *Greweln der Verwüstung* des H. Guarinonius'. *Theatrum Europaeum. Festschrift für Elida Maria Szarota,* edited by Richard Brinkmann, Karl-Heinz Habersetzer, Paul Raabe, Karl-Ludwig Selig and Blake Lee Spahr. München: Fink, 1982, 193–216.

Valentin, Jean-Marie, *Theatrum Catholicum. Les jésuites et la scène en Allemagne au XVIᵉ et au XVIIᵉ siècles*. Nancy: Presses Universitaires, 1990.

Veltruský, Jarmila F, 'The old Czech apothecary as clown and symbol'. *Festive drama: papers from the sixth triennial colloquium of the international society for the study of medieval theatre, Lancaster, 13–19 July, 1989*, edited by Meg Twycross. Cambridge: Brewer, 1996, 270–8.

[Vincent, William], *Hocvs Pocvs Ivnior: the anatomie of legerdemain, or, the art of Iugling set forth in his proper colours*. London: R M, 1634.

Vischer, Christoph, 'Die Stammbücher der Universitätsbibliothek Basel. Ein beschreibendes Verzeichnis'. *Festschrift Karl Schwarber: Beiträge zur schweizerischen Bibliotheks-, Buch- und Gelehrtengeschichte*. Basel: Schwabe, 1949, 247–66.

Vonach, Andreas, 'Die heilige Schrift als Heiligung der Gedanken. Anmerkungen zur Rezeption der Bibel im Werk des Hippolytus Guarinonius'. *Hippolytus Guarinonius*, edited by Amann and Siller, 289–98.

Wagner, Hans, *Kurtze doch gegründte beschreibung des Durchleuchtigen Hochgebornnen Fursten vnnd Herren / Herren Wilhalmen / Pfaltzgrauen bey Rhein / Hertzogen inn Obern und Nidern Bairen / Vnd derselben geliebsten Gemahel / der Durchleuchtigisten Hochgebornnen Fürstin / Frewlin Renata [...]*. München: Adam Berg, 1568.

Walker, Anita M. and Edmund H. Dickerman, '"A woman under the influence": a case of alleged possession in sixteenth-century France'. *Sixteenth Century Journal* 22.3 (1991): 534–54.

Walton, Michael T., 'Anthonius Margaritha – honest reporter?'. *Sixteenth Century Journal* 36.1 (2005): 129–41.

Watanabe-O'Kelly, Helen, 'Early modern European festivals – politics and performance, event and record'. *Court festivals of the European Renaissance: art, politics and performance*, edited by J. R. Mulryne and Elizabeth Goldring. Aldershot: Ashgate, 2002, 15–25.

Watanabe-O'Kelly, Helen, 'The iconography of German Protestant tournaments in the years before the Thirty Years War'. *Image et spectacle: actes du XXXIIᵉ colloque international d'etudes humanistes du Centre d'Etudes Supérieures de la Renaissance (Tours, 29 juin–8 juillet 1989)*, edited by Pierre Béhar. Amsterdam: Rodopi (Chloe: Beihefte zum Daphnis 15), 1993, 47–64.

Watanabe-O'Kelly, Helen, *Triumphall shews: tournaments at German-speaking courts in their European context 1560–1730*. Berlin: Gebr. Mann, 1992.

Watanabe-O'Kelly, Helen and Anne Simon, *Festivals and ceremonies: a bibliography of works relating to court, civic, and religious festivals in Europe 1500–1800*. London: Mansell, 2000.

Watson, Sara Ruth, 'Sidney at Bartholomew Fair'. *Publications of the Modern Language Association* 53.1 (1938): 125–8.

Weldon, Anthony, *The court and character of King James*. London: John Wright, 1650.

Wells, Stanley and Gary Taylor, *William Shakespeare, a textual companion*. Oxford: Clarendon Press, 1987.

Wenzel, Edith, 'The representations of Jews and Judaism in sixteenth-century German literature'. *Jews, Judaism, and the Reformation*, edited by Bell and Burnett, 393–417.

Wenzel, Siegfried, 'The seven deadly sins: some problems of research'. *Speculum* 43.1 (1968): 1–22.

Whetstone, George, *An Heptameron of Ciuill Discourses. Containing: The Christmasse Exercise of sundrie well Courted Gentlemen and Gentlewomen [...]*. London: Richard Iones, 1582.

Wier, Johannes, *De praestigiis daemonum et incantationibus ac veneficijs*. Basel: Ioannes Oporinus, 1563.

Wiesner-Hanks, Merry, *The marvelous hairy girls, the Gonzales sisters and their worlds*. New Haven: Yale University Press, 2009.

Wiles, David, *Shakespeare's clown: actor and text in the Elizabethan playhouse*. Cambridge: Cambridge University Press, 1987.

Wiley, W. L. *The early public theatre in France*. Cambridge, MA: Harvard University Press, 1960.

Wiley, W. L., 'The Hotel de Bourgogne. Another look at France's first public theatre'. *Studies in Philology* 70 (1973): 1–114.

Wiley, W. L. 'A royal child learns to like plays: the early years of Louis XIII'. *Renaissance News* 9.3 (1956): 135–44.

Williams, Alison, 'Sick humour, healthy laughter: the use of medicine in Rabelais's jokes'. *The Modern Language Review* 101.3 (2006): 671–81.

Williams, Clare, *Thomas Platter's travels in England, 1599*. London: Jonathan Cape, 1937.

Wilson, Arthur, *The history of Great Britain, being the life and reign of King James the First*. London: Richards Lownds, 1653.

Wilson, Richard, '"Is this a holiday?": Shakespeare's Roman carnival'. *English Literary History* 54.1 (1987): 31–44.

Wirre, Hainrich, *Ordenliche Beschreybung der Fürstlichen Hochzeyt*. Augsburg: Philipp Ulhart, 1568.

Wright, A. Dickson, 'Quacks through the ages', *Journal of the Royal Society of Arts* 105.4995 (1957): 161–78.

Yates, Frances A., 'English actors in Paris during the lifetime of Shakespeare'. *Review of English Studies* 1.4 (1925): 392–403.

Zapperi, Roberto, *Der wilde Mann von Teneriffa. Die wundersame Geschichte des Pedro Gonzalez und seiner Kinder*. München: Beck, 2004.

Welch, Anthony. *The Christian ... of Shakespeare.* London: John Wiley, 1850.

Wells, Stanley, and Gary Taylor. *William Shakespeare: a Textual Companion.* Oxford: Clarendon Press, 1987.

Wenzel, Edith. The representations of Jews and Judaism in sixteenth-century German literature ... and the Reformation, edited by itself and ... Brussels: 302–312.

Wood, Siegfried. The seven deadly sins: some problems of research. *Speculum* 43 (1968) 1–22.

Whetstone, George. An Heptameron of Civill Discourses. Containing: The Christmasse Exercise of sundrie well courted Gentlemen and Gentlewomen ... London: Richard Jones, 1582.

Index

botanical gardens 20, 64
Bottoni, Albertino 235
Bourges 33, 48, 123, 165–6
Bowers, John Z 177, 179
Bragato, Bragetta, Braghetta, Braquette,
    Broghetta *see* Alfieri
Bragatto see Martini
Brand, Peter 139
Brandauer, Christine 274
Brandenburg, von, Barbara Sophia 112,
    Diagram 5
    Georg Friedrich 286
    Joachim Friedrich 286
Brandstätter, Klaus 3
Brant, Sebastian, *Narrenschiff* 12, 267, 276,
    326
Brantôme, Pierre Bourdeille de *Recueil des
    Dames* 98, 175–6
Breslau (Wrocław) 132, Plate 8
Breuer, Dieter 31, 34, 40, 85
Briard, Monsieur 130
Brixen (Bressanone) 175, 256, Plate 6
Brockliss, Laurence 215, 224
Brome, Richard, *The Late Lancashire-
    Witches* 188–90
Brooke, George 133
    Henry, Lord Cobham 132–3
Brossier, Jacques and Marthe 'la
    démoniaque' 166
Brouwer, Francesco de Simone 238
Browe, Peter, 176, 178
Brown, Iain Gordon 260
Browne, Robert 139
Brückle, Wolfgang 37, 106
Brüggemann, Romy 246, 267
Brun, Pierre 224–5
Brunfels, Otto 18
Brussels 90, 100, 102–6, 112, 117,
    Diagram 5
Bucher, Andreas 132
Bücking, Jürgen 31, 35–6, 40–1, 89, 93,
    106, 113, 141, 196, 218, 233, 242,
    256, Diagram 3
Budapest Plate 37
Buggs, John 129
Buhlmeyer, Johannes and Anna Gertrud
    225–6
Bujok, Elke 20, 199

Bumiller, Casimir 16, 117, 283, 288
Burchard, Bishop of Worms 177
Burgundy 50, 173
Burnett, Mark Thornton 194, 201, 207–8,
    210
Burnett, Stephen G 77, 82
Burton, Robert, *The Anatomy of
    melancholy* 22, 236, 278
Bütikum, Ludwig von 283, 296, 301
Butterworth, Emily 164
Butterworth, Philip 162–3
Button, Mr 130
Buxtorf, Johannes the Elder
    Synagoga Ivdaica 27, 82–4, 303–13
    The Jewish Synagogue 82, 303–13
Buzzurui, Giovanni 224

'C', I, *The two merry milke-maids* 236
cabinets of curiosities 20, 78, 129, 131,
    134, 170, 172–3, 194, 199–201,
    298
Calabi, Donatella 81
Calais 132, 200
calendar, almanac 156–7, 176, 274
    Gregorian 25, 47
    Jewish 82
    Julian 25, 135
    reforms 25, 47–8, 101, 136
Calf, Joseph 133
Calvin, Jean 79
    Calvinists 146, 225, 292
Campion, Thomas, *The description of a
    maske* 182–3, 187–8
Campolongo, Emilio 235
Campos, Giulia 239
Canisius, Peter 31–2, 35
cannibalism *see* food
canon law *see* law
Cantecroy, François Perrenot de Granvelle,
    Comte de 70, 171, 173
Canterbury 133, 177, 182
Capozza, Nicoletta 169, 238–40, 249–61,
    270
Carcassonne 65
Cardoso, Aldonza, de Velasco 178
Carleton, Sir Dudley 182
Carnival and Lent *see* costume; festivals;
    food; stock roles